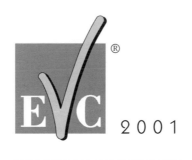

COMPLICATIONS IN VASCULAR AND ENDOVASCULAR SURGERY

PART I

Library of Congress Cataloging-in-Publication Data

Complications in vascular and endovascular surgery. Part I/[edited] by Alain Branchereau and
Michael Jacobs.
    p.; cm.
    Includes bibliographical references and index.
    ISBN 0-7993-4808- (hardcover: alk. paper)
    1. Blood-vessels--Surgery--Complications. 2. Blood-vessels--Endoscopic
surgery--Complications. I. Branchereau, Alain. II. Jacobs, Michael, MD.
    [DNLM: 1. Vascular Surgical Procedures. 2. Postoperative Complications. WG 170
C7369 2000]
RD598.5 .C635 2000
617.4'1301--dc21

                                                             00-067767

Published by
Futura Publishing Company, Inc.
135 Bedford Road
Armonk, NY 10504-0418

LC #: 00-067767
ISBN #: 0-87993-4808

Every effort has been made to ensure that the information in this book is as up to date and as accurate as
possible at the time of publication. However, due to the constant developments in medicine, neither the
author, nor the editor, nor the publisher can accept any legal or any other responsibility for any errors or
omissions that may occur.

Printed in France on acid-free paper.

COMPLICATIONS IN VASCULAR AND ENDOVASCULAR SURGERY

PART I

Edited by

ALAIN BRANCHEREAU, MD
University Hospital, Marseille, France

&

MICHAEL JACOBS, MD
University Hospital, Maastricht, The Netherlands

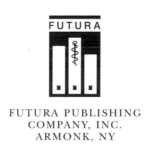

FUTURA PUBLISHING
COMPANY, INC.
ARMONK, NY

LIST OF CONTRIBUTORS

Angelo ANZUINI
Unita di Emodinamica
e Cardiologia Interventistica
Ospedale San Raffaele, Via Olgettina, 60
20145 Milano, Italy

Domenico ASTORE
Chirurgia Vascolare
Ospedale San Raffaele, Via Olgettina, 60
20145 Milano, Italy

Raouf AYARI
Department of Vascular Surgery
Hôpital Timone Adultes,
13385 Marseille Cedex 05, France

José Antonio BALLESTEROS
Departamento de Urología
Hospital de la Esperança
08003 Barcelona, Spain

Michel BARTOLI
Department of Vascular Surgery
Hôpital Timone Adultes
13385 Marseille cedex 05, France

Ahmed BESBISS
Department of Vascular Surgery
Hôpital Gabriel Montpied
CHU de Clermont-Ferrand, 63000, France

Franklin BONTEMPO
3636 Boulevard of the Allies
PA 15213 Pittsburg, USA

Thomas BOWER
Division of Vascular Surgery
Mayo Clinic, 200 First Street SW
MN 55905 Rochester, USA

Alain BRANCHEREAU
Department of Vascular Surgery
Hôpital Timone Adultes
13385 Marseille cedex 05, France

Piergiorgio CAO
Chirurgia Vascolare
Azienda Ospedaleria di Perugia
66122 Perugia, Italy

Gianfranco CARLINI
Chirurgia Vascolare
Azienda Ospedaleria di Perugia
66122 Perugia, Italy

Alain CARLIER
Hôpital Universitaire de Liège
Dom. Univ du Sart - Tilman, Bat B. 35
4000 Liège 1, Belgium

Renata CASTELLANO
Chirurgia Vascolare
Ospedale San Raffaele, Via Olgettina, 60
20145 Milano, Italy

Jocelyn CELERIEN
Department of Vascular Surgery
Hôpitaux Universitaires de Strasbourg
67000 Strasbourg, France

Nabil CHAKFÉ
Department of Vascular Surgery
Hôpitaux Universitaires de Strasbourg
67000 Strasbourg, France

Kenneth CHERRY
Division of Vascular Surgery
Mayo Clinic, 200 First Street SW
MN 55905 Rochester, USA

Roberto CHIESA
Chirurgia Vascolare
Ospedale San Raffaele, Via Olgettina, 60
20145 Milano, Italy

Albert CLARÁ
Cirugía Vascular
Hospital del Mar
08003 Barcelona, Spain

Marc COGGIA
Department of Vascular Surgery
Hôpital Ambroise Paré, 9, av. Ch. de Gaulle
92104 Boulogne Cedex, France

Massimo D'ADDATO
Chirurgia Vascolare
Universita di Bologna
40138 Bologna, Italy

Bas de MOL
Department of Cardiac Surgery
Academic Medical Center, PO Box 22660
1100DD Amsterdam, The Netherlands

Paola DE RANGO
Chirurgia Vascolare
Azienda Ospedaleria di Perugia
66122 Perugia, Italy

Charles DOILLON
Université Laval
Québec, Canada

Christer DROTT
Department of Surgery
Boras Hospital
50182 Boras, Sweden

Bernard DURAND
Department of Vascular Surgery
Hôpitaux Universitaires de Strasbourg
67000 Strasbourg, France

Bertrand EDE
Department of Vascular Surgery
Hôpital Timone Adultes,
13385 Marseille cedex 05, France

Ted ELENBAAS
Department of Cardiothoracic Surgery
University Hospital Maastricht, PO Box 5800
6202 AZ Maastricht, The Netherlands

Sillia FRIGERIO
Chirurgia Vascolare
Ospedale San Raffaele, Via Olgettina, 60
20145 Milano, Italy

Peter GAINES
Sheffield Vascular Institute
Herries Road
Sheffield S5 7AU, United-Kingdom

Luca GARRIBOLI
Chirurgia Vascolare
Ospedale San Raffaele, Via Olgettina, 60
20145 Milano, Italy

Bernard GASSER
Department of Anatomy and Pathology
Hôpitaux Universitaires de Strasbourg
67000 Strasbourg, France

Gian Pietro GESU
Laboratorio di Microbiologia
Ospedale San Raffaele, Via Olgettina, 60
20145 Milano, Italy

Gérard GLANDDIER
Department of Vascular Surgery
Hôpital Gabriel Montpied
CHU de Clermont-Ferrand, 63000, France

Peter GLOVICZKI
Division of Vascular Surgery
Mayo Clinic, 200 First Street SW
MN 55905 Rochester, USA

Olivier A. GOËAU-BRISSONNIÈRE
Department of Vascular Surgery
Hôpital Ambroise Paré, 9 av. Ch. de Gaulle
92104 Boulogne Cedex, France

Gilbert HABIB
Cardiologie B
Hôpital Timone Adultes,
13385 Marseille Cedex 05, France

John HALLET
Division of Vascular Surgery
Mayo Clinic, 200 First Street SW
MN 55905 Rochester, USA

George HAMILTON
Department of Surgery - Royal Free Hospital
and Royal Free and University
College School of Medicine
Pond Street, London NW3 2QG, United-Kingdom

Othman HASSANI
Department of Vascular Surgery
Hôpitaux Universitaires de Strasbourg
67000 Strasbourg, France

Roland HETZER
Deutsches Herzzentrum Berlin
Klinik für Herz-, Thorax-, and Gefässchirurgie
Augustenburger Platz 1
13353 Berlin, Germany

Herbert IMIG
II Department of Surgery
Allgemeines Krankenhaus Hamburg
Eissendorfer Pferdeweg 52
21075 Hamburg, Germany

Michael JACOBS
Department of Surgery
University Hospital Maastricht, PO Box 5800
6202 AZ Maastricht, The Netherlands

Jean-Michel JAUSSERAN
Department of Cardiovascular Surgery
Hôpital Saint Joseph, 26 bd de Louvain
13008 Marseille, France

John KAKISIS
Section of Vascular Surgery
"Laiko" General Hospital of Athens
Athens University School of Medicine
17 AG Thoma Street, 11527 Athens, Greece

Melina KIBBE
Division of Vascular Surgery
University of Pittsburgh, School of Medicine
A 1011-PUH, 200 Lothrop Street
Pittsburgh PA 15213, USA

Jean-Georges KRETZ
Department of Vascular Surgery
Hôpitaux Universitaires de Strasbourg
67000 Strasbourg, France

Hendrik LACROIX
Center for Vascular Diseases
University Clinic Gasthuisberg
Leuven, Belgium

Bernard LALANNE
Department of Cardiovascular Surgery
Hôpital Saint Joseph, 26 bd de Louvain
13008 Marseille, France

Dink LEGEMATE
Department of Surgery
Academic Medical Center, PO Box 22660
1100DD Amsterdam, The Netherlands

Karel LEUNISSEN
Department of Nephrology
University Hospital Maastricht
6202 AZ Maastricht, The Netherlands

Christos LIAPIS
Section of Vascular Surgery
"Laiko" General Hospital of Athens
Athens University School of Medicine
17 AG Thoma Street, 11527 Athens, Greece

Raymond LIMET
Hôpital Universitaire de Liège
Domaine Univ du Sart - Tilman, Bat B. 35
4000 Liège 1, Belgium

Heike LORCH
Department of Radiology
University Hospital, Ratzeburger Allee 160
23638 Lübeck, Germany

Bruno MACHEDA
Department of Vascular Surgery
Hôpital Gabriel Montpied
CHU de Clermont-Ferrand, 63000, France

Michel MAKAROUN
Division of Vascular Surgery
University of Pittsburgh, School of Medicine
A 1011-PUH, 200 Lothrop Street
Pittsburgh PA 15213, USA

Gaart MALEUX
Center for Vascular Diseases
University Clinic Gasthuisberg
Leuven, Belgium

Germano MELISSANO
Chirurgia Vascolare
Ospedale San Raffaele, Via Olgettina, 60
20145 Milano, Italy

André MERY
Department of Cardiovascular Surgery
Hôpital Saint Joseph, 26 bd de Louvain
13008 Marseille, France

Maria Luisa MIR
Departamento de Nefrología
Hospital del Mar,
08003 Barcelona, Spain

Michele MIRELLI
Chirurgia Vascolare
Universita di Bologna
40138 Bologna, Italy

Manuel MIRALLES
Cirugía Vascular
Hospital del Mar
08003 Barcelona, Spain

Bas MOCHTAR
Deparment of Cardiothoracic Surgery
University Hospital Maastricht, PO Box 5800
6202 AZ Maastricht, The Netherlands

Sameh MORCOS
Department of Diagnostic Imaging
Northern General, Herries Road
S5 7AU Sheffield, United-Kingdom

Michael MORLOCK
II Department of Surgery
Allgemeines Krankenhaus Hamburg
Eissendorfer Pferdeweg 52
21075 Hamburg, Germany

André NEVELSTEEN
Center for Vascular Diseases
University Clinic Gasthuisberg
Leuven, Belgium

Christoph NIENABER
Abteiliung für Kardiologie
Medizinische Klinik
Universitätsklinikum Rostok
Ernst-Heydemann-Strasse 6
18055 Rostok, Germany

Audra NOEL
Division of Vascular Surgery
Mayo Clinic, 200 First Street SW
MN 55905 Rochester, USA

Raymond PADOVANI
Department of Cardiovascular Surgery
Hôpital Saint Joseph, 26 bd de Louvain
13008 Marseille, France

Jean PANNETON
Division of Vascular Surgery
Mayo Clinic, 200 First Street SW
MN 55905 Rochester, USA

Miralem PASIC
Deutsches Herzzentrum Berlin
Klinik für Herz-, Thorax-, and Gefässchirurgie
Augustenburger Platz 1
13353 Berlin, Germany

Guiseppe PICCOLO
Centro Transfusionale
e di Immunologia dei Trapianti
Ospedale Maggiore, Policlinico IRCCS
20145 Milano, Italy

Mathieu POIRIER
Department of Vascular Surgery
Hôpital Gabriel Montpied
CHU de Clermont-Ferrand, 63000, France

Janet POWELL
Department of Vascular Surgery
Imperial College at Charing Cross
St Dunstan's Road
W6 8RP London, United-Kingdom

Jonathan REFSON
Regional Vascular Unit, St. Mary's Hospital
London W2, United-Kingdom

Michel REGGI
Department of Cardiovascular Surgery
Hôpital Saint Joseph, 26 bd de Louvain
13008 Marseille, France

Tim REHDERS
Abteiliung für Kardiologie
Medizinische Klinik
Universitätsklinikum Rostok
Ernst-Heydemann-Strasse 6
18055 Rostok, Germany

Lars REX
Department of Surgery
Boras Hospital
50182 Boras, Sweden

Jean-Pierre RIBAL
Department of Vascular Surgery
Hôpital Gabriel Montpied
CHU de Clermont-Ferrand, 63000, France

Gunnar RIEPE
II Department of Surgery
Allgemeines Krankenhaus Hamburg
Eissendorfer Pferdeweg 52
21075 Hamburg, Germany

Eugénio ROSSET
Department of Vascular Surgery
Hôpital Gabriel Montpied
CHU de Clermont-Ferrand, 63000, France

Mario SCALAMOGNA
Servizio per il Prelievo
e la Conservazione di Organi e Tissuti
Ospedale Maggiore, Policlinico IRCCS
20145 Milano, Italy

Marc SCHEPENS
Department of Cardiovascular
and Thoracic Surgery
St Antonius Hospital, Koekoekslaan 1
3435 CM Nieuwegein, The Netherlands

Geert-Willem SCHURINK
Department of Surgery
University Hospital Maastricht, PO Box 5800
6202 AZ Maastricht, The Netherlands

Girolamo SIRCHIA
Centro Transfusionale
e di Iimmunologia dei Trapianti
Ospedale Maggiore, Policlinico IRCCS
20145 Milano, Italy

Fabien THAVEAU
Department of Vascular Surgery
Hôpitaux Universitaires de Strasbourg
67000 Strasbourg, France

Henrik THOMSEN
Department of Diagnostic Radiology
Copenhagen University Hospital at Herlev
Herlev Ringvej 75, 2730 Herlev, Denmark

Jan TIJSSEN
Department of Epidemiology
Academic Medical Center, PO Box 22660
1100DD Amsterdam, The Netherlands

Jan TORDOIR
Department of Surgery
University Hospital Maastricht
6202 AZ Maastricht, The Netherlands

Nicolas VALERIO
Department of Cardiovascular Surgery
Hôpital Saint Joseph, 26 bd de Louvain
13008 Marseille, France

Wim-Jan van BOVEN
Department of Cardiovascular
and Thoracic Surgery
St Antonius Hospital, Koekoekslaan 1
3435 CM Nieuwegein, The Netherlands

Frank van de SANDE
Department of Nephrology
University Hospital Maastricht
6202 AZ Maastricht, The Netherlands

Francesco VIDAL-BARRAQUER
Cirugía Vascular
Hospital del Mar,
08003 Barcelona, Spain

John WOLFE
Regional Vascular Unit, St. Mary's Hospital
London W2, United-Kingdom

August YSA
Cirugía Vascular
Hospital del Mar
08003 Barcelona, Spain

Simona ZANETTI
Chirurgia Vascolare
Azienda Ospedaleria di Perugia
66122 Perugia, Italy

X

FOREWORD

The working field of the vascular specialist comprises arteries and veins in the whole human body, implying the wide range of pathologic vascular diseases, subsequently requiring an extensive armementarium of therapeutic modalities. Application of surgical and endovascular procedures entails the occurrence of complications, primarily affecting the patient but also concerning the vascular specialist, impinging upon hospital stay and financial resources.

Complications are not a popular subject of discussion and should obviously be limited as much as possible. However, the dominant function of complications is to understand the mechanism, discern preventive measures, determine causative factors and thereby master and improve future procedures. Development, assessment and evaluation of vascular and endovascular complications is not limited to procedural problems and failed patency but includes an extensive spectrum of interactive aspects which finally determine the outcome of the treatment.

This year's European Vascular Course addresses the subject of complications in vascular and endovascular surgery and this book contains twenty nine chapters covering the domain of definition and analysis of complications, assessment of preoperative risks, hypercoagulable and myointimal hyperplasia mechanisms, graft behaviour and infection. Furthermore, neurologic complications after cerebrovascular revascularization, renal failure, recurrent stenosis, and failures following first rib resection and sympathectomy are extensively discussed. Surgical and endovascular treatment of aortic arch and descending thoracic aortic aneurysms and dissections are highlighted as well as problems occurring during and after vascular access, kidney transplantation, reconstruction of the main venous trunks and surgery for varicose veins. Complications of treatment for abdominal and thoracoabdominal aortic disease, renal and visceral arterial pathology and upper and lower limb ischemia will be addressed in next year's book of the European Vascular Course.

The superb contribution of the authors is the basis of this textbook, which aims to provide a comprehensive update on important aspects of complications in vascular and endovascular surgery and we would like to thank the authors for their highly valuable input. Dirk Ubbink and Bertrand Ede have performed major editorial work, significantly contributing to the scientific level of the book. Jean-Pierre Jacomy is acknowledged as the medical artist wo prepared the drawings and illustrations. We express our sincere thanks to our secretaries and other collaborators from both departments: Annie Barral, Caroline Lorenzati and Claire Meertens. Marie France and the team of ODIM have succeeded again in printing the high quality English and French version of this book. Futura Publishing Company substantially contributed with editorial assistance of Kirstin Bellhouse and vital advice of Jacques Strauss.

The European Vascular Course and this textbook can only be realized with the support of the biomedical industry. We are very grateful to our major sponsors for their encouragement, collaboration and support.

Maastricht - Marseille, 2001

Michael Jacobs   Alain Branchereau

CONTENTS

XIV

1

DEFINITIONS AND ANALYSIS OF COMPLICATIONS IN RELATION TO THE BENEFITS OF TREATMENT

DINK A LEGEMATE, JAN G TIJSSEN

Although interventions are intended to benefit the patient, they also involve the danger of complications. Clinicians often encounter patients who are exposed to the risk of complications, and they have the difficult task of weighing the benefits of treatment against the risk of complications for a particular intervention. Balancing benefits against harm is sometimes easy, e.g. in a patient with a ruptured aneurysm. In such a case severe complications as a result of operation, although not desirable, are acceptable. In contrast, in a patient with an asymptomatic carotid stenosis, even minor complications as a result of intervention are hardly acceptable.

How should we approach the balance between benefit and harm? Clinicians are well aware of complications, but there is a lack of knowledge on the interpretation of harm as a consequence of complications in relation to the benefits of treatment. The literature concerning this matter is scarce. Some new terms, however, have emerged over recent years and these are useful to further understand the effect of complications.

Risk reduction

The outcomes of vascular interventions are often of a dichotomous nature, i.e. dead or alive, patent or occluded, limb salvage or amputation, stroke or no stroke. The clinician performs an intervention with

the aim of reducing the risk of a particular event. Useful terms to define the magnitude of the effect of treatment are the absolute risk reduction (ARR) and the number needed to treat (NNT). These terms have been developed primarily for the interpretation of the results of controlled randomized trials in which an experimental intervention is compared with standard treatment.

The ARR is the difference in risk between the treated or experimental event rate (EER) and the unexposed or control event rate (CER). The ARR can also be applied to surgical patients and be translated into the difference in risk for a particular event between a surgical and a nonsurgical patient. The NNT is defined as the number of patients that need to be treated over a specific period of time to prevent one bad outcome and is defined as the inverse of the absolute risk reduction: $\frac{1}{ARR}$. The advantage of the NNT is that it makes it easy to see how many patients will or will not benefit from a particular intervention.

Some examples from the literature might best explain how these terms should be used. In a systematic review of carotid endarterectomy for symptomatic carotid stenosis, the efficacy of surgery for a 70%-99% carotid stenosis was translated into an ARR for any disabling or fatal stroke or surgical death of 6.7% with a 95% confidence interval (CI) of 3.2%-10%. The NNT is therefore 1/0.067 = 15 with a CI between 1/0.10 and 1/0.032 = 10 to 31 [1]. In practical terms, this means that 15 patients need to be operated on in order to prevent one stroke (95% CI: 10 – 31). The NNT also tells us that 14 out of 15 patients will not benefit, despite the operation.

The UK small aneurysm trial has taught us that, in aneurysms up to a size of 5.5 cm, there is no benefit from early prophylactic surgery when compared to watchful waiting and ultrasonographic surveillance, therefore defining the NNT for the surgical treatment of small aneurysms as infinite [2]. As in this trial patients with aneurysms greater than 5.5 cm were not included; we do not know the NNT for larger aneurysms.

It is important to realize that tradition coupled with empirical evidence from case series dictate the way in which we perceive indications and consequently treat a patient, and also that clear evidence from randomized trials is often lacking. For these reasons the NNT for many interventions is unknown, thus limiting our knowledge of the real benefits of treatment. We will probably never know the NNT of some diseases because they will never be the subject of randomized trials. However, a good guess can often be made in the treatment of ruptured abdominal aneurysm, for example. If we assume that all patients with this condition arriving at the hospital alive have a 100% risk of dying if we do not intervene, and that operation reduces the risk of mortality by 50%, then the ARR is 50% and the NNT is 2.

Risk increase (complications)

The disadvantage of a surgical or radiological intervention is that harm may be done. Terms which define the magnitude of harm are, the absolute risk increase (ARI) and the number needed to harm (NNH). In controlled randomized trials, the ARI is defined as the absolute difference in the risk of an adverse outcome between an experimental and a control patient. This term can also be applied to complications occurring as a result of intervention in surgical patients and is defined as the difference in the rate of complications between a surgical and a nonsurgical patient. The NNH is the number of patients who, if they receive treatment, would lead to one additional patient being harmed and is defined as the reciprocal of the ARI: $\frac{1}{ARI}$.

For example a patient might experience a complication immediately or shortly after aneurysm surgery, such as death, a myocardial infarction or a wound infection. In the case of a 5% mortality rate for the treatment of an asymptomatic abdominal aneurysm, the ARI is 5% which translates into an NNH of 20 (1/0.05). In the case of survival accompanied by a 5% risk of a disabling and undesirable myocardial infarction we can add another 5% risk increase for the remaining 95 patients. This translates into an aggregate absolute risk increase of 0.05 + 0.05 x 0.95 = 0.0975% which in turn translates into a total NNH of 1/0.0975 = 10.

The question is, which particular complications should be included in the definition of risk increase and NNH? Of course this depends on the severity of the disease, the severity of the complication and the trade-offs made by both the patient and the doctor. When defining complications we should differentiate between the acceptable and the unacceptable. In the aforementioned example it is probably inappropriate to include a wound infection in the definition of harm, but very appropriate to include a disabling myocardial infarction. As there is also a risk of a bad outcome in the long run, such as dying from a ruptured false aneurysm at a vascular anastomosis site or from an infected prosthesis, delayed complications should also be included in the definition of absolute risk increase.

A sensible way to judge whether a complication should be included in the definition of unacceptable or acceptable harm is to ask both the patient and ourselves if we would embark upon an intervention if we knew that it would result in a complication, the consequences of which the patient would find unacceptable and for this reason would refuse to undergo the intervention. It is conceivable that a patient with intermittent claudication would accept a hematoma, a blood transfusion, and suturing of a puncture hole as a complication of percutaneous transluminal angioplasty. Contrast this for example, with a patient with a type II thoracoabdominal aneurysm who would probably abandon any thought of operation if he knew that he would be the unlucky patient with postoperative paraplegia.

The risk to surgical patients of complications immediately or shortly following intervention is fairly well known from case series and to a much lesser extent, from randomized experiments. The inclusion of delayed complications in the definition of harm is limited by the fact that data on late complications are often imprecise or even absent as a result of inadequate follow-up.

The effect of complications on the benefit of treatment

Weighing the balance between the benefits of treatment and the risk of complications is often difficult. The NNT and NNH are very helpful here and the combination of these two parameters can improve insight into the effect of treatment and treatment related complications. Unqualified success, defined as a successful intervention with no complications, and unmitigated failure, defined as a failed intervention accompanied by one or more complications, are at each end of the spectrum. In between are a variety of combinations of benefit and complications (such as the patient treated successfully for an asymptomatic aneurysm, but complicated by a myocardial infarction or a wound infection).

The method by which we would be able to arrange the entire spectrum into methodological and easily understandable models still has to take definite shape, although some concepts have recently been proposed [3-6]. One proposal, put forward by the *Evidence Based Medicine Working Group*, is the calculation of the likelihood of being helped versus harmed (LHH) [7]. The LHH is defined as the ratio of the absolute risk reduction and the absolute risk increase (ARR/ARI) or alternatively the aggregate ratio of $\frac{1}{NNT}$ and $\frac{1}{NNH}$. In the previously mentioned systematic review of carotid endarterectomy, the ARR for the endpoint of death or major disability from stroke was 6.7% and the NNT was 15 [1]. In this review 6.7% is the combined result of both the prevented strokes and deaths and the induced strokes and deaths as a result of surgery. The review also showed that the 30-day postoperative risk of death or major disability from stroke was 3%. If we assume that all these deaths and strokes are directly related to the surgical intervention and would not have happened if it were possible to operate without complications, the ARR as a result of surgery would have been 6.7% + 3% = 9.7%, which can be translated into an NNT of 10.3. From this data the point estimate of the LHH can be calculated from the ratio of the ARR and the ARI: 9.7%/3% being 3.2. This number tells us that carotid endarterectomy is 3.2 times more likely to help than harm the patient. The NNT and NNH also provide the opportunity for an alternative look at the data: if we operate on a hundred patients for a more than 70% symptomatic carotid stenosis, we will prevent stroke in approximately 10 patients and induce stroke and/or death in 3. About 87 patients will neither benefit nor seriously be harmed by the operation. Calculation of probability shows that the one who is most harmed by the operation is probably also the one who otherwise would have remained asymptomatic. This example shows that a perioperative complication can have a major effect on the balance between benefit and harm.

The higher the NNT and the lower the NNH the smaller the therapeutic window. The therapeutic window for the treatment of asymptomatic disease is small, sometimes very small, and the effect of complications might completely erase the potential benefit of a particular intervention. This is one of the reasons for the controversy concerning the operative treatment of asymptomatic carotid artery disease following the publication of the results of the ACAS trial [7]. As the treatment of asymptomatic aortic aneurysms is often accompanied by serious perioperative complications and the NNT is unknown, we are left with much uncertainty about the balance between benefit and harm. The lower the NNH, as in more complex aneurysms, the higher this uncertainty.

In the discussion on complications, two other aspects should be mentioned: the assessment of the benefit-risk ratio for an individual patient and the incorporation of the patients values and preferences. Some patients are at a higher risk of developing a complication than others, which results in a more unfavorable benefit-risk ratio. A patient with a symptomatic carotid stenosis, a contralateral carotid occlusion, diabetes, impaired renal function, two previous myocardial infarctions and hypertension is at higher risk as the average vascular patient. By introducing a correcting factor for the higher risk, we can adjust the benefit-risk ratio. Let us assume a hypothetical situation in which this patient is being considered for carotid endarterectomy because of an 80% symptomatic stenosis and carries a risk of developing a serious complication which is four times higher than that of the average patient in the systematic review of carotid endarterectomy. The

ARI increases to 12% (4 x 3%). Accordingly, the LHH of 3.2 changes to an adjusted LHH of 0.8 (9.7%/12%). It is clear from the adjusted LHH that the patient has a greater chance of being harmed than helped by an endarterectomy. In many cases information concerning risks is not available and it is not always possible to tailor the benefit-risk ratio to a particular patient. This leaves us with uncertainty about the effectiveness of the treatment and the extent to which it is influenced by the effects of complications. In such circumstances best clinical judgment, although subjective, must estimate the correcting factor.

The patients' value is the other factor that has to be incorporated into the calculation of the adjusted LHH. Patients value complications differently. A complication that is unacceptable to one patient might be acceptable to another. This directly influences the definition of NNH, and accordingly the

Table	GLOSSARY OF DEFINITIONS
Absolute risk reduction (ARR)	**In randomized trials:** the difference in risk between the treated or experimental event rate (EER) and the unexposed or control event rate (CER). The ARR can also be applied to a surgical patient and translated into the difference in risk for a particular event between a surgical and a nonsurgical patient. ARR = EER – CER.
Absolute risk increase (ARI)	**In randomized trials:** the absolute difference in the risk of getting an adverse outcome between an experimental and a control patient. The ARI can also be defined as the difference in the rate of complications between a surgical and a nonsurgical patient.
Benefit-risk ratio	The ratio of the absolute risk reduction and absolute risk increase ($\frac{ARR}{ARI}$) See also *likelihood of being helped versus harmed*.
Complications	Adverse events as a result of treatment. Surgical complications can be divided into *perioperative* and *delayed* complications and *acceptable* and *unacceptable* complications.
Likelihood of being helped versus harmed (LHH)	The ratio of the absolute risk reduction and absolute risk increase ($\frac{ARR}{ARI}$) or the aggregate ratio of $\frac{1}{NNT}$ and $\frac{1}{NNH}$ An alternative term is the *benefit-risk ratio*.
Number needed to treat (NNT)	The number of patients that need to be treated to prevent one bad outcome and is defined as the reciprocal of the absolute risk reduction ($\frac{1}{AAR}$)
Number needed to harm (NNH)	The number of patients who, if they receive the treatment, would lead to one additional patient being harmed. The NNH is the reciprocal of the absolute risk increase ($\frac{1}{ARI}$)
Patient values	What a patient believes in and holds dear about the way he/she lives.
Risk aversion	The aversion of a patient to running the risk of complications as a result of an intervention that intends to prevent a future outcome.

LHH. One term that needs to be mentioned in relation to the risk of complications is *risk aversion*. This is the aversion of the patient to running the risk of complications as a result of an intervention that intends to prevent a future event. Risk aversion is particularly important when treating asymptomatic disease. To date the value the patients put on a complication has been insufficiently studied and an objective and validated scale is lacking. It should further be realized that assessment of a complication does not always involve a straightforward choice between two determinants, but often a choice on a sliding scale.

This procedure resembles the steps in a formal clinical decision analysis. In a clinical decision analysis, a patient has probabilities and choices with regard to a particular outcome. Clinical decision analysis is an alternative way to approach and assessing outcomes of treatment and complications. Clinical decision analysis, although useful, is a rather complicated method to use in daily clinical practice and the approach as outlined in this chapter might be more practical.

Conclusion

Achieving a balance between the benefits of treatment and treatment-induced complications is often difficult. The literature concerning the evaluation of this balance is scarce. However, over the past few years methodological insight has improved and new terms and definitions have been introduced. These definitions are useful for the interpretation of treatment induced complications in relation to the benefits of treatment. A summary of definitions is shown in the Table. Knowledge of these definitions and their applications in daily practice will improve the care of the vascular patient.

REFERENCES

1 Cina CS, Clase CM, Haynes BR. Refining the indications for carotid endarterectomy in patients with symptomatic carotid stenosis: a systematic review. *J Vasc Surg* 1999; 30: 606-617.

2 Anonymous. Mortality results for randomised controlled trial of early elective surgery or ultrasonographic surveillance for small abdominal aortic aneurysms. The UK Small Aneurysm Trial Participants. *Lancet* 1998; 352: 1649-1655.

3 Levine M, Walter S, Lee H et al. Users' guides to the medical literature. IV. How to use an article about harm. Evidence Based Medicine Working Group. *JAMA* 1994; 271: 1615-1619.

4 Schulzer M, Mancini GB. "Unqualified success" and "unmitigated failure": number-needed-to-treat-related concepts for assessing treatment efficacy in the presence of treatment-induced adverse events. *Int J Epidemiol* 1996; 25: 704-712.

5 Mancini GB, Schulzer M. Reporting risks and benefits of therapy by use of the concepts of unqualified success and unmitigated failure. Application to highly cited trials in cardiovascular medicine. *Circulation* 1999; 99: 377-383.

6 McAlister FA, Straus SE, Guyatt GH, Haynes RB. Users' guides to the medical literature: XX. Integrating research evidence with the care of the individual patient. Evidence Based Medicine Working Group. *JAMA* 2000; 283: 2829-2836.

7 Anonymous. Endarterectomy for asymptomatic carotid stenosis. Executive Committee for the Asymptomatic Carotid Atherosclerosis Study. *JAMA* 1995; 273: 1421-1428.

2

MANAGEMENT OF CARDIAC DISEASE AND CARDIAC RISK IN THE VASCULAR ATHEROSCLEROTIC PATIENT

GILBERT HABIB

Peri-operative cardiac complications are the most important cause of mortality and morbidity after major vascular surgery. Patients undergoing major non-cardiac vascular surgery are known to be at high risk of both peri-operative and long-term cardiac events. Although the risk of myocardial infarction after vascular surgery has declined, it remains relatively high, especially because of the increasing age of the operated patients. Non-cardiac vascular disease is an increasingly important problem in patients over age 60, whose numbers in Europe are expected to increase over 60% to 224 million by 2025 [1]. In addition, the preoperative evaluation of these patients may take into account not only their peri-operative risk, but also their long-term cardiac risk. The preoperative assessment of the cardiac risk in vascular patients therefore aims to reduce the immediate risk of surgery and to reduce the long-term cardiac morbidity and mortality.

Preoperative cardiac risk assessment

Ideally, preoperative assessment should stratify patients into three groups: patients with low surgical risk in whom surgery can be performed without additional investigation; patients at high risk in whom surgery may be postponed so that cardiac assessment and treatment may be performed before surgery; and patients at intermediate risk, in whom the cardiac peri-operative risk may be reduced by a specific intervention [1]. Usually, a combination of a clinical evaluation and of non-invasive tests allows such a classification.

The most frequent approach of the risk of vascular surgery is a combination of clinical assessment, functional capacity, and specific surgical risk [1-5]. Based on clinical assessment, patients may be at high risk of peri-operative cardiac events in case of recent myocardial infarction, unstable angina, decompensated heart failure, significant arrhythmias, and severe valvular disease [2]; these conditions justify an immediate management of cardiac disease and may result in delay or cancellation of surgery unless it is emergent. Intermediate predictors of increased risk are mild angina, prior myocardial infarction, compensated heart failure, and diabetes mellitus. These conditions justify a careful evaluation of patients before surgery. Other markers of increased surgical risk include advanced age, abnormal electrocardiogram and uncontrolled hypertension [2].

Functional capacity is another important marker of surgical risk. Patients with very low capacity are at higher risk of subsequent cardiac event; functional capacity may be assessed either by history of daily activities or by exercise stress testing, when possible [1].

Finally, peri-operative risk of non-cardiac surgery depends on the type of surgery. Surgery associated with severe modifications in blood pressure, cardiac rhythm, and bleeding are at higher risk for cardiac events; high-risk surgery includes aortic and peripheral vascular surgery, while cardiac risk is only intermediate for carotid endarterectomy [6-7].

This clinical evaluation is of high value for preoperative prediction of peri-operative cardiac risk and management. Patients with minor or no clinical predictors of cardiac risk and with good functional capacity may be operated on regardless of type of surgical procedure, whereas patients with poor functional capacity and intermediate clinical risk may undergo functional testing [2]. Several classifications of peri-operative risk have been proposed based on clinical evaluation [3-5]. However, despite a multifactorial approach to clinical stratification, these clinical risk indices lack sensitivity to detect silent coronary artery disease, especially in patients with severely limited exercise capacity [8]. This explains the increased reliance by clinicians on non-invasive tests that detect underlying coronary artery disease not requiring physical exercise [8].

Specific non-invasive tests

EXERCISE ELECTROCARDIOGRAPHY

The aim of exercise electrocardiography before surgery is to reproduce the increase in myocardial consumption provoked by the surgical trauma.

Cardiac events are frequently associated with sinus tachycardia, increased myocardial oxygen consumption, and myocardial ischemia, that may be reproduced by exercise electrocardiography. Electrocardiographic response to exercise, and probably more important exercise tolerance, are both helpful predictors of cardiac events [9]. Unfortunately, the value of exercise electrocardio-graphy in predicting events is relatively low and vary among studies. Furthermore, patients assessed before vascular surgery frequently cannot perform maximal exercise testing because of their clinical status or the presence of severe peripheral arterial disease [10]. Similarly, ambulatory electrocardiographic detection of silent ischemic changes is a marker of adverse outcome in some studies, but suffers from relatively low sensitivity [11].

ECHOCARDIOGRAPHY

Echocardiography in patients undergoing vascular surgery has the same indications as in other patients. Predictors of peri-operative cardiac morbidity are the presence of severe left ventricular dysfunction, valvular disease, or pulmonary hypertension. However, the additional value of resting echocardiography to the conventional clinical data is only modest [1,9]. Nevertheless, resting echocardiography must be performed preoperatively when clinically indicated by abnormal clinical findings.

Stress echocardiography plays a much more important role in these patients. Stress echocardiography, using either dobutamine [8], exercise, or dipyridamole [12], increases the myocardial oxygen consumption and induces myocardial ischemia in patients with significant coronary artery disease. Dobutamine stress echocardiography (DSE) has been the most frequently used method in the pre-operative assessment of cardiac risk [8,13-14]. Dobutamine is administered at progressively increasing doses beginning at 5 mg/kg/min up to 40 or 50 mg/kg/min. Atropine may be added when the target rate is not reached. New wall motion abnormality during dobutamine infusion is observed in the presence of significant coronary stenosis causing ischemia. The value of dobutamine echocardiography in detecting coronary artery disease has been proven by numerous studies [15-17]. In addition, dobutamine echocardiography has been shown to be safe, both in non-selected patients and in patients with aortic aneurysm [18-19]. In a study of 98 patients with aortic aneurysm, Pellikka et al. observed no case of aneurysm rupture during

DSE [18]. Thus, dobutamine echocardiography may be considered as a safe test for the evaluation of the coronary risk before surgery.

The value of DSE in predicting peri-operative events has been assessed in several studies [8,13-14]. The largest series included 300 consecutive patients undergoing DSE before major vascular surgery. In this series, Poldermans et al. [13] showed that all 27 postoperative cardiac complications occurred in the 72 patients with positive DSE. Moreover, the combination of clinical assessment and DSE allows ideal risk assessment in these patients; in the study from Poldermans, 100 out of 300 patients had no clinical risk factor and DSE provided no additional information in these patients. Patients with one or more clinical risk factors had a 13% peri-operative complication rate, and were further stratified by DSE; in these patients, peri-operative event rate was 43% when DSE was positive, and 0% in patients with negative DSE. Patients with positive DSE at lower heart rate were at higher risk.

DIPYRIDAMOLE THALLIUM SCINTIGRAPHY

The technique of dipyridamole thallium scintigraphy (DTS) has been extensively used in patients undergoing vascular surgery [20]. Dipyridamole mimics the coronary vasodilatator response associated with exercise [9]. Patients presenting with perfusion defects during DTS are at increased risk of subsequent cardiac events during surgery. Generally, early studies showed that DTS was both sensitive and specific for the assessment of surgical risk [21-25]. More recently, the extent of perfusion defects and the increased lung thallium uptake were also shown to be prognostic markers [26].

However, the true value of DTS for the evaluation of peri-operative risk has been questioned by several authors. Mangano et al. [27] noted a sensitivity of 46% and a negative predictive value of 82% for DTS. Baron et al. [28] suggested that DTS results were not predictive for subsequent cardiac events. The causes for discrepancies between studies include the fact that, in most earlier studies, the physicians were not blinded to the preoperative result of DTS, so that all consecutive patients scheduled for surgery were not included, but rather only selected patients [1].

On the other hand, it may be argued that studies of Mangano and Baron included consecutive patients which represent a low-risk population and that the value of DTS may be better in an intermediate-risk selected population [29]. Vanzetto et al. [26] confirmed this hypothesis, showing that a positive DTS performed in an intermediate-risk population had a good prognostic value for cardiac events. Furthermore, this study showed that, in this population, DTS added to the risk determination provided by the clinical risk factors. In this study, 134 patients were selected for the presence of two or more risk factors (age above 70, history of myocardial infarction, angina, congestive heart failure, diabetes mellitus, hypertension with severe ventricular hypertrophy, or abnormal electrocardiogram at rest) and underwent DTS. DTS accurately discriminated between high-risk and low-risk patients; the major event rate was 23% and 1% when a reversible defect was present or absent, respectively.

Practical approach and guidelines for non-invasive evaluation of cardiac patients before surgery

When assessing a patient's risk for major cardiac events, the first step is the clinical assessment. Using clinical risk indices, patients may be classified in according to a risk scale of three categories [8-9]. High-risk patients may be identified in the presence of three or more clinical risk factors; in these patients, the risk of cardiac events is 10% to 15%, and surgery must be delayed if possible; careful cardiac evaluation and treatment may be performed before surgery.

Low-risk patients are identified in the presence of zero or one risk factors; in the study of Poldermans et al. [13], patients with none of the clinical risk factors defined by Eagle had a 1% peri-operative risk. Additional cardiac testing is not necessary in these patients. Between these two populations, a large number of patients (between 30% to 60% having vascular surgery) are at intermediate risk for peri-operative cardiac events. Dobutamine echocardiography and DTS both provide useful information for the peri-operative risk of these patients and may be recommended for further risk stratification. In summary, clinical assessment and DTS or dobutamine echocardiography allow correct assessment of the cardiac risk of the majority of patients referred for vascular surgery.

Management of specific cardiovascular conditions

CORONARY HEART DISEASE

Peri-operative cardiac events are principally caused by myocardial ischemia due to coronary artery disease [8]. Patients presenting for major vascular surgery have a high incidence of coronary artery disease. Hertzer et al. [30] using coronarography in all vascular surgical candidates found a 37% prevalence of coronary stenosis even in the absence of clinical evidence of coronary artery disease. The goal of peri-operative stratification is to detect intermediate risk patients in whose increased risk may be reduced by preoperative therapeutic interventions. As previously described, this risk may be assessed by the combination of clinical assessment and results of non-invasive tests. Once the risk status of the patient is known, therapeutic strategies may be applied.

In high-risk patients, with unstable coronary syndromes, surgery may be delayed if not urgent, and cardiac catheterization performed; if possible, the patient will be revascularized either by surgical coronary artery bypass grafting or by percutaneous angioplasty. In low-risk patients, the patient may be operated on without other investigation; similarly, patients with recent (i.e., within one year) coronary revascularization do not need further testing. In intermediate risk patients, the therapeutic strategies may be based on the results of the non-invasive testings (DSE or DTS). Patients with a negative test have a very low event-rate and may be sent for surgery.

The optimal treatment for patients with a positive test is still debated. The benefit of *preventive* revascularization has not been prospectively evaluated [8]; the potential benefit of coronary revascularization may be counterbalanced by the risk of bypass coronary surgery and percutaneous angioplasty [1]. The lack of demonstrable benefit and the risk of invasive procedures have influenced the *American College of Physicians* [29] to recommend not to revascularize such patients. A better recommendation would be to perform revascularization in the same patients as one would have done if no surgery was planned [1]. Finally, the decision to revascularize or not a patient with a positive non-invasive test may be influenced by the degree of ischemia. Patients with severe ischemia at low heart rate are a particularly high-risk subset and would undergo revascularization before surgery [8].

The optimal medical therapy in patients with ischemia who do not need revascularization is based on use of beta-blocker agents. Mangano et al. in 1996 [31] and more recently Poldermans et al. [32] underlined the major value of beta-blocker therapy before vascular surgery in reducing peri-operative cardiovascular events. In the series of Poldermans, 846 patients with one or more risk factors underwent DSE, with positive results in 173; 59 patients were randomly assigned to receive bisoprolol, and 53 received standard care. Cardiac mortality was higher in the standard care group than in the bisoprolol group (17 % vs. 3.4%, p = 0.02). Beta-blockers may thus be recommended in patients with risk factors and positive dobutamine tests.

HYPERTENSION

Moderate hypertension is not an independent risk factor for peri-operative cardiovascular complications. However, intra-operative blood pressure variations are associated with myocardial ischemia during surgery [33]. In mild to moderate hypertension, surgery must not be delayed. Adequate antihypertensive medications may be continued during the peri-operative period. In more severe hypertension, blood pressure must be controlled before surgery. Beta-blockers appears particularly indicated in these patients.

CONGESTIVE HEART FAILURE

Congestive heart failure carries a high risk in the peri-operative period. Care must be taken to obtain a stabilization of the clinical status of the patient before surgery. The diagnosis of the underlying disease may be very important because of different management strategies. Echocardiography must be performed in this setting to differentiate between hypertrophic and dilated cardiomyopathy, and to detect features of ischemic cardiomyopathy.

VALVULAR HEART DISEASE

In most patients, valvular disease may be known by the patient or easily diagnosed by clinical examination. Mitral valve stenosis is very rare, and must be recognized and treated if severe before surgery. Aortic regurgitation is more frequent and even severe regurgitations are usually asymptomatic and without left ventricular dysfunction; these patients may be operated on without cardiac problem; aortic insufficiency with left ventricular dysfunction or clinical heart failure may be treated specifically before surgery. Mitral regurgitation is now the more frequent valve disease. The severity and etiology of mitral regurgitation may be evaluated before surgery; transthoracic and transesophageal echocardiography are both useful in this setting. In fact, aortic stenosis poses the greater risk for non-cardiac surgery [4]. Aortic stenosis may be detected by clinical examination and quantified by doppler echocardiography. In case of severe aortic stenosis, aortic valve replacement may be performed prior to vascular surgery.

ARRHYTHMIAS AND CONDUCTION DISTURBANCES

Arrhythmias and conduction disturbances are frequently observed before vascular surgery. Arrhythmias detected before surgery do not necessitate a different approach than other arrhythmias. The presence of an arrhythmia frequently justifies a search for an underlying cardiac or pulmonary disease, a drug toxicity, or a metabolic abnormality [2].

Patients with conduction abnormalities may be treated as in the absence of surgery. Temporary pacing is exceptionally necessary. In case of symptomatic severe conduction abnormality, a permanent pacemaker must be proposed.

Long-term cardiac prognosis in vascular patients

Late cardiac events occur as frequently as 19% in the two years following vascular surgery [34], essentially because of the high prevalence of coronary artery disease in these patients [30]. Therefore the preoperative assessment of vascular patients may include the risk of late events.

As for immediate events, the onset of a late cardiac event may be predicted by clinical markers and non-invasive tests. Patients with history of coronary artery disease or heart failure have worse prognoses than others [8]. Positive DSE as well as DTS have been shown to be very good markers of further cardiac events [35-36]. In a recent study of 318 survivors of major vascular surgery [35], 32 cardiac events occurred during a 10-month follow-up period. Univariate predictors of cardiac events include history of angina, myocardial infarction or diabetes mellitus, non-fatal peri-operative cardiac event, and a positive stress test. Multivariate predictors of events were nonfatal peri-operative events, new wall motion abnormality during stress, and a history of myocardial infarction.

Dobutamine stress echocardiography may thus be performed preoperatively in all patients with one or more risk factors. This will provide both peri-operative risk stratification and prediction of late cardiac events after successful surgery [8]. Interestingly, Poldermans et al. [36] recently reported that the benefit of early beta-blockade in these patients persists as long as 22 months after surgery. In this series, the incidence of late cardiac events was 8.8% in the 57 patients randomized to bisoprolol, and 27% in the 44 patients in the standard care group (p< 0.001).

Conclusion

Although the cardiac risk of vascular surgery has declined in the recent years, coronary and cardiac events are still the main cause of mortality and morbidity in the peri-operative period. The increasing age of the surgical population and the limitations of the clinical risk assessment justify the use of non-invasive diagnostic tests in a selected intermediate-risk population. Dipyridamole thallium scintigraphy and dobutamine stress echocardiography are both useful markers of an increased risk. Combination of clinical markers and either DTS or DSE results provides an optimal assessment of the peri-operative as well as the long-term cardiac risk of patients undergoing vascular surgery. Optimal management of intermediate-risk patients with a positive diagnostic test remains to be precisely defined. Beta-blocker therapy seems to play an important role in the prevention of both peri-operative and late cardiac events.

R E F E R E N C E S

1 Poldermans D, Bax JJ, Thomson IR et al. Role of dobutamine stress echocardiography for preoperative cardiac risk assessment before major vascular surgery : a diagnostic tool comes of age. *Echocardiography* 2000 ; 17 : 79-91.

2 Eagle KA, Brundage BH, Chaitman BR et al. Guidelines for peri-operative cardiovascular evaluation for non cardiac surgery. Report of the American College of Cardiology/American Heart Association Task Force on practice guidelines. *J Am Coll Cardiol* 1996 ; 27 : 910-948.

3 Detsky AS, Abrams HB, Forbath N et al. Cardiac assessment for patients undergoing non-cardiac surgery. A multi factorial clinical risk index. *Arch Intern Med* 1986 ; 146 : 2131-2134.

4 Goldman L, Caldera DL, Nussbaum SR et al. Multifactorial index of cardiac risk in non-cardiac surgical procedures. *N Eng J Med* 1977 ; 297 : 845-850.

5 L'Italien GJ, Paul SD, Hendel RC et al. Development and validation of a Bayesian model for peri-operative cardiac risk assessment in a cohort of 1081 vascular surgical candidates. *J Am Coll Cardiol* 1996 ; 27 : 779-786.

6 Taylor LM Jr., Yeager RA, Moneta GL et al. The incidence of peri-operative myocardial infarction in general vascular surgery. *J Vasc Surg 1994* ; 15 : 52-61.

7 L'Italien GJ, Cambria RP, Cutler BS et al. Comparative early and late cardiac morbidity among patients requiring different vascular surgery procedures. *J Vasc Surg* 1995 ; 21 : 935-944.

8 Poldermans D, Rambaldi P, Fioretti PM et al. Prognostic value of dobutamine – atropine stress echocardiography for peri-operative and late cardiac events in patients scheduled for vascular surgery. *Eur Heart J* 1997 ; 18 suppl D : D86-D96.

9 Mangano DT, Goldman L. Preoperative assessment of patients with known or suspected coronary disease. *N Eng J Med* 1995 ; 333 : 1750-1756.

10 Rose EL, Liu XJ, Henley M et al. Prognostic value of non invasive cardiac tests in the assessment of patients with peripheral vascular disease. *Am J Cardiol* 1993 ; 71 : 40-44.

11 Fleisher LA, Rosenbaum SH, Nelson AH et al. Preoperative dipyridamole thallium imaging and ambulatory electro-cardiographic monitoring as a predictor of peri-operative cardiac events and long term outcome. *Anesthesiology* 1995 ; 83 : 906-917.

12 Sicari R, Picano E, Lusa AM et al. The value of dipyridamole echocardiography in risk stratification before vascular surgery : a multicenter study. *Eur Heart J* 1995 ; 16 : 842-847.

13 Poldermans D, Arnese M, Fioretti PM et al. Improved cardiac risk stratification in major vascular surgery with dobutamine-atropine stress echocardiography. *J Am Coll Cardiol* 1995 ; 26 : 648-653.

14 Lane RT, Sawada SG, Segar DS et al. Dobutamine stress echocardiography for assessment of cardiac risk before non-cardiac surgery. *Am J Cardiol* 1991 ; 68 : 976-977.

15 Segar DS, Brown SE, Sawada SG et al. Dobutamine stress echocardiography : correlation with coronary lesion severity as determined by quantitative angiography. *J Am Coll Cardiol* 1992 ; 19 : 1197-1202.

16 Previtali M, Lanzarini L, Fetiveau R et al. Comparison of dobutamine stress echocardiography, dipyridamole stress echocardiography and exercise stress testing for diagnosis of coronary artery disease. *Am J Cardiol* 1993 ; 72 : 865-870.

17 Marwick T, D'Hondt AM, Baudhuin T et al. Optimal use of dobutamine stress for the detection and evaluation of coronary artery disease : combination with echocardiography, or scintigraphy or both ? *J Am Coll Cardiol* 1993 ; 22 : 159-167.

18 Pellikka PA, Roger VL, Oh JK et al. Safety of performing dobutamine stress echocardiography in patients with abdominal aortic aneurysms > or 4 cm in diameter. *Am J Cardiol* 1996 ; 77 : 413-416.

19 Picano E, Mathias W Jr, Pingitore A, Bigi R et al. Safety and tolerability of dobutamine-atropine stress echocardiography : a prospective, multicentre study. Echo Dobutamine International Cooperative Study Group. *Lancet* 1994 ; 344 : 1190-1192.

20 Shaw L, Eagle KA, Gersh B, Miller D. Meta-analysis of intravenous dipyridamole thallium 201 imaging (1985 to 1994) and dobutamine echocardiography (1991 to 1994) for risk stratification before vascular surgery. *J Am Coll Cardiol* 1996 ; 27 : 787-798.

21 Lette J, Waters D, Lapointe J et al. Usefulness of the severity and extent of reversible perfusion defects during thallium-dipyridamole imaging for cardiac risk assessment before non-cardiac surgery. *Am J Cardiol* 1989 ; 64 : 276-281.

22 Eagle KA, Coley CM, Newell JB et al. Combining clinical and thallium data optimizes preoperative assessment of cardiac risk before major vascular surgery. *Ann Intern Med* 1989 ; 110 : 859-866.

23 Boucher CA, Brewster DC, Darling RC et al. Determination of cardiac risk by dipyridamole-thallium imaging before peripheral vascular surgery. *N Engl J Med* 1985 ; 312 : 389-394.

24 Stratmann HG, Younis LT, Wittry MD et al. Dipyridamole-technetium 99m sestamibi myocardial tomography in patients evaluated for elective vascular surgery : prognostic value for peri-operative and late cardiac events. *Am Heart J* 1996 ; 131 : 923-929.

25 Cutler BS, Hendel RC, Leppo JA. Dipyridamole-thallium scintigraphy predicts peri-operative and long-term survival after major vascular surgery. *J Vasc Surg* 1992 ; 15 : 972-981.

26 Vanzetto G, Machecourt J, Blendea D et al. Additive value of thallium single-photon emission computed tomography myocardial imaging for prediction of peri-operative events in clinically selected high cardiac risk patients having abdominal aortic surgery. *Am J Cardiol* 1996 ; 77 : 143-148.

27 Mangano DT, London MJ, Tubau JF et al. Dipyridamole-thallium 201 scintigraphy as a preoperative screening test. A reexamination of its predictive potential. Study of peri-operative Ischemia Research Group. *Circulation* 1991 ; 84 : 493-502.

28 Baron JF, Mundler O, Bertrand M et al. Dipyridamole-thallium scintigraphy and gated radionuclide angiography to assess cardiac risk before abdominal aortic surgery. *N Eng J Med* 1994 ; 330 : 663-669.

29 Palda VA, Detsky AS. Peri-operative assessment and management of risk from coronary artery disease. *Ann Intern Med* 1997 ; 127 : 313-328.

30 Hertzer NR, Beven EG, Young JR et al. Coronary artery disease in peripheral vascular patients. A classification of 1000 coronary angiograms and results of surgical management. *Ann Surg* 1984 ; 199 : 223-233.

31 Mangano DT, Layug EL, Wallace A, Tateo I. Effect of atenolol on mortality and cardiovascular morbidity after non-cardiac surgery. Multicenter Study of Peri-operative Ischemia Research Group. *N Eng J Med* 1996 ; 335 : 1713-1720.

32 Poldermans D, Boersma E, Bax JJ et al. The effect of bisoprolol on peri-operative mortality and myocardial infarction in high-risk patients undergoing vascular surgery. Dutch Echocardiographic Cardiac Risk Evaluation Applying Stress Echocardiography Study Group. *N Eng J Med* 1999 ; 341 : 1789-1794.

33 Stone JG, Foex P, Sear JW et al. Risk of myocardial ischaemia during anaesthesia in treated and untreated hypertensive patients. *Br J Anaesth* 1988 ; 61 : 675-679.

34 Krupski WC, Layug EL, Reilly LM et al. Comparison of cardiac morbidity rates between aortic and infra-inguinal operations : two-year follow-up. Study of Peri-operative Ischemia Research Group. *J Vasc Surg* 1993 ; 18 : 609-617.

35 Poldermans D, Arnese M, Fioretti P et al. Sustained prognostic value of dobutamine stress echocardiography for late cardiac events after major non cardiac vascular surgery. *Circulation* 1997 ; 95 : 53-58.

36 Poldermans D, Fioretti PM, Boersma E et al. Dobutamine-atropine stress echocardiography and clinical data for predicting late cardiac events in patients with suspected coronary artery disease. *Am J Med* 1994 ; 97 : 119-125.

37 Steinberg EH, Madmon L, Patel CP et al. Long-term prognostic significance of dobutamine echocardiography in patients with suspected coronary artery disease : results of a 5-year follow-up study. *J Am Coll Cardiol* 1997 ; 29 : 969-973.

38 Poldermans D, Boersma E, Bax JJ. Bisoprolol reduces long-term cardiac events in high-risk patients after successful major vascular surgery (abstract). *Circulation* 2000 ; 102 II : 373.

3

HYPERCOAGULABLE STATES AND UNEXPLAINED VASCULAR THROMBOSIS

FRANKLIN A BONTEMPO, MELINA R KIBBE, MICHEL S MAKAROUN

Recent advances in the diagnosis of hypercoagulability have made the testing for underlying causes of thrombosis more fruitful. This has been an area of active interest for hematologists who specialize in coagulation and is becoming increasingly important for vascular surgeons.

The traditional concept of hypercoagulability was put forth by Virchow over 100 years ago. He proposed that vascular thrombosis was associated with either 1) damage to the vessel wall 2) blood stasis or 3) hypercoagulability of the blood. This concept remains a reasonable starting point for determining the cause of thrombosis. In particular, advances have been made in the understanding of the underlying defects that lead to hypercoagulability in the circulation. However, vascular wall damage and venous stasis frequently occur concomitantly to further enhance the risk of vascular thrombosis.

Thrombosis remains a complicated process that is a balance between the procoagulant clotting cascades, the anticoagulant fibrinolytic mechanism, and the naturally occurring anticoagulant proteins. Any congenital or acquired disorder of clotting may upset this balance and lead to thrombosis. The basic outline of these pro and anticoagulant forces is shown in the figure. The major procoagulant forces are the intrinsic and extrinsic coagulation pathways and the major anticoagulant forces are the plasminogen based fibrinolytic mechanism along with the natural clot inhibitors antithrombin III, protein C, and protein S.

In vascular surgery, because the therapeutic approach to arterial and venous thromboses frequently differ, the common causes of both arterial and venous thromboses are discussed separately.

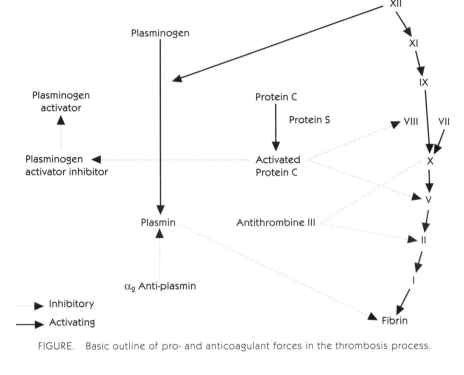

FIGURE. Basic outline of pro- and anticoagulant forces in the thrombosis process.

Arterial thrombosis

Common causes of arterial thrombosis in vascular surgery are listed in Table I.

ATHEROSCLEROSIS, HYPERLIPIDEMIA, TOBACCO

Atherosclerosis associated with hyperlipidemia remains one of the most common causes of vascular wall damage and subsequent thrombosis in vascular surgery. In the United States, approximately 40%-50% of deaths are related to atherosclerosis and hyperlipidemia when both heart disease and stroke are included [1]. In approximately 80%-85% of patients with heart disease and stroke, a thrombotic event is usually associated with the formation of atherosclerotic plaques. When underlying atherosclerotic disease is present with a hypercoagulable state, the risk of thrombosis including graft thrombosis after vascular bypass surgery may be increased. Cigarette smoking remains an additional complicating factor in patients with arterial thrombosis due to the increased rate of atherosclerotic plaque formation, direct damage to the arterial wall, vasoconstriction, and platelet hyper-reactivity. While the

prevalence of cigarette smoking in adults in the United States has declined, smoking rates in Europe have remained higher and the prevalence of smoking among teenagers in the United States is again

Table I	COMMON CAUSES OF ARTERIAL THROMBOSIS

➤ Atherosclerosis/hyperlipidemia

➤ Cigarette smoking

➤ Lupus anticoagulant/antiphospholipid antibody

➤ Heparin-induced thrombocytopenia

➤ Prothrombin gene variant

➤ MTHFR homozygotes

➤ Vasculitis

➤ Oral contraceptives/estrogens

➤ Myeloproliferative disorders

➤ Factor V Leiden mutation

on the rise [2]. Recent improvements in therapies aimed at helping patients to stop smoking should be more strongly encouraged in the management of patients with vascular disease.

LUPUS ANTICOAGULANTS (LACS)

LACs are found in approximately 2%-4% of the patients in the general population and are associated with venous as well as arterial thrombosis [3,4]. The exact risk of thrombosis in patients with LACs remains unclear, as does the mechanism for causation of thrombosis. However, because of the high incidence of LACs, testing for them in patients with arterial thrombosis may be fruitful. Additionally, LACs have a significant impact on anticoagulant therapy since the level of required anticoagulation is often higher and the duration of anticoagulant therapy may need to be longer. In a study of Nielsen et al., antibodies to cardiolipin were identified in 9% of patients undergoing infrainguinal vein bypass surgery and appeared to be associated with increased risk of bypass failure [5]. In contrast, in the report of Lee et al., there was minimal difference in graft primary patency rates, and no difference in assisted primary patency, limb salvage, and survival rates between patients with and without antiphospholipids (APLs) who underwent leg bypass grafting procedures [6]. It is therefore possible that the lack of a difference between the groups can be explained by the difference in use of anticoagulation with warfarin.

HEPARIN-INDUCED THROMBOCYTOPENIA

Heparin-induced thrombocytopenia (HIT) is one of the most feared complications of heparin therapy. Approximately 4%-5% of patients who receive standard unfractionated heparin develop thrombocytopenia [7]. Of those cases, approximately 20% of them have an associated venous or arterial thrombosis [7]. This may lead to the white clot syndrome where platelet-fibrin thrombi form in the arterial circulation leading to loss of a limb, particularly, but not exclusively, in the four to six day period after commencement of heparin therapy. During this critical time period as well as throughout the duration of heparin therapy, monitoring of the platelet count is recommended. Low molecular weight heparins (LMWHs) are associated with an approximately 2% incidence of HIT [8]. However, if a patient taking standard unfractionated heparin develops HIT and is switched to LMWHs, the cross reactivity is 50%-80%; therefore, LMWHs are not

recommended for treatment in patients with HIT [9]. Danaparoid is a heparin-like substance that only has a 5%-10% cross reactivity with heparin and may be used when HIT is present [9]. Lepirudin, which has been recently introduced in the United States, has no cross reactivity with heparin and may be used in patients with HIT [10]. Danaparoid is monitored by use of the anti-factor X activity assay and lepirudin is monitored by either the APTT or the ecarin clotting time. More recently another direct thrombin inhibitor, argatroban, has been introduced which has no cross reactivity with regular heparin, is monitored with the APTT, and may also be used in patients with HIT [11].

PROTHROMBIN GENE VARIANT

The prothrombin gene variant (20210 G to A) is one of the more common genetic disorders (Table II) that may predispose to arterial thrombosis [12]. This is a genetic abnormality of the untranslated portion of the gene for clotting factor II, resulting in an increase in the normal circulating level of factor II (prothrombin) [13]. This leads to an increased risk of thrombosis. Reports have indicated that there is a four to six-fold increase in mild myocardial infarction in females who are heterozygous for this gene [14]. Additionally, an odds ratio of 3 to 6 for the development of myocardial infarction has been reported in carriers of the prothrombin gene mutation who also possess one of the following risk factors: diabetes mellitus, smoking, hypertension, or obesity [15]. Current testing for this gene variant is by direct detection using polymerase chain reaction (PCR).

Table II	RELATIVE FREQUENCY OF CONGENITAL THROMBOTIC DISORDERS
Antithrombin III deficiency	1: 4 000
Protein C deficiency	1: 16 000
Protein S deficiency	1: 16 000
Thrombotic dysfibrinogens	1: 1 000 000
Plasminogen deficiency	1: 1 000 000
Factor V Leiden mutation	1: 17
Prothrombin variant	1: 50-100
Homocysteine homozygotes	1: 12

HYPERHOMOCYSTEINAEMIA, METHYLENETETRAHYDROFOLATE REDUCTASE GENE MUTATION

Homocysteine is a sulfhydryl-containing amino acid that is formed by the demethylation of methionine. Homocysteine is also remethylated to methionine by methionine synthase, a vitamin B12 dependent enzyme and by methylenetetrahydrofolate reductase (MTHFR). Environmental factors such as folate, or vitamin B12, or vitamin B6 deficiencies and genetic defects such as cystathionine beta-synthase or abnormality of MTHFR or some vitamin B12 metabolism defects may contribute to increasing plasma homocysteine levels [16]. Though it is now well known that homocysteine is an independent risk factor for premature vascular disease [17], the pathogenesis of homocysteine-induced vascular damage is, for the most part, unknown. It may be multifactorial, including direct homocysteine damage to the endothelium, an enhanced low-density lipoprotein peroxidation, an increase of platelet thromboxane A2, or a decrease of protein C activation [18]. Patients with classic congenital homocysteinuria who are deficient in cystathionine beta-synthase, are known to have a very high incidence of arterial thrombosis before the age of 30 [19]. Homozygosity for the MTHFR gene is found in approximately 9%-17% of the United States and Canadian population [20]. Current estimates describe a two-fold increase in thrombosis risk in patients who are homozygous for the MTHFR gene [21]. Different reports suggested that hyperhomocysteinaemia is a risk factor for vein graft stenosis from intimal hyperplasia [22,23] and appear to confer a graded, independent increased risk for hemodialysis access thrombosis [24]. Hyperhomocysteinaemia is also associated with cardiovascular disease in renal-transplant recipients [25]. Treatment with folic acid at a dose of 1-2 mg daily or at a dosage able to decrease the circulating level of plasma homocysteine to a more normal range may be associated with a decrease in risk of arterial thrombotic events including myocardial infarction and stroke. Current studies are ongoing that examine this important issue.

VASCULITIS

Vasculitis has also been associated with an increased risk of arterial thrombosis. The different forms include lupus vasculitis, rheumatoid vasculitis, hypocomplementemic vasculitis, Takayasu's-vasculitis, as well as the vasculitis associated with Behcet's disease. Many of these patients may have other evidence of auto-immune dysfunction, including anti-nuclear antibodies (ANA), low levels of serum complement, and increased erythrocyte sedimentation rates. Treatment with corticosteroids may reduce the thrombotic risk, but therapy is usually aimed at the specific type of vasculitis.

ORAL CONTRACEPTIVES AND ESTROGENS

Oral contraceptives and estrogens have long been associated with an increase in risk in arterial thrombosis including myocardial infarction and stroke [26]. The frequency of these events has varied over the years depending on the dose of estrogens used. Current oral contraceptive formulations in the United States use lower doses of estrogens and are probably associated with a lower risk of arterial thrombotic events. Of concern, however, is the increase in risk of thrombotic events that may occur when oral contraceptives are given to patients who have underlying prothrombotic tendencies. Further elucidation of these risks awaits the outcome of ongoing studies. Currently, recommendations for the use of oral contraceptives and post-menopausal estrogens do not include routine genetic testing. However, before commencing either therapy, all patients should be questioned for a prior history of thrombotic events or of a family history of thrombotic events. Under these circumstances, genetic testing may be warranted.

MYELOPROLIFERATIVE DISORDERS

Myeloproliferative disorders such as essential thrombocytosis and polycythemia vera may be associated with an increased risk of arterial thrombotic events and should be considered in patients with the abnormalities of cell counts found in these disorders.

FACTOR V LEIDEN MUTATION

Activated protein C (APC) resistance, caused by factor V R506Q gene mutation (factor V Leiden mutation) has been clearly associated with venous thrombosis in the best studies done to date [27]. Several studies have suggested that there is no increased risk of arterial thrombosis with this mutation. However, Eskandari et al. have reported evidence suggesting that the factor V Leiden mutation may be associated with arterial thrombotic events, particularly in younger patients [28]. The factor V Leiden gene mutation and abnormal APC ratios are significantly increased in patients with lower extremity peripheral vascular disease [29,30] and could be a risk factor for failure of infrainguinal bypass [31].

Venous thrombosis

Venous thrombosis is less often cared for primarily by vascular surgeons who are more likely to be asked to see patients with deep venous thrombosis (DVT) only after they have become advanced or are recurrent. Venous thrombotic problems differ from arterial in that they tend to involve the clotting cascade more than platelets, and take more time to develop compared to arterial clots. Common causes of venous thrombosis are provided in Table III.

FACTOR V LEIDEN MUTATION

The factor V Leiden mutation is one of the most common genetic prothrombotic tendencies, particularly for venous thrombosis in European populations [27] (Table II). This mutation causes the factor V molecule to be insensitive to the normal anticoagulant action of activated protein C and thereby increases thrombotic risk. Estimates from several centers suggest that 20% of all patients presenting with venous thrombosis have the factor V

Leiden mutation [27]. Of interest, the frequency of the factor V Leiden gene has been shown to be 6% in the United States and between 3.5 and 7% in most European population [27,32]. Of further interest, factor V Leiden is essentially absent in black Africans and in Chinese, Japanese, and Korean populations [32]. Black Americans have a rate of factor V Leiden mutation that is approximately a quarter of the rate in the U.S. population as a whole [33]. The presence of the factor V Leiden mutation has been associated with a seven-fold increase in venous thrombosis [34]. There also appears to be a synergistic effect of factor V Leiden mutation with oral contraceptives where the combination of the two increases the risk of venous thrombosis 30 times the general population [35]. In patients using third generation desogestrel containing contraceptives the risk is 42-fold [36]. Screening for the factor V Leiden mutation may be done with the activated protein C resistance test, which is less expensive than polymerase chain reaction (PCR) testing; the latter will confirm the presence of the mutation and indicate whether the gene is present in the heterozygous or homozygous state. Venous thrombotic risk associated with the homozygous state is reported to be 79 times higher than the general population [37]. The current recommendations for patients presenting with a DVT and the factor V Leiden mutation suggest that in the absence of other risk factors, a six month course of oral anticoagulant therapy, followed by observation is acceptable rather than committing the patient to life-long anticoagulant therapy. Should a second, unprovoked event occur, life-long therapy should be considered.

PROTHROMBIN GENE VARIANT

The second most common genetic cause of venous thrombosis is the prothrombin gene variant or mutation of clotting factor II [13]. It is also referred to as the prothrombin variant 20210 G to A. This mutation, located in the untranslated portion of the factor II gene, causes an overproduction of the normal factor II molecule. In patients of the European population, the frequency of this gene in the heterozygous condition is approximately 1%-2% [13]. While there is a definite association of arterial thrombotic events with the prothrombin variant, the risk of venous thrombosis is at least 2 to 3 times greater than in a general population [13]. Estimates suggest that approximately a quarter of all the patients who present with DVTs have the factor V

Table III	CAUSES OF VENOUS THROMBOSIS

➤ Factor V Leiden mutation

➤ Prothrombin gene variant

➤ Antithrombin III deficiency

➤ Protein C deficiency

➤ Protein S deficiency

➤ Lupus anticoagulant

➤ Stasis

➤ Obesity

➤ Nephrotic syndrome

➤ Paroxysmal nocturnal hemoglobinuria

➤ Plasminogen deficiency

➤ Dysfibrinogens

Leiden mutation, the prothrombin variant, or both [38]. Current testing for the prothrombin gene variant is by PCR. Patients with the prothrombin gene variant without other risk factors may also be treated with six months of warfarin therapy, followed by observation. The current recommendation for patients having both the prothrombin gene variant and the factor V Leiden mutation is that these patients should be committed to indefinite anticoagulation because of a higher risk of recurrent thrombosis than with either gene mutation alone.

ANTITHROMBIN III DEFICIENCY

A deficiency of the natural anticoagulant antithrombin III is one of the earliest described prothrombotic tendencies and approximately 70%-80% of patients with antithrombin III deficiency will develop a venous thrombotic event during their lifetime [39]. This increased risk occurs because of a loss of the natural anticoagulant action of antithrombin III, which is primarily directed against factors II and X. Older reports suggest the frequency of antithrombin III deficiency is as common as 1: 4 000 in the general population [40]. However, clinical coagulation centers fail to find clinically significant antithrombin III deficiency this commonly. Patients with antithrombin III deficiency usually have a strong family history of recurrent thrombosis and may be difficult to anticoagulate with heparin. A plasma derived antithrombin III concentrate is available to aid in the treatment of patients with congenital antithrombin III deficiency who must withhold their anticoagulation therapy for surgery. Antithrombin III deficiency may also be acquired in patients who have nephrotic syndrome and who may lose antithrombin III in the urine [41]. Not all patients with nephrotic symdrome will lose antithrombin III in the urine but those who do may lower the antithrombin III level sufficiently to cause venous thrombosis.

PROTEIN C DEFICIENCY

Congenital deficiency of protein C was described in the 1980's as a cause of venous thrombosis [42]. The prevalence of this deficiency in a health population is approximately 0.2% [43]. If protein C is deficient, its natural anticoagulant activity against clotting factors V and VIII is reduced and predisposes patients to venous thrombosis. Of particular interest is the dependence of protein C on vitamin K, which may lead to warfarin-induced skin necrosis, usually, but not exclusively, seen during

the initiation of warfarin therapy [44]. The mechanism is thought to be that, following the initiation of warfarin, both protein C antigen and activity levels drop rapidly, compared with levels of other vitamin K-dependent factors such as factors IX and X, and prothrombin. This observed rapid early fall in protein C level prompted the hypothesis that the administration of warfarin to protein C-deficient individuals causes a temporary exaggeration of the imbalance between procoagulant and anticoagulant pathways, that is, the early suppressive action of warfarin on protein C may not be counterbalanced by the anticoagulant effect created by the decline in other vitamin K-dependent factors, thereby leading to a relative hypercoagulable state at the start of treatment. This leads to thrombotic occlusions of the microvasculature with resulting necrosis. Protein C deficiency is also associated with a 70%-80% incidence of venous thrombosis throughout a patient's life [39]. Homozygosity for protein C has been associated with neonatal purpura fulminans and an occasional patient has survived with aggressive therapy and/or liver transplantation [45]. However, historically, homozygosity for protein C deficiency has been incompatible with life. Protein C concentrate is currently available in some European countries, but it is not currently licensed for use in the United States.

PROTEIN S DEFICIENCY

A deficiency of protein S presents similarly to a deficiency of protein C and may also be associated with warfarin-induced skin necrosis [44]. Once again, approximately 80% of the patients with protein S deficiency will have a venous thrombotic event in the their lifespan [39]. The prevalence of protein S deficiency has not been determined in a healthy unselected population, however, in patients presenting with thrombotic events, the prevalence has been reported to be approximately 1%-2% [38]. Currently, protein S concentrates are not available in Europe or in the United States.

LUPUS ANTICOAGULANTS

As described previously in the section on arterial thrombotic events, lupus anticoagulants are also major causes of venous thrombosis [3]. Commonly, they are present in patients who have other known risk factors for thrombosis and may appear and disappear at various times over a patient's medical course. They may appear during pregnancy and may be associated with complications in pregnancy such as pre-eclampsia, abruptio placentae, intrauterine growth retardation, and stillbirth. Laboratory testing for the presence of a LACs requires documentation of the presence of inhibition in the clotting cascade as well as demonstration of phospholipid dependency of this inhibition. No single test adequately rules in or out the presence of a LACs and many laboratories offer panels of tests that are designed to more effectively diagnose the presence of LACs. Many clinicians currently recommend that inpatients with LACs and a DVT should have their anticoagulant therapy intensified, with the international normalized ratio (INR) maintained at a level of 2.5 to 3.5 instead of the more standard 2.0 to 3.0 in patients without LACs. Alternative and possibly more accurate monitoring of patients on oral anticoagulants who have LACs may be obtained with the use of chromogenic factor X assays.

CONGENITAL DYSFIBRINOGENS

Congenital dysfibrinogens may be associated with bleeding but many are associated with thrombosis or thrombosis and bleeding, depending on how the molecule has been genetically altered through mutation. These patients may also have a family history of thrombosis and may present in the laboratory with abnormalities of immunologic or kinetic fibrinogen testing, as well as abnormalities of the thrombin and reptilase times on clotting profiles. Treatment for these patients must be individualized.

PAROXYSMAL NOCTURNAL HEMOGLOBINURIA (PNH)

This is a rare disorder that is due to a complement sensitive clone of RBCs that is predisposed to thrombosis. The mechanism of the prothrombotic tendency has only recently been elucidated and is related to abnormalities in the walls of the red cells and platelets in a clone of CD59 negative cells [46]. Patients with paroxysmal nocturnal hemoglobinuria develop thromboses in low flow systems, particularly in hepatic veins and many patients with PNH have been found to have intra-abdominal thrombosis at the time of death [47]. They may also have cerebral venous thrombosis. Diagnosis of paroxysmal nocturnal hemoglobinuria should be suspected in patients who are iron deficient and show evidence for hemolysis and pancytopenia, particularly when they have a history of intra-abdominal thrombosis. Standard tests for making this diagnosis in the labo-

ratory include the finding of a low leukocyte alkaline phosphatase score and positive sucrose lysis or Ham's tests.

MYELOPROLIFERATIVE DISORDERS

Myeloproliferative disorders may also be associated with intra-abdominal venous thrombosis and therefore a diagnosis of an essential thrombocytosis or polycythemia vera should be considered in those patients. A high index of suspicion must be maintained since not all patients with essential thrombocytosis or polycythemia vera.

OTHER RISK FACTORS

Other common but less well-defined risk factors for thrombosis include stasis, obesity, and indwelling catheters. Static conditions that may predispose to thrombosis include the post-operative state, immobilized medical patients with congestive heart failure or stroke, and patients taking extended airplane flights or automobile trips. Obesity appears to be a risk factor for thrombosis but the actual degree of risk is poorly defined. Indwelling catheters may also be a cause of static flow, particularly in pediatric patients, where indwelling catheters appear to be a major cause of thrombosis. Less common causes of venous thrombosis include a deficiency of plasminogen or an abnormal plasminogen molecule, but we currently do not recommend routine checking for this deficiency because of its rarity. The abnormalities should be considered, however, in patients who have negative hereditary prothrombotic testing but a strong family history for thrombosis.

Laboratory

Testing recommendations for the diagnosis of hypercoagulable states vary. We currently recommend checking for LACs, deficiencies of ATIII, protein C and protein S, activated protein C resistance, the prothrombin gene variant, and the MTHFR gene in patients with venous thrombosis under the age of 50 or 60. Selected patients over the age of 60 should have similar testing performed depending on family history and index of suspicion.

Vascular bypass patency

Recently, we presented preliminary data that prospectively examined the effect of the factor V Leiden, prothrombin gene, and the MTHFR gene mutations on vascular bypass patency. Two hundred forty-four randomly selected volunteers participating in the *U.S. Veterans Affairs Cooperative Study #362* were tested for the presence of these three gene mutations by polymerase chain reaction. The frequency of pre- and postoperative thrombo-embolic events as well as primary, assisted primary, and secondary patency rates were compared among carriers of the various mutations.

Fourteen patients (5.7%) were heterozygous for the factor V Leiden mutation, 7 (2.9%) were heterozygous for the prothrombin gene variant, and 108 (44.6%) were heterozygous and 15 (6.2%) homozygous for the MTHFR gene mutation. Of the preoperative variables examined, including a history of a prior transient ischemic attack, reversible ischemic neurologic deficit, stroke or myocardial infarction, no statistically significant trend was noted among the patients with the different gene mutations. Postoperatively, there was a trend toward increased graft thrombosis for patients homozygous for the MTHFR gene mutation (33.3%), however,

patients heterozygous for the MTHFR mutation experienced fewer graft thromboses (11.1% vs. 24.4%, p=0.01) and fewer below knee amputations (BKA) than controls (0.9% vs. 7.6%, p=0.02). Patients homozygous for the MTHFR mutation exhibited lower primary, assisted primary, and secondary patency rates compared to heterozygous carriers, while heterozygous carriers exhibited higher primary, assisted primary, and secondary patency rates compared to wild-type controls. Patients with either the factor V Leiden or prothrombin gene variant were not at an increased risk for postoperative graft occlusion or thrombo-embolic events.

These data provide important yet preliminary information about the risk of thrombosis of infrainguinal vascular reconstructions (Table IV). Prothrombin gene mutation did not appear to confer an increased risk of graft thrombosis. In our study, in opposition to Sampram et al. [29], the factor V Leiden mutation is not associated with an increased risk of graft thrombosis. Hyperhomocysteinaemia seems to be a risk factor for vein graft stenosis from intimal hyperplasia [22,23], and our results showed that the presence of the homozygous MTHFR gene mutation did confer an increased risk of graft thrombosis while the heterozygous MTHFR provided an unexpected benefit with regard to graft

Table IV	EFFECT OF ACTIVATED PROTEIN C RESISTANCE, FACTOR V LEIDEN, PROTHROMBIN GENE VARIANT, HYPERHOMOCYSTEINAEMIA AND MTHFR GENE MUTATION ON VASCULAR BYPASS THROMBOSIS					
	Irvine [22] 1996	*Ouriel* [31] 1996	*Donaldson* [30] 1997	*Sampram* [29] 1998	*Beattie* [23] 1999	*Personal experience* 2001
Activated protein C resistance	-	Yes	Yes	Yes	-	-
Factor V Leiden mutation	-	-	-	Yes	-	No
Prothrombin gene variant	-	-	-	-	-	No
Hyperhomocysteinaemia	Yes	-	-	-	Yes	-
MTHFR homozygotes	-	-	-	-	-	Yes
MTHFR heterozygotes	-	-	-	-	-	No

MTHFR: methylenetetrahydrofolate reductase

patency. The mechanisms for these observed effects are unclear but may be due to altered homocysteine and/or folate levels, or other factors related to the MTHFR gene. Future efforts aimed at substantiating these findings will require a large prospective randomized study. When such studies are completed, the additional information may support recommendations regarding screening for the MTHFR mutation preoperatively in order to identify patients who could benefit from close postoperative surveillance and possibly anticoagulation therapy to maintain graft patency.

REFERENCES

1 Anonymous. Decline in deaths from heart disease and stroke- United States, 1900-1999. *Morb Mortal Wkly Rep (MMWR)* 1999; 48: 649-656.
2 Cummings KM, Hyland A, Pechacek TF et al. Comparison of recent trends in adolescent and adult cigarette smoking behaviour and brand preferences. *Tob Control* 1997; 6 Suppl 2: S31-S37.
3 Ginsburg KS, Liang MH, Newcomer L et al. Anticardiolipin antibodies and the risk for ischemic stroke and venous thrombosis. *Ann Intern Med.* 1992; 117: 997-1002.
4 Tanne D, Triplett DA, Levine SR. Antiphospholipid-protein antibodies and ischemic stroke: not just cardiolipin any more. *Stroke* 1998; 29: 1755-1758.
5 Nielsen TG, Nordestgaard BG, von Jessen F et al. Antibodies to cardiolipin may increase the risk of failure of peripheral vein bypasses. *Eur J Vasc Endovasc Surg* 1997; 14: 177-184.
6 Lee RW, Taylor LM Jr, Landry GJ et al. Prospective comparison of infrainguinal bypass grafting in patients with and without antiphospholipid antibodies. *J Vasc Surg* 1996; 24: 524-533.
7 Kibbe MR, Rhee RY. Heparin-induced thrombocytopenia: pathophysiology. *Semin Vasc Surg* 1996; 9: 284-291.
8 Fabris F, Luzzatto G, Stefani PM, et al. Heparin-induced thrombocytopenia. *Haematologica* 2000; 85: 72-81.
9 Ramakrishna R, Manoharan A, Kwan YL, Kyle PW. Heparin-induced thrombocytopenia: cross-reactivity between standard heparin, low molecular weight heparin, dalteparin (Fragmin) and heparinoid, danaparoid (Orgaran). *Br J Haematol* 1995; 91: 736-738.
10 Greinacher A, Eichler P, Lubenow N et al. Heparin-induced thrombocytopenia with thromboembolic complications: meta-analysis of 2 prospective trials to assess the value of parenteral treatment with lepirudin and its therapeutic aPTT range. *Blood* 2000; 96: 846-851.
11 Lewis BE, Walenga JM, Wallis DE. Anticoagulation with Novastan (argatroban) in patients with heparin-induced thrombocytopenia and heparin-induced thrombocytopenia and thrombosis syndrome. *Semin Thromb Hemost* 1997; 23: 197-202.
12 Seeburger JL, Stepak M, Fukuchi SG et al. Multiple arterial thromboembolisms in a patient with the 20210A prothrombin gene mutation. *Arch Surg* 2000; 135: 6, 721-722.
13 Poort SR, Rosendaal FR, Reitsma PH, Bertina RM. A common genetic variation in the 3'-untranslated region of the prothrombin gene is associated with elevated plasma prothrombin levels and an increase in venous thrombosis. *Blood* 1996; 88: 3698-3703.
14 Rosendaal FR, Siscovick DS, Schwartz SM et al. A common prothrombin variant (20210 G to A) increases the risk of myocardial infarction in young women. *Blood* 1997; 90: 1747-1750.
15 Doggen CJ, Cats VM, Bertina RM, Rosendaal FR. Interaction of coagulation defects and cardiovascular risk factors: increased risk of myocardial infarction associated with factor V Leiden or prothrombin 20210 A. *Circulation* 1998; 97: 1037-1041.

16 Selhub J, Jacques PF, Rosenberg IH et al. Serum total homocysteine concentrations in the third National Health and Nutrition Examination Survey (1991-1994): population reference ranges and contribution of vitamin status to high serum concentrations. *Ann Intern Med* 1999; 131: 331-339.
17 Taylor LM Jr, Moneta GL, Sexton GJ et al. Prospective blinded study of the relationship between plasma homocysteine and progression of symptomatic peripheral arterial disease. *J Vasc Surg* 1999; 29: 8-19.
18 Nicolas JP, Chango A. Deregulation of homocysteine metabolism and consequences for the vascular system. *Bull Acad Natl Med* 1997; 181: 313-329.
19 Gaustadnes M, Rudiger N, Rasmussen K, Ingerslev J. Familial thrombophilia associated with homozygosity for the cystathionine beta-synthase 833 T to C mutation. *Arterioscler Thromb Vasc Biol* 2000; 20: 1392-1395.
20 Deloughery TG, Evans A, Sadeghi A et al. Common mutation in methylenetetrahydrofolate reductase. Correlation with homocysteine metabolism and late-onset vascular disease. *Circulation* 1996; 94: 3074-3078.
21 Margaglione M, D'Andrea G, d'Addedda M et al. The methylenetetrahydrofolate reductase TT677 genotype is associated with venous thrombosis independently of the coexistence of the FV Leiden and the prothrombin A 20210 mutation. *Thromb Haemost* 1998; 79: 907-911.
22 Irvine C, Wilson YG, Currie IC et al. Hyperhomocysteinaemia is a risk factor for vein graft stenosis. *Eur J Vasc Endovasc Surg* 1996; 12: 304-309.
23 Beattie DK, Sian M, Greenhalgh RM, Davies AH. Influence of systemic factors on pre-existing intimal hyperplasia and their effect on the outcome of infrainguinal arterial reconstruction with vein. *Br J Surg* 1999; 86: 1441-1447.
24 Shemin D, Lapane KL, Bausserman L et al. Plasma total homocysteine and hemodialysis access thrombosis: a prospective study. *J Am Soc Nephrol* 1999; 10: 1095-1099.
25 Ducloux D, Ruedin C et al. Prevalence, determinants and clinical significance of hyperhomocysteinaemia in renal-transplant recipients. *Nephrol Dial Transplant* 1998; 13: 2890-2893.
26 Sherif K. Benefits and risks of oral contraceptives. *Am J Obstet Gynecol* 1999; 180: S 343-S 348.
27 Bertina RM, Koeleman BP, Koster T et al. Mutation in blood coagulation factor V associated with resistance to activated protein C. *Nature* 1994; 369: 64-67.
28 Eskandari MK, Bontempo FA, Hassett AC et al. Arterial thromboembolic events in patients with the factor V Leiden mutation. *Am J Surg* 1998; 176: 122-125.
29 Sampram ES, Lindblad B, Dahlback B. Activated protein C resistance in patients with peripheral vascular disease. *J Vasc Surg* 1998; 28: 624-629.

30 Donaldson MC, Belkin M, Whittemore AD et al. Impact of activated protein C resistance on general vascular surgical patients. *J Vasc Surg* 1997; 25: 1054-1060.

31 Ouriel K, Green RM, DeWeese JA, Cimino C. Activated protein C resistance: prevalence and implications in peripheral vascular disease. *J Vasc Surg* 1996; 23: 46-51.

32 Pepe G, Rickards O, Vanegas OC et al. Prevalence of factor V Leiden mutation in non-European populations. *Thromb Haemost* 1997; 77: 329-331.

33 Gregg JP, Yamane AJ, Grody WW. Prevalence of the factor V Leiden mutation in four distinct American ethnic populations. *Am J Med Genet* 1997; 73: 334-336.

34 Koster T, Rosendaal FR, de Ronde H et al. Venous thrombosis due to poor anticoagulant response to activated protein C: Leiden Thrombophilia Study. *Lancet* 1993; 342: 1503-1506.

35 Vandenbroucke JP, Koster T, Briet E et al. Increased risk of venous thrombosis in oral-contraceptive users who are carriers of factor V Leiden mutation. *Lancet* 1994; 344: 1453-1457.

36 Bloemenkamp KW, Rosendaal FR, Helmerhorst FM et al. Enhancement by factor V Leiden mutation of risk of deep-vein thrombosis associated with oral contraceptives containing a third-generation progestagen. *Lancet* 1995; 346: 1593-1596.

37 Rosendaal FR, Koster T, Vandenbroucke JP, Reitsma PH. High risk of thrombosis in patients homozygous for factor V Leiden (activated protein C resistance). *Blood* 1995; 85: 1504-1508.

38 Rosendaal FR. Venous thrombosis: a multicausal disease. *Lancet* 1999; 353: 1167-1173.

39 Martinelli I, Mannucci PM, De Stefano V et al. Different risks of thrombosis in four coagulation defects associated with inherited thrombophilia: a study of 150 families. *Blood* 1998; 92: 2353-2358.

40 Tait RC, Walker ID, Perry DJ et al. Prevalence of antithrombin deficiency in the healthy population. *Br J Haematol* 1994; 87: 106-112.

41 Kauffmann RH, Veltkamp JJ, Van Tilburg NH, Van Es LA. Acquired antithrombin III deficiency and thrombosis in the nephrotic syndrome. *Am J Med* 1978; 65: 607-613.

42 Broekmans AW, Veltkamp JJ, Bertina RM. Congenital protein C deficiency and venous thromboembolism. A study of three Dutch families. *N Engl J Med* 1983; 309: 340-344.

43 Tait RC, Walker ID, Reitsma PH et al. Prevalence of protein C deficiency in the healthy population. *Thromb Haemost* 1995; 73: 87-93.

44 Chan YC, Valenti D, Mansfield AO, Stansby G. Warfarin induced skin necrosis. *Br J Surg* 2000; 87: 266-272.

45 Marciniak E, Wilson HD, Marlar RA. Neonatal purpura fulminans: a genetic disorder related to the absence of protein C in blood. *Blood* 1985; 65: 15-20.

46 Rother RP, Rollins SA, Mennone J et al. Expression of recombinant transmembrane CD59 in paroxysmal nocturnal hemoglobinuria B cells confers resistance to human complement. *Blood* 1994; 84: 2604-2611.

47 Ray JG, Burows RF, Ginsberg JS, Burrows EA. Paroxysmal nocturnal hemoglobinuria and the risk of venous thrombosis: review and recommendations for management of the pregnant and nonpregnant patient. *Haemostasis* 2000; 30: 103-117.

4

GRAFT HEALING
AND GRAFT INCORPORATION

NABIL CHAKFÉ, FABIEN THAVEAU, GUNNAR RIEPE
OTHMAN HASSANI, JOCELYN CELERIEN, BERNARD GASSER
CHARLES DOILLON, BERNARD DURAND, JEAN-GEORGES KRETZ

The development of grafting techniques has been a major step in modern vascular surgery. This technique requires the use of arterial substitutes. In 1906 Goyanes for the first time performed an arterial bypass procedure in man by means of an autologous venous graft. In the first part of the 20th century, both numerous and diverse materials, like glass, metal and allograft materials have been proposed to construct vascular prostheses with a caliber greater than the saphenous vein. Yet, the implantation of solid tubes were continually complicated by anastomotic ruptures, distal embolizations, and thrombosis, mainly due to the failure of incorporation into the host tissues. The first modern surgical vascular reconstruction was performed in 1951 by Oudot, who implanted an arterial allograft in a human at the level of the abdominal aorta.

A second important step was made when Voorhees, Jaretzki and Blakemore [1] implanted the first conduit made from a synthetic, porous fabric in Vinyon-N. The porosity of vascular prostheses has since been recognized as one of the essential factors of tissue incorporation and healing of prostheses. The experimental and clinical studies of Wesolowski et al. allowed assessment of the influence of the geometric characteristics of the textile structure and, in particular, its porosity on its healing capacity. [2] Wesolowski et al. showed that an increase of the porosity facilitated tissue infiltration, whereas a decrease promoted the development of calcifications in the wall of the prosthesis. After these initial studies the manufacturers and researchers have recognized the importance of tissue incorporation for the performance of vascular prostheses, and it was in the form of a highly porous fabric that Soyer et al. in 1972 launched the use of microporous Teflon® prostheses [3].

Introduction

Ideally, a vascular prosthesis should have a performance comparable to that of a native artery. To attain this goal, its characteristics after implantation should also be comparable to those of the artery. The mechanical properties of the prosthesis are determined by its composition. The fundamental characteristic of the native artery, being the thrombotic resistance of the luminal surface, will theoretically be seen in the prosthesis only after incorporation into the host tissues, which should allow for the development of a biologically active neo-endothelium.

In this chapter we will only address the historical description of graft healing of vascular prostheses that are actually in use in clinical practice, and we will not elaborate on the interactions of the various humoral and cellular mediators of the inflammatory reaction. The interactions of the mediators are complex and still poorly understood. They have been rarely studied in the healing process of vascular prostheses, except in the process of intimal hyperplasia, which is the topic of another chapter in this book (see chapter 7).

The implantation of a synthetic vascular prosthesis causes a nonspecific inflammatory response at the interface between host tissue and prosthesis, which follows the classical phases of the inflammatory response. The acute phase is characterized by an edematous congestion, an inflammatory exudate formed by fibrin, and an infiltration by neutrophil leukocytes, some macrophages and lymphocytes. Then a cleaning phase is seen, characterized by an increased number of macrophages clearing the necrosis, the appearance of an inflammatory response around the foreign body, including syncytial cells (giant cells) through the contact with the prosthetic material, and an increasing lymphocytic infiltration. Subsequently, the healing phase is observed. This phase is characterized by capillary neogenesis with proliferation and migration of fibroblasts, which cause a collagen secretion that gradually replaces the zone of fibrin and leukocytes we described before. The remaining prosthesis may induce a sustained phase of cleaning and healing, characterized by a chronic infiltration by macrophages around the prosthesis. At the internal interface the relative thrombogenicity of the biomaterial invokes platelet aggregation and local activation of the coagulation cascade. Thus, the luminal surface is covered by fibrin, which will progressively organize itself to form an internal layer. Ideally, the healing response should continue starting from the external layer by producing granulation tissue, which allows for the colonization of the prosthesis and its incorporation into the host tissues. The endothelialization of the luminal surface should take place through the support of transmural neocapillaries.

Experimental data

POLYESTER PROSTHESES

In canine experiments with thoracoabdominal bypasses using polyester and knitted polyester we observed the following healing sequence [4-6]. Four and 24 hours after implantation the mesh of the knitted prostheses is still filled with the preclotting matrix applied during the procedure. Numerous neutrophil leukocytes, indicating an acute inflammatory response, are observed in the fibrin (Fig. 1). Forty-eight hours after implantation the acute inflammatory response is still present and most frequently a beginning organization is seen of the thrombotic material at the luminal surface. Two weeks after implantation the first signs of collagen formation are observed at the external layer with sometimes a beginning infiltration of the mesh. At the luminal surface, the internal layer is formed by means of a more compact fibrin layer during the organization phase. The first endothelial cells are observed on the luminal surface, but only at the anastomosis sites. One month after implantation the external layer is formed of collagen tissue over the whole length of the prosthesis. The graft mesh is infiltrated by collagen from the external layer (Fig. 2). The internal layer is also infiltrated with collagen tissue. This tissue is smooth and covered partially by endothelial cells. Two months after implantation the external layer is organized; it is the seat of a chronic, low-cellular inflammatory response. The internal layer is also organized and becomes thinner and covered more regularly with endothelial cells (Fig. 3).

We have been able to evaluate the functionality of the neo-endothelium by measuring the local secretions of prostaglandin PGI2 and thromboxane A2 (TXA2). We have shown that one month after implantation, the organization of the internal layer was accompanied by an increase of the PGI2 secretion with a PGI2/TXA2 ratio above one.

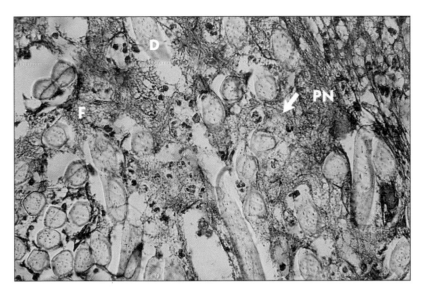

FIG. 1 Preclotted, woven polyester prosthesis implanted for 4 hours as a thoracoabdominal bypass in the canine model (Weigert staining, magnification 40x). The mesh is penetrated by fibrin infiltrated by numerous neutrophil leukocytes. (D: polyester filament; F : fibrin; PN: polynuclear neutrophil)

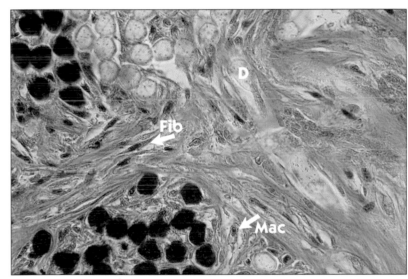

FIG. 2 Preclotted, woven polyester prosthesis implanted for one month as a thoracoabdominal bypass in the canine model (Masson trichrome staining, magnification 40x). The mesh is invaded with collagen together with a moderate occurrence of fibroblasts and macrophages. (D: polyester filament; Fib : fibroblast; Mac: macrophage)

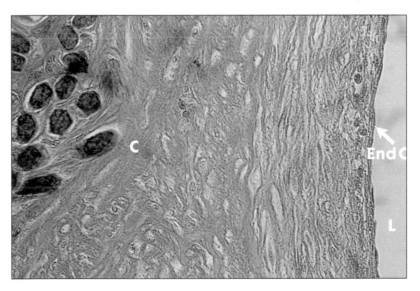

FIG. 3 Preclotted, woven polyester prosthesis implanted for five months as a thoracoabdominal bypass in the canine model (Masson trichrome staining, magnification 40x). The internal layer consists of collagen and is covered with neo-endothelial cells. (C: collagen; EndC: endothelial cell; L: vascular lumen)

The healing process, as we observed in the polyester and knitted polyester prostheses presently offered by the manufacturers, should be modified depending on the characteristics of the fabric of the prostheses [7,8]. The tightly woven prostheses show a lesser infiltration due to their lower porosity. This reduced infiltration considerably reduces the attachment quality of the internal layer, which may detach from the prosthetic wall and cause peripheral embolization or thrombosis of the prosthesis [9]. The recent, less tightly woven and soft fabrics have healing properties comparable to those of knitted fabrics [10]. The addition of a softening effect at the level of the external layer of the prosthesis increases experimentally the attachment quality and incorporation of the prosthesis. The impact of the softening effect on the internal surface is much more uncertain.

The polyester prostheses, which were initially implanted after preclotting, have been replaced during the 1980s by impregnated prostheses that are presently used by the large majority of surgeons [11]. The impregnation matrix of these prostheses plays a hemostatic role during the first days after implantation. Subsequently this matrix breaks down, thereby allowing the incorporation of the prosthesis by means of the healing process. This degrading corresponds with the cleaning phase of the inflammatory response and activates the phagocytes, especially in the acute phase. Hence, a chronic inflammatory response is initiated. The speed of resorption of the prosthetic matrix does not seem to change the quality of incorporation of the prosthesis. In a study comparing the healing process of a *Vasculour II Albumine*® prosthesis versus a *Vasculour II*®, we found a delayed healing of the prosthesis impregnated with albumin of two weeks to one month after implantation. The infiltration with collagen of the internal layer of the nonimpregnated prosthesis occurred more rapidly with an earlier appearance of a regular endothelial surface. These histological data were corroborated by an earlier prostaglandin synthesis and a PGI2/TXA2 ratio that rose quicker above one in the nonimpregnated *Vasculour II*® prosthesis. This healing difference disappeared two months after implantation. This delayed healing response can be explained by the delayed degradation of the albumin, which, like in other studies, occurs between two weeks and one month after implantation in the dog. This delayed healing was observed in other animal models in which the albumin degradation occurred with vari-

able delays, because traces of albumin could still be found after three months in the pig [12] and after six months in the sheep [13]. These variations in degradation speed probably illustrate the differences in the cleaning phase of the inflammatory response between different animal species. The healing sequence in the dog with the *Gelseal*® prosthesis impregnated with gelatin was very similar to that of the preclotted *Triaxial*® prosthesis, especially because the degradation of gelatin takes place within one or two weeks, which is the same delay as the cleaning of the thrombofibrin matrix of the *Triaxial*® prosthesis.

The healing process of the *Unigraft*® prosthesis that is coated with gelatin braided by a carbodiimid was delayed as compared with the preclotted *Protegraft*® prosthesis, because of the delayed degradation of the gelatin, which occurred between two weeks and one month. The healing process of the *Hemashield*® prosthesis was slightly delayed as compared with the same, nonimpregnated prosthesis, as the degradation of the collagen occurred also between two weeks and one month.

We could conclude that the healing process of the currently commercially available prostheses is at best similar or mostly delayed as compared with those without a impregnated and preclotted skeleton. The type of protein and meshing agent do not seem to influence the healing, since these different protein matrices all coalesce after their meshing and their only role is to assure impermeability of the prosthesis at the implantation.

The optimum resorption delay of the protein matrix appears to be between one and two weeks, which is in accordance with the cleaning phase of the thrombofibrin matrix of preclotted prostheses. The type of distribution of the protein matrix within the textile structure, either in the form of complete impregnation of the mesh, or on the other hand in the form of internal and/or external coating layers, may influence tissue infiltration. Progressive matrix degradation allows for a more regular and progressive external attachment of the prosthesis because it is impregnated, while the coatings form a hindrance for infiltration of the mesh so long as they are not resorbed.

Data concerning polyester prostheses that are modified by means of surface treatments, such as silver salts, pyrolytic carbons or a fluoropolymer, are still insufficient to draw reliable conclusions.

ePTFE PROSTHESES

ePTFE prostheses are produced with micropores, formed by nodes, oriented in a transversal direction across the prosthesis, connected by longitudinal microfibers. The average distance between the nodes, or mean internode distance, defines the porosity. The greater the internodal distance, the more important is the porosity. The construction of these prostheses varies with the manufacturer, except for the *Gore-Tex®* prostheses, which are covered by a Teflon® film on the external side.

Experimentally, the cellular and tissue infiltration of the microporous structure with collagen and the neo-endothelialization of the luminal surface are influenced by the mean internodal distance and the presence or absence of an external sheath.

Florian et al. [14] showed that in *Gore-Tex®* prostheses, a mean internodal distance of 100 μm caused an intense fibrous infiltration and intimal hyperplasia in the dog. The fibrous infiltration had a fatal effect on the prosthesis, because there foci of hemorrhagic necrosis were seen and also a fragmentation of the fiber structure of the prosthesis. In contrast, a reduction of the mean internodal distance to 10 μm prevented the desired infiltration, except at the holes in the external sheath, which correspond with the anchoring points on the external side of the prosthesis.

Hanel et al. [15] compared healing of the *Impra®* and *Gore-Tex®* prosthesis and found no differences in healing in the dog after three months. The infiltration of the micropores during the healing process occurred only from the external layer, except at the anastomoses, and with a large variability between different areas of the prosthesis. The central part of the prosthetic wall was filled with nearly acellular eosinophil protein deposits. These authors also stressed that the infiltration process occurred mainly across the anchoring points of the external sheath of *Gore-Tex®* prostheses.

Golden et al. [16] attempted to appreciate the optimum mean internodal distance in relation with the incorporation of PTFE prostheses. They implanted in the baboon aortoiliac prostheses of 4 mm in diameter and 6 to 8 mm in length, of which the mean internodal distance was 10, 30, 60 or 90 μm. The found that the neo-endothelialization was never completed three months after implantation in prostheses with a mean internodal distance of 10μm and 30 μm, while it was at least one month when the internodal distance was 60 or 90 μm. The authors showed that the neo-intima was less stable and seat of areas with localized de-endothelialization in prostheses with a mean internodal distance of 90 μm. They concluded that increasing the internodal distance to 30 or 60 μm allowed for an improved incorporation of the ePTFE prostheses by facilitating the transmural proliferation of capillaries from the external layer.

This concept of the importance of transmural proliferation of capillaries in the incorporation of ePTFE prostheses was re-investigated by Contreras et al. [17]. These authors studied the impact of the mean internodal distance (30μm and 60 μm) on the incorporation of prostheses with an internal diameter of 2 mm and a length of 2 cm, implanted in the carotid area in the rabbit. Half of both types of prostheses received an external polyurethane coating, in order to prevent tissue penetration form the external layer. Eight months after implantation the internal layer looked the same in every prosthesis, except for the thickness, which was slightly better in prostheses without an external polyurethane coating. The infiltration of the microporous structure during the healing process was also comparable, except for the most external part of the prostheses with a polyurethane coating. The authors concluded that increasing the mean internodal distance of ePTFE prostheses did not improve the permeability and healing.

POLYURETHANE PROSTHESES

The vascular prostheses made from polyurethane are constructed with either closed or open micropores. Only those with open micropores actually allow normal infiltration. The only prosthesis that has become commercially available is a prosthesis composed of Corethane® fibers, which are simultaneously wound around a mandrin with a controlled transversal displacement and rotation speed. The fibers have a mean diameter of 10-15 μm and the pores a diameter of 30-60 μm. This cylinder is then impregnated with gelatin and re-inforced by means of a external polyester mesh. Wilson et al. [18] have implanted this prosthesis in the dog. Six months after implantation they observed a well-developed external layer with a chronic inflammatory response at the level of the polyester mesh. The healing response at the level of the polyurethane micropores consisted of a moderate inflammatory infiltrate. The internal layer was formed by collagen covered with endothelial cells.

The healing process in humans

POLYESTER PROSTHESES

Our own observations in humans corroborate those of the literature [19,20]. During the first week after implantation the preclotted prostheses are infiltrated with neutrophil leukocytes at the level of the thrombofibrin matrix. The protein matrix of preclotted prostheses is most often virtually intact. The external layer diminishes to form a fine thrombotic sheath between the host tissues and the prosthesis. The internal layer is covered with fibrin, which is not yet organized. After the first week after implantation the prosthesis is the seat of a healing inflammatory response. Between one and six weeks after implantation, the inflammatory infiltrate is mainly localized on the external side of the prosthesis and consists exclusively of neutrophil leukocytes. The external layer starts presenting collagen around the prosthesis, but without infiltrating the mesh. The fibrin of the luminal surface is organized and becomes more regular, but often remains scattered with fresh thrombi. Between two and six months the external layer is always present; it consists of collagen in which neutrophil leukocytes reside in a cellular infiltrate with predominantly macrophages and T-lymphocytes. B-lymphocytes are always seen, but rare. The infiltration of the mesh begins to be formed, but is mostly scanty. The internal layer is formed by organized fibrin scattered with thrombi. Six months after implantation the external layer consists of collagen with a cellular infiltrate predominantly comprising macrophages and multinuclear giant cells in direct contact with the polyester fibers. (Fig. 4). The fraction of lymphocytes in the infiltrate consists mainly of T-lymphocytes with few B-lymphocytes (Fig. 5). The infiltration of the mesh is scanty, but varies greatly. The internal capsule always consists of organized fibrin, except at the anastomoses, where it consists of collagen covered with endothelial cells in connection with the artery. Away from the anastomoses the organized fibrin is never covered with endothelial cells, except for some rare cases reported in the literature (Fig. 6). In these rare cases we observed collagen at the level of the internal layer, at a distance from an anastomosis, starting from a transmural infiltration of the prosthesis originating from the external layer, at the level of the hollow part of the crimped surface.

The study in humans on the incorporation of impregnated prostheses shows no difference as compared with preclotted, nonimpregnated prostheses. However, in case of a *Vasculour II Albumine*® prosthesis we found that the resorption of the albumin was even more delayed, which was observed in animal models since the albumin was still present in large quantities between two and six months and traces at 22 months.

ePTFE PROSTHESES [21]

The external layer usually appears in the first month following implantation. It consists of frequently thick collagen. Around the prosthesis it is very often the seat of a chronic inflammatory response, characterized by the presence of macrophages and multinuclear giant cells (Fig. 7). This inflammatory response is variable and not related to the duration of implantation. It is frequently intense and very rarely absent. The infiltration of the micropores in the prosthesis consists only of blood in the first days after implantation (Fig. 8). After the first week following implantation the micropores are filled with various protein deposits, like fibrin or hemosiderin, which have crossed the luminal surface. An inflammatory response is not seen in the prosthetic structure itself (Fig. 9). Collagen infiltration is especially observed after the first month following implantation and occurs mainly from the external layer. Tissue infiltration of the micropores is very variable and its stimulating factors are poorly understood. Important infiltration differences exist between prostheses explanted after an identical period of implantation, but also between neighboring areas of the same prosthesis. Apparently, the role of the interface between external layer and prosthesis is very important. Indeed, even in cases where a clear chronic inflammatory response is observed at the level of this interface, one can frequently find an absence of inflammatory cells and collagen in the prosthesis, whether or not the prosthesis is coated. Therefore, the integrity of the coating appears not to be the only factor limiting tissue infiltration. Nevertheless, tissue infiltration of prosthesis models with an external coating seems to occur, as is observed experimentally, mainly where the external coating loses its integrity, i.e. anchor points or iatrogenic traumatic lesions. Finally we have observed that the incidence of morphological lesions of the external layer, as well as the decomposing as seen by light microscopy, increased with an increased intensity of tissue infiltration of

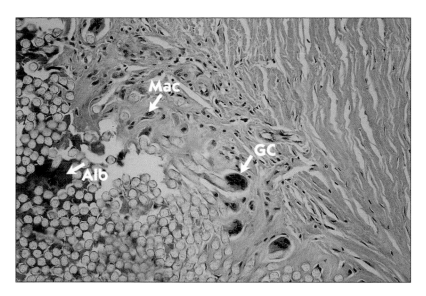

FIG. 4 Woven polyester prosthesis pretreated with albumin and implanted for 21 months in the human model (Hematoxylin eosin staining, magnification 20x). The external layer consists of collagen with a cellular infiltrate comprising mainly of macrophages and multinuclear giant cells in direct contact with the polyester fibers. Traces of the impregnation matrix are still visible in the polyester mesh. (Alb: albumine; GC: giant cells; Mac: macrophage)

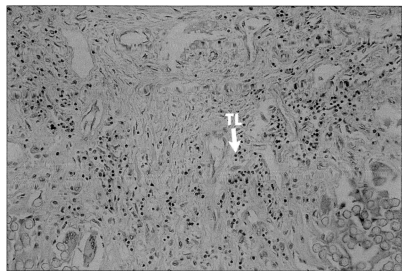

FIG. 5 Woven polyester prosthesis pretreated with albumin and implanted for 24 months in the human model (Immuno-histochemical staining with anti-CD45RO, magnification 50x). The lymphocytic component of the infiltrate consists mainly of T-lymphocytes. (TL: T-lymphocyte)

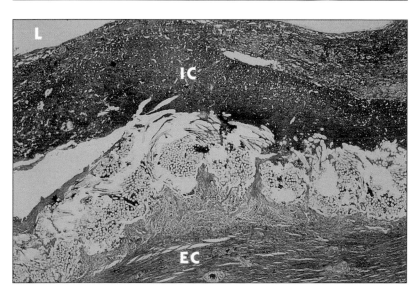

FIG. 6 Woven polyester prosthesis pretreated with albumin and implanted for nine months in the human model (Masson trichrome staining, magnification 5x). The external layer consists of collagen and shows a considerable cellular infiltrate comprising mainly of macrophages and multinuclear giant cells in direct contact with the polyester fibers. The collagen hardly invades the polyester mesh. The internal layer merely consists of a layer of organized fibrin. (EC: external capsule; IC: internal capsule; L: lumen)

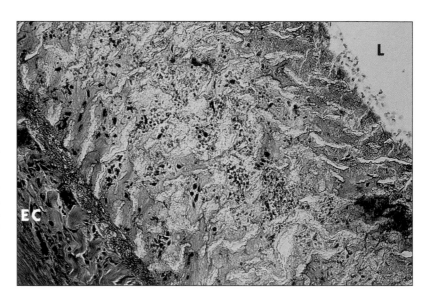

FIG. 7 ePTFE prosthesis implanted for nine months in the human model. (Masson trichrome staining, magnification 50x). To the left, the external layer consists of collagen on the prosthesis with a chronic, resorbing inflammatory response, characterized by the presence of macrophages and multinuclear giant cells. The collagen partly invades the most external part of the micropore structure. To the right, the luminal surface is covered with fibrin. (EC: external capsule; L: lumen)

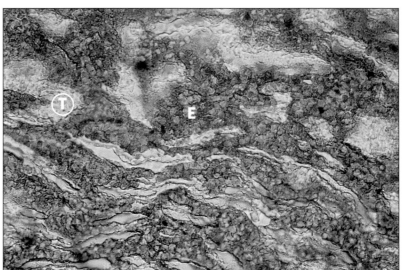

4

30

FIG. 8 ePTFE prosthesis implanted for one day in the human model (Masson trichrome staining, magnification 400x). The infiltration of the micropores in the prosthesis merely consists of blood. (E: erythrocytes; T: teflon modules)

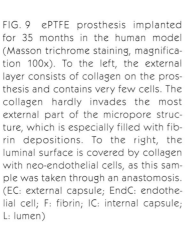

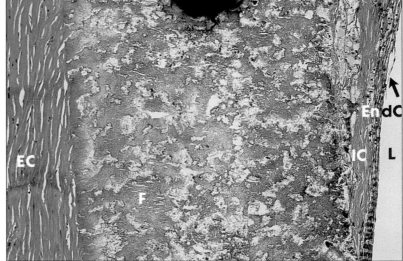

FIG. 9 ePTFE prosthesis implanted for 35 months in the human model (Masson trichrome staining, magnification 100x). To the left, the external layer consists of collagen on the prosthesis and contains very few cells. The collagen hardly invades the most external part of the micropore structure, which is especially filled with fibrin depositions. To the right, the luminal surface is covered by collagen with neo-endothelial cells, as this sample was taken through an anastomosis. (EC: external capsule; EndC: endothelial cell; F: fibrin; IC: internal capsule; L: lumen)

the micropores (Fig. 10). In this case one can hypothesize that these lesions may be secondary to tissue infiltration. Contrary to observations in animal models is the luminal surface of ePTFE prostheses never covered with collagen nor neo-endothelium, except for the first millimeters next to the anastomosis. Most often the internal layer consists of a more or less regular fibrin layer, which is organized with time.

Perspectives

The healing and incorporation of vascular prostheses is a complex phenomenon still incompletely understood. One of the major factors that facilitate the healing of prostheses is undoubtedly the possibility to apply porous materials allowing tissue colonization. In experimental experiments the healing and tissue incorporation of vascular prostheses is satisfactory, because it allows the formation of an internal layer, consisting of collagen and covered by a biologically functional endothelium. However, this result was never observed in man because, as we have seen, the healing starts mostly with the incorporation of the external part of the prosthesis in its external layer without complete colonization of the prosthetic structure and the internal layer. Hence, the luminal surface never possesses the antithrombotic properties of the vascular endothelium.

The vascular healing invokes multiple mechanisms that should normally result in a complete restoration of the vascular damage. The incomplete character of the healing and incorporation process of vascular prostheses in humans is not yet elucidated. Clearly, differences exist between the different species of the various experimental models and the human model [19]. The factors explaining these differences are unknown and various research routes may be proposed. Differences in cellular content of the inflammatory response among the different species might be responsible. The pathology inherent in the human model undergoing a vascular reconstruction, and in particular the promoting factors for atherosclerotic disease, like hyperlipidemia, smoking, hypertension and diabetes may also influence the healing of vascular prostheses in man. However, typically atherosclerotic histological findings [22] are rare in our experience, even in explanted prostheses after very long periods of implantation.

Pathologic healing

The complexity of vascular healing presents itself through pathological processes that are incompletely known and manageable, like neo-intimal hyperplasia and periprosthetic seromas. Neo-intimal hyperplasia shows the phenomenon of an overshooting healing process in areas of vascular restoration, such as the anastomoses of prosthesis and artery. It causes stimulation of inflammatory cells, which produce growth factors that initiate

4

31

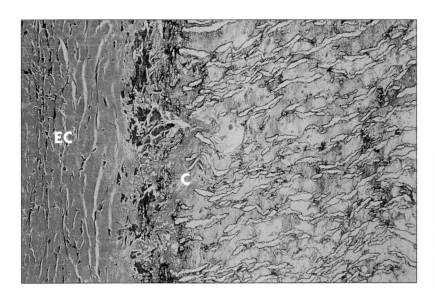

FIG. 10 ePTFE prosthesis implanted for 48 months in the human model (Masson trichrome staining, magnification 50x). To the left the external layer consists of collagen. A loss of structure is seen of the external ribbon wrapping of the prosthesis where the collagen invades the most external part of the micropore structure. (C: collagen; EC: external capsule)

cellular proliferation and apposition of extracellular matrix. Inversely, periprosthetic seromas show a phenomenon of non-healing, which leads to a disturbed incorporation of the prosthesis into the host tissues: the prosthesis floats freely in a serous pocket. Numerous etiologies have been proposed to explain the periprosthetic seromas. For some seromas occurring directly postoperatively are thought to be secondary to physicochemical modifications of ePTFE prostheses that are normally hydrophobic, but become hydrophilic and, thus, allow a transudation through the wall, causing a fluid collection around the prosthesis. Mechanical factors, like crawling movements of axillofemoral bypasses due to the cardiac cycle, might foster disturbed incorporation of the prosthesis and the formation of a periprosthetic collection. Some authors have imputed this pathology to serum factors inhibiting fibroblast proliferation, which may be responsible for non-healing after rather long implantation delays. We have not been able to find evidence for these factors in our experience. We observed a considerable activation of the fibroblast metalloproteinase system in patients presenting with a periprosthetic seroma. The activation of the metalloproteinases might induce lysis of the external layer and cause, together with other factors, a disturbed incorporation of the prosthesis. The causative factors of a periprosthetic seroma are probably multiple and hamper the vascular healing mechanisms in humans.

Conclusion

The best understanding of vascular healing mechanisms in various experimental and human models is necessary to introduce future vascular prostheses with healing properties and improved performance. The impact of a biomaterial and its structure on the healing properties are certainly very important and has probably been underestimated as new models of vascular prostheses were generated. The healing process can be influenced by the implantation site of the biomaterial, but also by its structure. Salzmann et al. [23] showed that the implantation site of a given biomaterial in subcutaneous or adipose tissue considerably influences its healing. Hence, one could hypothesize that in the future it is important to study the healing process of a vascular biomaterial in the tissues for which it is meant in the

clinical setting. The intensity of the cellular inflammatory response secondary to the implantation of a biomaterial is influenced by the polymer used for its construction, but also, for any type of polymer, by the way the prosthesis is constructed.

These differences in inflammatory response may be explained in several ways. The inflammatory response is influenced by the type of proteins absorbed onto the surface of the polymer. In the first phase, the protein absorption onto the polymer depends on the relative concentrations of the different proteins in the environment (Vroman effect). In the next phase these proteins are gradually replaced by proteins that have the greatest affinity to this polymer. The inflammatory response induced by the polymer may also vary with time. The structure of the polymer surface may also influence the inflammatory response through its impact on protein absorption or by means of the direct interactions between the receptors of the inflammatory cells and the polymer. The release of impurities introduced during the manufacturing process could also influence the inflammatory response. The intensity of the cellular part of the inflammatory response plays a role in the neovascularization of the prosthesis. The neovascularization may be more important in biomaterials that induce an inflammatory response with a limited cellular contribution. The quality of the angiogenic response around an implant as well as its capacity to infiltrate its micropores is almost certainly the most important factor in the colonization of the external layer by a healing tissue covered by neo-endothelial cells. This healing approach should hopefully lead to better results than those of direct endothelialization of vascular prostheses at the time of implantation.

Thus, in the future the improvement of the healing and incorporation of vascular prostheses could be realized via two main routes:
1 - the development of new concepts of vascular prostheses using new microporous structures, whether or not textile, that can control the cellular inflammatory response and thus improve its healing properties;
2 - the incorporation of protein matrices more or less connected to cellular elements or growth factors, allowing modulation of the inflammatory response or the characteristics of the healing process [24,25].

4
32

REFERENCES

1 Voorhees AB, Jaretzki III A, Blakemore AH. The use of tubes constructed from Vinyon N cloth in bridging arterial defects. *Ann Surg* 1952; 135: 332-336.

2 Wesolowski SA, Fries CC, Karlson KE et al. Porosity: primary determinant of ultimate fate of synthetic vascular grafts. *Surgery* 1961; 50: 91-96.

3 Soyer T, Lempinen M, Cooper P et al. A new venous prosthesis. *Surgery* 1972; 72: 864-872.

4 Chakfé N, Marois Y, Guidoin R et al. Biocompatibility and biofonctionality of a gelatin impregnated polyester arterial prosthesis. *Polym Comp Polym* 1993; 1: 229-251.

5 Marois Y, Chakfé N, Deng X et al. Carbodiimide cross-linked gelatin, a new coating for polyester arterial prostheses. *Biomaterials* 1995; 16: 1131-1139.

6 Marois Y, Chakfé N, Guidoin R, et al. An albumin-coated polyester arterial graft: in vivo assessment of biocompatibility and healing characteristics. *Biomaterials* 1996; 17: 3-14.

7 Mathisen SR, Wu HD, Sauvage LR et al. An experimental study of eight current arterial prostheses. *J Vasc Surg* 1986; 4: 33-41.

8 White RA. The effect of porosity and biomaterial on the healing and long-term mechanical properties of vascular prostheses. *ASAIO Trans* 1988; 34: 95-100.

9 Hokken RB, Spitaels SEC, Hagenouw RR, Bogers AJ. Dissection in a right sided porcine-valved Dacron conduit. *J Cardiovasc Surg* 2000; 41: 57-59.

10 Chakfé N, Chaput C, Douville Y et al. Woven velour polyester arterial grafts with polypropylene wrap: in vivo evaluation. In: M. Szycher (ed). *High performance biomaterials: a comprehensive guide to medical/pharmaceutical applications*. Lancaster, Technomic Publishing Co, 1991, pp 105-424.

11 Chakfé N, Bizonne SC, Beautigeau M et al. Impregnated polyester arterial prostheses: performances and prospects. *Ann Vasc Surg* 1999; 13: 509-523.

12 Hake U, Gabbert H, Iversen et al. Healing parameters of a new albumin coated knitted Dacron graft. *Thorac Cardiovasc Surgeon* 1991; 39: 208-213.

13 Kadoba K, Schoen FJ, Jonas RA. experimental comparison of albumin-sealed and gelatin-sealed knitted Dacron conduits. Porosity control, handling, sealant resorption, and healing. *J Thorac Cardiovasc Surg* 1992; 103: 1059-1067.

14 Florian A, Cohn LH, Dammin GJ, Collins JJ. Small vessel replacement with Gore-Tex (expanded polytetrafluoroethylene). *Arch Surg* 1976; 111: 267-270.

15 Hanel KC, McCabe C, Abbott WM et al. Current PTFE grafts: a biomechanical, scanning electron, and light microscopic evaluation. *Ann Surg* 1982; 195: 456-463.

16 Golden MA, Hanson SR, Kirkman TR et al. Healing of polytetrafluoroethylene arterial grafts is influenced by graft porosity. *J Vasc Surg* 1990; 11: 838-845.

17 Contreras MA, Quist WC, Logerfo FW. Effect of porosity on small-diameter vascular graft healing. *Microsurgery* 2000; 20: 15-21.

18 Wilson GJ, MacGregor DC, Klement P et al. The composite Corethane/Dacron vascular prosthesis. Canine in vivo evaluation of 4 mm diameter grafts with one year follow-up. *ASAIO Trans* 1991; 37: M475-M476.

19 Sauvage LR, Berger KE, Wood SJ et al. Interspecies healing of porous arterial prostheses: observations, 1960 to 1974. *Arch Surg* 1974; 109: 698-705.

20 Chakfé N, Gasser B, Lindner V et al. Albumin as a sealant for a polyester vascular prosthesis: its impact on the healing sequence in humans. *J Cardiovasc Surg* 1996; 37: 431-440.

21 Guidoin R, Chakfé N, Maurel S et al. Expanded polytetrafluoroethylene arterial prostheses in humans: histopathological study of 298 surgically excised grafts. *Biomaterials* 1993; 14: 678-693.

22 Walton KW, Slaney G, Ashton F. Atherosclerosis in vascular grafts for peripheral vascular disease. Part 2. Synthetic arterial prostheses. *Atherosclerosis* 1986; 61: 155-167.

23 Salzmann DL, Kleinert LB, Berman SS, Williams SK. Inflammation and neovascularization associated with clinically used vascular prosthetic materials. *Cardiovasc Pathol* 1999; 8: 63-71.

24 Fréchette E, Dion YM, Cardon A et al. Fat- and bone marrow-impregnated small diameter PTFE grafts. *Eur J Vasc Endovasc Surg* 1999; 18: 308-314.

25 Cardon A, Chakfé N, Thaveau F et al. Sealing of polyester prostheses with autologous fibrin glue and bone marrow. *Ann Vasc Surg* 2000; 14: in press.

4

33

5

DILATATION AND DURABILITY
OF POLYESTER GRAFTS

GUNNAR RIEPE, NABIL CHAKFÉ
MICHAEL MORLOCK, HERBERT IMIG

In the absence of autologous material for the replacement of the aorta and the iliac arteries, the use of synthetic graft material is unavoidable. In the years after World War II military surgeons experimented with various materials. First attempts with glass and metal tubes failed due to poor handling, high thrombosis rate and compliance mismatch. Reasonable experiences were made with parachute textiles. Experience obtained during surgical application revealed deficiencies of the different materials: vinyon-N was damaged by autoclaving, nylon degraded within a year duration in the human body, teflon and orlon showed poor ingrowth characteristics, fortisan and stainless steel were too thrombogenic and fiberglass grafts were difficult to manufacture. Polyester appeared to have the right balance of biochemical resistance, tissue incorporation and handling properties. Polyester fibers from E.I. Dupont de Nemours & Company, Inc. (USA), called dacron, *were the first to attain the acceptance of the FDA (Food and Drug Administration). This resulted in the exclusive, worldwide distribution of dacron in vascular grafts until their withdrawal from the medical market by the company a few years ago. Today various polyester fibers are in use [1,2].*

Textile grafts

The first self-made grafts were rigid woven textiles with a broad, thrombogenic seam. Specialized industrial manufacturing processes improved the graft properties. In 1956 Meadox Medicals (USA) produced the first commercially available woven graft, the *Meadox Medi-Graft.* Woven grafts were primarily blood-proof, but difficult to handle and frayed at cut edges. Knitted textiles, well known to clothing industry, were less rigid and easier to handle. They were not blood-proof, needing preclotting and dilated under pressure. The first commercially available knitted graft was the

DeBakey standard, introduced in 1957. Until today, many alterations have lead to improved material characteristics. Warp knitting, an industrial knitting technique, increased the strength of the textile wall, reducing the radial dilatation and preventing a raveling of the yarns at cut edges and holes. Texturization of the fibers, additional velour yarns and a higher porosity improved the ingrowth of the grafts. Coating by gelatin, collagen or albumin made warp-knitted grafts blood-proof [1].

The *childhood* of textile vascular grafts was dominated by fiber degradation and textile dilatation. The choice of polyester fibers (dacron) reduced the degradation, the improvement of warp knitting techniques minimized radial graft dilatation. Almost half a century later we were astonished to observe graft dilatation during postoperative sonography and severe degradation leading to graft aneurysms after 10 to 20 years duration in the human body.

Dilatation

The Second Department of Surgery at the General Hospital of Harburg performed 284 infrarenal abdominal aortic aneurysm (AAA) operations between 1981 and 1985. Exceptionally warp-knitted dacron grafts were used. In a follow-up study, abdominal sonography was performed in 127 patients (44.7%) one to six years postoperatively. Another 105 patients surgically treated for an AAA between 1985 and 1987 were examined within 7 to 32 days postoperatively by ultrasonography.

The following findings were encountered.

1 - Filling of the aneurysm sack, which is the result of the in-lay technique of the aortic surgery. The thrombus is removed, the aneurysm sack sutured and periprosthetic hematoma or seroma fills the emptied sack. Early postoperative ultrasonography showed a filled aneurysm sack in 89.5% of the examinations and after one to six years filling persisted in only 11% of the patients.

2 - Dilated ureters were observed in 4.7% of the late postoperative sonographies. In one case a re-operation was necessary after a CT-scan had proven that the retroiliac crossing of the ureter was the cause of the stenosis and subsequent hydronephrosis.

3 - In 97% of the early postoperative and 93% of the late postoperative ultrasonographies graft dilatation was shown. The diameter of the graft, defined by the manufacturer, had increased by a mean of 17.4% in 7 to 32 days (mean 12 days) and 34.8% in 1 to 6 years (mean 3 years) (Fig. 1).

Degradation

In 1992 we started with the investigation of explanted grafts in cooperation with the Section of Biomechanics and the Section of Polymer & Composites of the Technical University of Hamburg-Harburg. Matter of interest in our examinations were chemical and physical aspects of material alteration leading to the observed failure of polyester vascular grafts and their correlation to the period

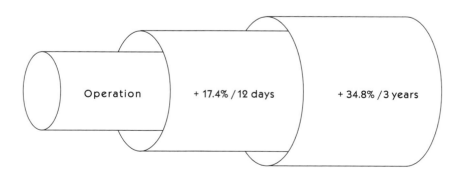

FIG. 1 Dilatation of polyester vascular grafts as seen during sonography in an early (7-32 days) and late (1-6 years) postoperative follow-up.

of implantation in the human body. Until the end of 1995 a number of 170 explanted polyester vascular grafts were obtained from surgeons in Germany, Austria and Great Britain. Sixty-five of the explants were examined intensively by the methods explained below. The majority, 63 grafts, was warp-knitted, one graft was woven, one was weft-knitted. The examined 65 grafts had been implanted between 1971 and 1994, the time of implantation ranging between zero and 23 years. They were explanted because of suture aneurysms in 18 cases (28%), occlusion in 12 cases (18%), graft infection in 12 cases (18%), rupture of graft material in 7 cases (11%) and post mortem in 16 cases (25%). Graft infections occurred within the first years of implantation, the majority of occlusions was seen between 5 and 10 years, suture aneurysms were already found after 4 years, reaching a peak of frequency around 10 years whereas graft aneurysms and ruptures were scattered between 9 and 23 years after implantation. The graft ruptures mostly were sealed ruptures developing pseudo-aneurysms. All explants were cleaned with an enzyme-detergent called Terg-a-zyme (Alconox, New York, USA) as proposed for polyester grafts by Berger and Sauvage [3].

ELECTRON MICROSCOPY

Scanning electron microscopy (SEM) allowed the observation of filament surfaces of the explanted grafts. Images were acquired on a Hitachi S-4500 cold field emission instrument (Hitachi, Kobe, Japan) using an accelerating voltage of 1kV. Several filaments were retrieved from every cleaned, dried graft and separately examined. Gold sputtering was not necessary.

Fig. 2 shows an SEM image of a thirteen-year old filament. This image is representative for the observations made on the 25 more than seven year-old specimens of the 65 examined grafts [4]. In the center of the picture a typical brittle fracture with torsion of the filament can be seen. On the right side the smooth surface of the intact fiber is still visible. Multiple fractures of filaments seen in SEM of elderly grafts were accompanied by general loosening of the textile structure.

PHYSICAL TESTING

The probe puncture test, described in ISO 7198-2 for cardiovascular implants and tubular vascular prostheses [5], is used by graft manufacturers to survey material quality. Due to the circular penetration hole and the hemispherical indenter the orientation

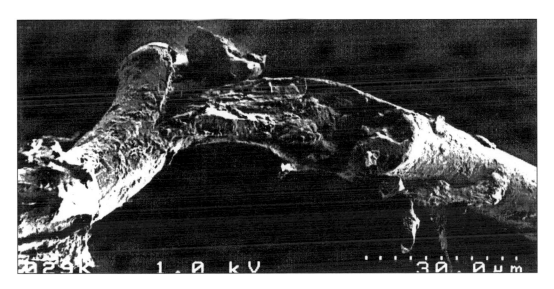

FIG. 2 Filament of a 13 year-old vascular graft showing a fracture in the center and the relatively smooth surface of the filament on the right side. *(Reprinted from Eur J Vasc Endovasc Surg, 13, Riepe G et al. Long-term in-vivo alterations of polyester vascular grafts in humans. pp 540-548, 1997, by permission of publisher WB Saunders).*

of textile yarns does not have to be regarded. This test was modified for use on a Bionix 858 MTS hydraulic testing machine (MTS Systems, Berlin) and the indenter was reduced to 48 millimeters in diameter, in order to cope with the mostly small pieces of explanted grafts. The velocity of the traverse was 70 mm/min. A minimum of three tests was performed. In 11 cases of the 65 explants discussed in this paper mechanical testing was not possible due to insufficient size of explanted material.

The probe puncture testing of various types of unused grafts showed differences in the maximum burst strength between graft-types and manufacturers ranging from 95 to 215 Newton. Mechanical testing of 54 explanted grafts revealed a decrease of maximum bursting strength with duration in the human body. Regarding the differences between unused grafts, the change of maximum burst strength was plotted against the time of implantation (Fig. 3), showing the normalized loss of strength with duration (adjusted $R^2=0.52052$). The change of bursting strength could only be calculated in 45 of the 65 cases. In 11 cases the explanted amount of material was not sufficient to be tested by probe puncture. In further 9 cases either the manufacturer or the type of graft implanted remains unknown or an unused graft of the same type could not attained for testing.

CHEMICAL EXAMINATION

Polyester (polyethyleneterephthalate, PET) consists of monomers of terephthalic acid and ethylene glycol. The synthesis of such a linear chain of carbonyl groups by extraction of water is called polycondensation. Hydrolysis, the reversed reaction, leads to chain scissions due to water uptake (Fig. 4). This re-exposes the carboxylic acid end groups of the monomers. The characteristic absorption of infrared light allows the identification of carbonyl groups and carboxylic acid end groups by infrared spectroscopy.

Fourier transformed infrared spectroscopy (FTIR) was performed using a Bio-Rad 650 instrument (Bio-Rad Laboratories GmbH, USA) on tablets of pulverized polyester material in transmission mode between 1800 cm^{-1} and 1400 cm^{-1} wave number of IR-light, with a resolution of 2 cm^{-1}. The mean of three values was attained. Differences in the quantity of examined material explain the different intensities of absorbance of the entire IR-spectra. It was therefore necessary to set the measured intensities of absorbance of infrared light of

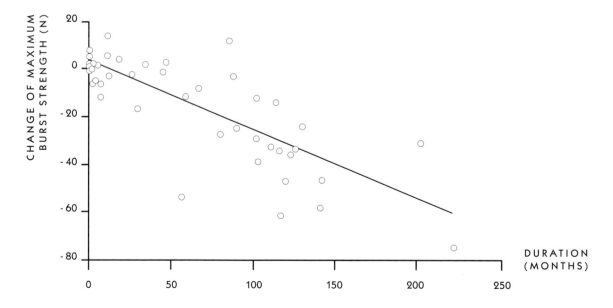

FIG. 3   Change of maximum bursting strength [N] in the probe puncture test with duration of PET-grafts in the human body (adjusted R²=0,52052). The measured maximum burst strength was related to the maximum burst strength of new grafts of the same type. (Reprinted from Eur J Vasc Endovasc Surg, 13, Riepe G et al. Long-term in-vivo alterations of polyester vascular grafts in humans. pp 540-548, 1997, by permission of publisher WB Saunders).

the carboxylic acid end group at 1640 cm^{-1} and the carbonyl groups at 1710 cm^{-1} in relation to the stable benzol group peak at 1510 cm^{-1} in order to obtain comparable, normalized intensities.

The IR-spectrograms of the 65 explanted grafts showed an increase of the carboxylic acid end-group peak at 1640 cm^{-1} and a stabile peak of the carbonyl

group at 1710 cm^{-1}. The normalized intensities of the carboxylic acid end-groups increase with duration of implantation (R^2=0.223). The increase of carboxylic end groups is due to chain scission of carbonyl groups. The normalized intensity of the carbonyl peak did not decrease considerably (R^2=0.005) (Fig. 5).

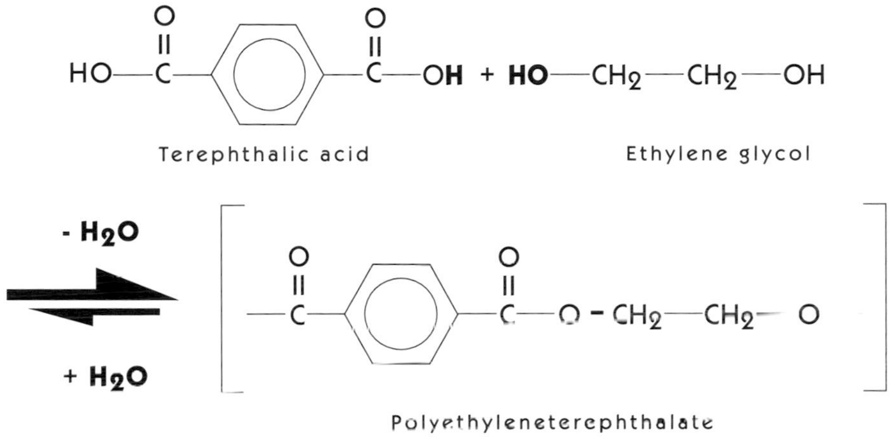

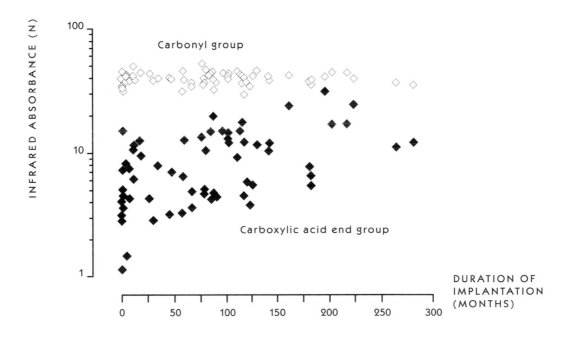

FIG. 4   Simplified synthesis of polyethyleneterephthalate (PET).

FIG. 5   Decrease of enthalpy of fusion with duration of PET-grafts in the human body (R^2=0,269). *(Reprinted from Eur J Vasc Endovasc Surg, 13, Riepe G et al. Long-term in-vivo alterations of polyester vascular grafts in humans. pp 540-548, 1997, by permission of publisher WB Saunders).*

Discussion

DILATATION

Dilatation of grafts specifically occurs in knitted textiles [6]. Woven textiles have a high radial and longitudinal strength. This is due to the dense structure of the warp and weft yarns, crossing each other in a rectangular fashion. In knitted textiles the yarns are far less dense. The fabric is less rigid but also has a lower longitudinal and radial stability allowing dilatation. Warp knitted fabrics reduce this tendency due to their dense structure and the interlinking meshes. Special techniques such as double tricot, locknit, reverse locknit or multilayer warp knits increase the radial strength by mesh-jumping yarns. These fabrics allow only very little dilatation [7].

The dilatation we observed is a question of diameter definition. The nominal diameter of a crimped polyester prosthesis given by the manufacturers consists in the internal diameter measured over a conus without internal pressure and longitudinal tension. An increase of the internal pressure, as in vivo, expands the fabric. In fact, our works on in vitro dilatation of polyester textile prostheses demonstrated that the internal pressure must by applied to the internal surface of the prosthesis without any compliant membrane in order to simulate the in vivo behavior. Under such conditions, the increase of the internal pressure leads to a displacement of the inner crests of the crimps from inside to outside until reaching the level of the outer crests. Consequently, the increase of the internal diameter after declamping a prosthesis has to be considered as an obligatory phenomenon, as proven by early postoperative in vivo measurements [8,9]. The percentage of unavoidable immediate dilatation of textile prostheses seems to range between 15% to 30%. After longer terms of implantation, we observed a maximum expansion of 34.8%, compared with the manufacturer's diameter definition on the graft package, after one to six years. Consecutive follow-up, carried out in some of the patients up to nine years later, showed no further dilatation. The main factors and the incidence of delayed prosthetic dilatation are not still defined since this topic has been exceptionally studied in the literature.

The time in which the maximum dilatation is reached depends on the arterial pressure. Hypertension or poor peripheral runoff increase the speed of expansion. Nunn et al. observed a 15% dilation under normotension and 21% under hypertension. The mean dilatation among their 95 patients after 2 months to 11 years was 17.6% [10]. Nunn et al. demonstrated that delayed dilatation of a polyester textile prosthesis was not a uniform phenomenon along the overall length the prosthesis [11]. The percentage of dilatation on the three parts of the prosthesis (body and/or the limbs) was most often different. Moreover, these parts did not dilate uniformly too. They observed a major dilatation (100% or greater) of at least one part of the prosthesis on 12 of the 32 (37.5%) prostheses followed for an average of 175 months, with a maximum percentage of dilatation of 367%. Only three patients (9.4%) with generalized and saccular dilatation required replacement of their prosthesis with woven dacron.

It is crucial to know that the early dilatation of modern warp knitted polyester grafts has no clinical relevance if it does not exceed 20%-40% compared with the manufacturer's unpressurized measurement of the internal diameter. It would be helpful for surgeons if the graft producers would determine the diameter under an average pressure or, as some companies already do, display the estimated maximum diameter under different pressures on the package. However, we believe that we must try to develop mechanical tests more relevant to appreciate the tendency of a textile structure to dilate. Such tests will analyze the response of a prosthesis simultaneously submitted to different stresses in order to determine its mechanical law behavior. Using this strategy, surgeons can adjust their choice of a fitting graft size.

DEGRADATION

Long-term degradation of polyester vascular prostheses is probably related to multiple factors such as the design of the textile structure, alterations of the prosthesis during its manufacturing process, or during its implantation by handling or application of clamps, or to secondary physico-chemical alterations when exposed to the systolic-diastolic arterial stress [4]. The first cases of rupture of textile polyester vascular prostheses occurred on weft-knitted structures. Weft-knit is the simplest form of knitting since a single yarn travels in the weft direction forming each row of stitches. These ruptures consisted in holes, transversal and longitudinal tears and were more often multiple and observed on the overall prosthesis. These prostheses have been discarded because of their poor stability, and replaced by warp-knit structures. Warp-knit structures are more complex than weft-knits. Yarns are assembled in the warp or machine direction. A series of needles interact with the yarns to form the stitches. Warp-knit structures, mainly lock-knit structures, demonstrated good mechanical performances in terms of long-term stability. However, sporadic cases of ruptures of warp-knit structures have been reported in the literature. They consisted sometimes in general degeneration of the textile structure with huge degradation of the fibers and complete destructuration of the prosthesis with multiple holes and tears. These kind of degradation were observed mainly on the first generation of prostheses incorporating trilobar filaments. The true incidence of degeneration of vascular prostheses is very difficult to estimate because of the following additional reasons. The number and the models of prostheses implanted in a specific population remains unknown in our countries. Most patients are not followed for long periods, and few undergo periodic appropriates studies, like ultrasonography and/or CT scanning, to evaluate graft integrity. It is also quite probable that fewer cases are reported because of the fear of litigation. At least, there is no suitable means of determining how many patients have died of graft failure since autopsies are not always performed and death may have been attributed to other causes. Longitudinal ruptures of warp-knit prostheses have also been reported. However, these cases exceptionally provided a precise description of the morphology of the rupture, or the model of prosthesis involved. Regarding these published cases, ruptures of prostheses seems extremely rare. Wilson et al. [12] reported in 1997 that 68 cases of degradation of polyester prostheses were reported to the FDA, which is obviously in all likelihood far from accurate since many cases are not reported to avoid an investigation. As a part of our European collaborative retrieval program we collected 20 cases of longitudinal ruptures occurring on two similar models of warp-knitted prostheses. We found the ruptures to occur on two specific areas of weakness of the prosthesis: the guide line and the remeshing line. Physical and chemical tests performed on virgin prostheses of the same models allowed us to demonstrate that the manufacturing process severely impaired the mechanical properties of the filaments knitted on these areas, and that these may have been considered as predictable. Our data demonstrate the importance of the manufacturing process on the long-term stability of textile prostheses. The filaments can be damaged during

the different steps of the manufacturing process. These steps are the texturization of the yarns by a thermal and mechanical treatment order to create a velour effect to the prosthesis where they will be incorporated. The yarns are then knitted or woven in order to construct a tubular or bifurcated prosthesis. The prosthesis is compacted by a chemical treatment in order to decrease its porosity. It is then crimped by thermal treatment and chemically cleaned. These treatments may modify the molecular structure, the orientation, and the cristalinity of the polymer. The prosthesis may also be damaged during its implantation by unprotected clamps of surgical instruments. All the damages occurring during the manufacturing process or the implantation may enhance the risk of long-term degradation of a prosthesis after its implantation. The polymer degradation is probably multifactorial and may be related to lipid adsorption, to the chemical characteristics of the surrounding host tissues such as its pH or its enzymatic activity.

Hydrolytic degradation of PET in watery mediums is well known [14,15] and is one of the reasons for the change of PET grafts in the human body. Despite the apparent simplicity of the basic mechanism, the hydrolysis of polyesters is a very complex process, which is still not fully understood, even in the case of linear polymers such as PET [14].

In an infrared spectrogram the characteristic peaks of IR absorption of not dissected carbonyl groups at 1710 cm^{-1} and carboxylic acid end groups at 1640 cm^{-1} allow the observation of the outcome of the hydrolytic chain scission. The reason of hydrolysis remains unknown. Autocatalytic mechanisms as well as catalyzation by metal ions are described in vitro [14,15]. The role of enzymes and lymphatic cells is not known. Attenuated total reflection (ATR) FTIR presented advanced hydrolysis on the luminal surface of grafts, the region in close contact to the watery medium blood [4,16]. The chain scissions, as the product of hydrolysis, lead to a shortening of macromolecules. In vitro examinations proved the predominance of terminal group scissions with extraction of short chain segments rather than internal chain scissions. The shortening of macromolecules results in change of physical properties [14]. These are evident in the brittleness of the material leading to fractures as seen in SEM. The change of physical properties is demonstrated by the probe puncture test. Although this test has little resemblance with physiological loading, it has the advantage of being a well reproducible method for examining the graft materials, independent of the orientation of yarns in the textile structure. These results do not inform about the quality of a graft for surgery. Unimplanted grafts from different manufacturers show differences in maximum burst strength ranging from 90 to 215 Newton. The results of implant examinations needed to be related to measurements of unused grafts of the same type. Because of the small number of specimens available from different manufacturers, a comparison of grafts types was not possible. Furthermore we were not able to match explants with unused grafts of the same batch number. This may explain the variation of our results. More precise mechanical evaluations such as the examination of single filaments and dynamic testing of entire tubes are necessary [4].

Conclusion

The early dilatation of modern warp knitted polyester grafts has no clinical relevance if it does not exceed 20%-40% compared with the manufacturers unpressurized measurement of the internal diameter. The mechanism of degradation is more complex than the process of dilatation. Chemical degradation by hydrolysis, possibly catalyzed by cell bounded enzymes as well as fatigue of the fibers under constant pulsation and joint movement are the suspected initiators of degradation within the body. A weakening of the polymer fiber during graft production by sterilization, texturization, compaction, crimping, coating and other procedures or even by surgical instruments such as vascular clamps or forceps during the operation itself must also be regarded [7,17-24]. Probably the truth of polyester degradation is a multifactorial process in an individual human *black box*. Relevant material deterioration presumably only occurs in 2% to 3% of the patients [3,25]. The earliest graft failure observed in our group was after 9 years, the latest after 23 years [4]. The rareness of graft failure may be due to the reduced life expectancy of elderly patients with atherosclerotic disease. The great majority of vascular patients needing artificial grafting is older than 60 years. The symptoms of graft failure varied amongst our patients. Coincidental findings of an asymptomatic graft aneurysm were observed as well as sudden pain attacks leading to emergency operation or even death. This variation of symptoms makes standardized diagnostic procedures for follow-up impos-

sible. The mere knowledge of possible degeneration after many years of implantation implicates the necessity of observing these patients, preferably by vascular surgeons themselves. In our opinion, the surveillance of a polyester vascular prosthesis requires annual ultrasonography investigation, not only for the research of anastomotic pathology but also for a complete analysis of the overall prosthesis since dilatation or degeneration may be localized on a restricted part. Duplex-scanning should include precise measurements of the prosthetic diameter for further comparisons, and look for mural thrombus in case of dilatation. The observation of a degenerative complication on a prosthesis requires a complete analysis of the overall prosthesis to look for associated lesions, mainly if the prosthesis has been implanted for a long time. Indications for re-operation may be summarized as follow. A false aneurysm either located on an anastomosis or on the body of the prosthesis requires a re-operation for a partial prosthetic replacement. Multiple simultaneous false aneurysms require a total replacement of the prosthesis since it always correspond to a major degeneration of the prosthesis. Moreover, we believe that an endovascular treatment of a proximal aortic false aneurysm using a covered stent should be avoided since in our opinion it may enhance the degenerative process of a weakened prosthesis and create secondary leaks. In order to consider the extent of graft alteration, the precise documentation of employed graft material by the implanting surgeon is a prior condition. This is not always granted, especially not as far as very old explants are concerned. It should be considered to supply patients with some form of material passport, comparable to cardiac pacemaker carriers.

It seems also very important to propose an information program to the surgeons about material surveillance. Material surveillance has been well defined in Europe. The first directive concerning medical devices was approved on June 20th 1990 (90/385/C.E.E., J.O.C.E. n° L 189/17) and was modified on June 14th 1993 (93/42/C.E.E., J.O.C.E. n° C 172, July 12th 1993). This directive clearly established the obligation to declare all failures of the characteristics or the performances of a medical device which was potentially susceptible to lead to the death or to a major degradation of the health of a patient. All these incidents have to be declared to the competent authorities that will take necessary measures in order to inform the manufacturer of the involved device, or its dealer in the European community. An evaluation of the device is required, if possible involving the manufacturer, in order to allow to the sanitary authorities to propose the measures that have to be taken. Consequently, all surgeons have to declare all incidents and to store the explanted devices in order to allow investigations, ideally performed by an independent laboratory. Only a systematic declaration of all cases of degenerated polyester vascular prostheses will allow to get in the future suitable epidemiological data on the models involved. Moreover, the investigations performed on the complicated explanted

prostheses will enhance the knowledge about long-term mechanical stability of polyester vascular prostheses and allow to develop new concepts in the future.

For the meantime, because of short-coming alternatives, we still employ PET grafts in the aortic and iliac segments. We take care to avoid any artificial grafts wherever possible, especially on younger patients, and have intensified interventional techniques such as wire-guided retrograde thrombo-endarterectomies performed in our hospital by a team of surgeons and radiologists.

REFERENCES

1 Voorhees AB. How it all began. In: Sawyer, Kaplitt eds. *Vascular grafts* New York: Appleton-Century-Crofts, 1978 p 3.

2 King MW, Marois Y, Guidoin R et al. Evaluating the dialine vascular prosthesis knitted from an alternative source of polyester yarns. *J Biomed Mater Res* 1995; 29: 595-610.

3 Berger K, Sauvage LR. Late fiber deterioration in dacron arterial grafts *Ann Surg* 1981; 193: 477-491.

4 Riepe G, Loos J, Imig H et al. Long-term in vivo alterations of polyester vascular grafts in humans. *Eur J Vasc Endovasc Surg* 1997; 13: 540-548.

5 International organization for standardization. Cardiovascular implants - Tubular vascular prostheses - Part 2. sterile vascular prostheses of biological origin - specification and methods of tests. *Committee Draft* ISO/CD 7198-2, 1994; 30-31.

6 Kim GE, Imparato AM, Nathan I, Riles TS. Dilatation of synthetic grafts and junctional aneurysm. *Arch Surg* 1979; 114: 1296-1303.

7 Koopmann MDE, Brands LC. Degenerative changes in dacron external velour vascular prostheses. *J Cardiovasc Surg* 1980; 21: 159-162.

8 Goëau-Brisonnière OA, Qanadli SD, Ippoliti A et al. Can knitting structure affect dilation of polyester bifurcated prostheses? A randomized study with the use of helical computed tomography scanning. *J Vasc Surg* 2000; 31: 57-163.

9 Alimi Y, Juhan C, Morati N et al. Dilatation of woven and knitted aoric prosthetic grafts: CT scan evaluation. *Ann Vasc Surg* 1994; 8: 238-242.

10 Nunn DB, Freemann MH, Hudgins PC. Postoperative alterations in size of dacron aortic grafts. *Ann Surg* 1978: 189: 741-744.

11 Nunn DB, Carter MM, Donohue MT, Hudgins PC. Postoperative dilation of knitted dacron aortic bifurcation graft. *J Vasc Surg* 1990; 12: 291-297.

12 Wilson SE, Krug R, Mueller G, Wilson L. Late disruption of dacron aoric grafts. *Ann Vasc Surg* 1997; 11: 383-386.

13 Chakfé N, Riepe G, Diéval F et al. Longitudinal ruptures of polyester knitted vascular prostheses. *J Vasc Surg*, in press.

14 Ballara A, Verdu J. Physical aspects of the hydrolysis of polyethylene terephtalate. *Polymer degradation and stability* 1989; 26: 361-374.

15 Zimmerman H, Kim NT. Investigations on thermal and hydrolic degradation of PET. *Polymer Eng Sci* 1980; 20: 680-683.

16 Fahrenort J. Attenuated total reflection. A new principle for the production of useful infrared reflection spectra of organic compounds. *Spectrochimica Acta* 1961; 17: 698-709.

17 King MW, Guidoin R, Blais P et al. Degradation of polyester arterial prostheses: a physical or chemical mechanism? In: Fraker AC, Griffin CD (eds) *Corrosion and degradation of implant materials: second symposium.* Philadelphia, ASTM STP 1985; 859 pp 294-307.

18 Nucho RC, Gryboski WA. Aneurysms of a double velour aortic graft. *J Cardiovasc Surg* 1987; 28: 723-726.

19 Friedmann M, Zelikovski A, Mor C, Reiss R. True aneurysm in a prosthetic aorto-femoral dacron graft. *J Cardiovasc Surg* 1989; 30: 136-137.

20 Clagett GP, Salander JM, Eddlemann WL et al. Dilation of knitted dacron aortic prostheses and anastomotic false aneurysms: etiologic considerations. *Surg* 1983; 193: 699-709.

21 Watanabe T, Kusaba A, Kuma H et al. Failure of dacron arterial prostheses caused by structural defects. *J Cardiovasc Surg* 1983; 24: 95-100.

22 Maarek JM, Guidoin R, Aubin M, Prudhomme RE. Molecular weight characterization of virgin and explanted polyester arterial prostheses. *J Biomed Mater Res* 1984; 18: 881-894.

23 Vinard E, Eloy R, Descotes J et al. Stability of performances of vascular prostheses. Retrospective study of 22 cases of human implanted prostheses. *J Biomed Mater Res* 1988; 22: 633-648.

24 Rudakova TE, Zaikov GE, Voronka OS et al. The kinetic specifity of polyethylenterephthalate in the living body. *J Polymer Sci* 1979; 66: 277-281.

25 Sladen JG, Gerein AN, Miyagishima RT. Late rupture of prosthetic aortic grafts. *Am J Surg* 1987; 153: 453-458.

6

ADAPTIVE CHANGES OF VEIN GRAFTS IN THE ARTERIAL CIRCULATION

JANET T POWELL

The saphenous vein graft remains the best conduit for bypass surgery in the lower limb, particularly when the distal anastomosis is below the knee. Many changes occur in the vein graft in its new environment within the arterial circulation. These early changes include healing responses, with regeneration of the injured endothelium and the obliterated vasa vasorum. *The vein also adapts to the new hemodynamic situation with thickening of the vessel wall and changes in diameter [1]. The thickening of the vessel wall is a complex process of vascular remodeling involving both medial and intimal thickening. For most patients this adaptive process results in renewed blood supply to the lower leg and perhaps limb salvage. For the less fortunate, the process of intimal thickening is not adequately controlled, leading to the development of discrete graft stenoses, altered flow and eventually thrombotic occlusion of the graft (Fig. 1). Further hospitalization, further procedures and perhaps limb loss are the sequelae. For all these reasons it is important to understand and control the adaptive processes in the newly implanted vein graft.*

Factors influencing arterialized vein grafts

There are at least nine separate mechanical factors that are altered by exposing veins to the arterial circulation. These include circumferential deformation, circumferential stress, longitudinal deformation, longitudinal stress, radial deformation, radial stress, pulsatile deformation, pulsatile stress, blood flow velocity, and shear stress. The increased shear stress has important effects on the endothelium [2]. The other forces have effects on the remodeling of the muscular part of the vessel wall. The elegant experiments of Dobrin et al. [1] in canine vein grafts indicated the important effects of circumferential deformation and blood flow velocity on the vascular remodeling. Using ligatures and external Marlex cuffs, these workers identified that both

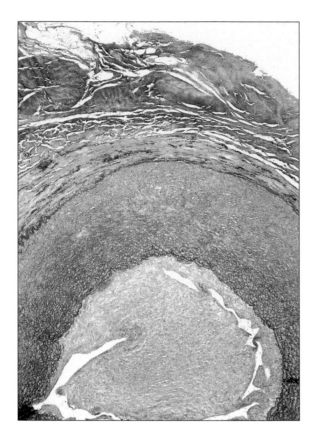

FIG. 1 Thrombosed vein graft. The lumen, at the bottom, is filled thrombus and connective tissue. The attempted recanalization by small vessels in the lumen has failed. The lumen is surrounded by a very thick intima.

lar surgeons, and overdistension of the vein and/or papaverine infusion are often used to overcome this problem. A more selective and gentler approach to this problem could be to block the potassium channels that appear to regulate myogenic tone [6]. We have developed an in vitro bypass circuit in which the early responses of saphenous vein to simulated arterial flows can be assessed [7]. Again, we have observed that external stenting of the vein, to abolish circumferential deformation, may have beneficial effects on the endothelium by preventing the upregulation of cell adhesion molecules such as ICAM-1 [7]. The beneficial effects of high blood flows also relate to the changing balance of anti-thrombotic molecules on saphenous vein endothelium, when vein is exposed to arterial flow conditions [8].

The development of vein graft pathology, with reduction of limb blood flow, usually occurs within the first few months after graft implantation (Fig. 2). After about 10 years there may be recurrent problems with atherosclerosis developing within the graft. With the increasing use of statins to lower the circulating cholesterol, these late complications, together with the progression of proximal and distal atherosclerosis, may become less common.

Early changes in vein graft endothelium

Preparation of saphenous vein for grafting, whether with valvulotomes or by excision and reversal of flow, injures the endothelial layer, often with 50% or more of the endothelial cells being lost. The increased shear stress to which the remaining endothelium is subject alters gene expression to increase the production of endothelial cell growth factors and under optimal circumstances a continuous endothelial cell lining can be regenerated within 7-14 days. This interim period leaves the vein graft very vulnerable to thrombosis. There is accumulating evidence that anticoagulation with warfarin improves vein graft patency [9]. The increased shear stress at the endothelial cell surface causes the altered expression of several proteins controlling the anticoagulant surface of the vein graft. The antithrombogenic properties of the protein thrombomodulin include the sequestration of thrombin and the activation of protein C by the thrombomodulin-thrombin complex (Fig. 3). In cultured

high flows and limitation of circumferential deformation by external vein cuffs attenuated the development of intimal hyperplasia. The Marlex cuffs also reduced the medial thickening. In a more recent extension of the Marlex cuff experiments, the research group of Angelini has confirmed that external stenting of porcine vein grafts reduced the development of intimal hyperplasia [3,4]. The potential use of stiff, prosthetic external stents in clinical practice is likely to be technically difficult, as well as increasing the long-term risk of infection. For these reasons there is discussion of biodegradable external supports for vein grafts [5].

Extrapolation of information obtained from experimental vein grafts is limited by the unique properties of human saphenous vein. Human saphenous vein exhibits myogenic tone, meaning that increased pressure loading causes vasoconstriction [6]. This phenomenon is well-known to vascu-

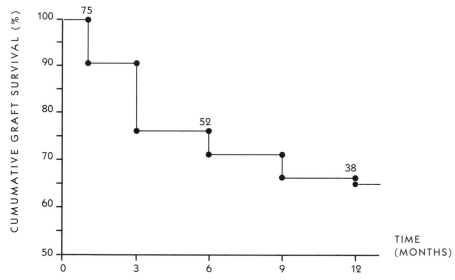

FIG. 2   Development of vein graft stenosis or occlusion in 79 consecutive femorodistal vein grafts. The indications for surgery included popliteal aneurysm (10), critical ischaemia (56) and incapacitating claudication (13). Graft surveillance, with color flow doppler ultrasonography was performed at 1, 3, 6, 9 and 12 months. The data are derived from reference 19.

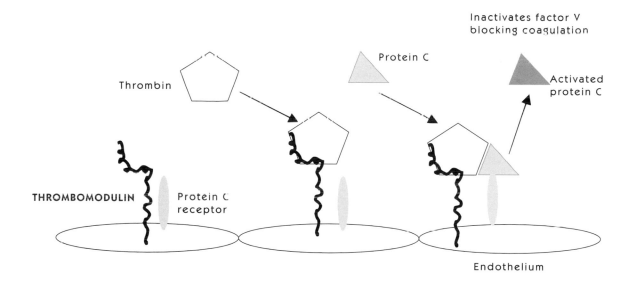

FIG. 3   The anticoagulant function of thrombomodulin.

6
47

cells, the thrombomodulin-protein C pathway has been shown to regulate the thrombogenic properties of endothelium under shearing conditions both venous and arterial circulations [10]. Cook et al. have demonstrated that preparation of saphenous vein for coronary artery bypass grafting diminishes the ability of thrombomodulin to activate protein C [11]. We have shown that within 90 minutes of being exposed to arterial flow conditions there was a 3-fold reduction in the amount of thrombomodulin on the endothelial cell surface (Fig. 4), together with a 3-fold reduction in the

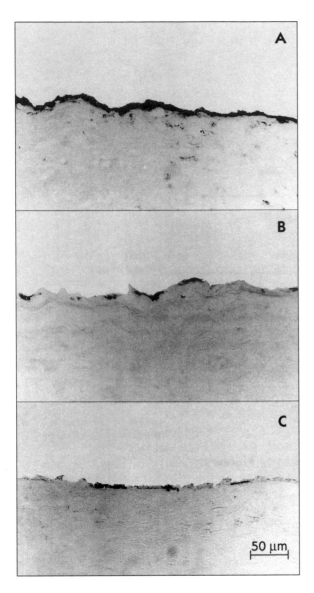

FIG. 4 Immunostaining for thrombomodulin on saphenous vein endothelium is reduced after arterial flow conditions. A - Freshly excised vein. B - Vein exposed to arterial flow conditions for 45 minutes. C - Vein exposed to arterial flow conditions for 90 minutes. The scale bar shows 50mm.

more modest, with only a 50% increase in endothelial staining for nitric oxide synthase and a similar increase in endothelium-dependent relaxation [7]. The upregulation of nitric oxide synthase may assume greater functional importance in the mature vein graft.

Many have assumed that femorodistal vein grafts are always maximally dilated, with no capacity for further dilatation in response to increase flow. Dilatation, by about 10%-15%, in response to increased flow is an important property of healthy arteries, including the femoral arteries, and underlies the phenomenon of reactive hyperemia [12]. This dilatation depends on the presence of functional endothelium and is known as endothelium-dependent relaxation. The biology underlying this phenomenon is the flow-induced release of endothelial-derived nitric oxide, which activates guanylate cyclase in the underlying smooth muscle to cause relaxation with vessel dilatation. Once the vascular remodeling is complete, patent vein grafts preserve this property of dilating in response to increased flow. In post-occlusion hyperemia the diameter of vein grafts in the thigh increased by 12%, with a maximal increase in diameter of 17% being observed after administration of the nitric oxide donor glyceryl trinitrate [13]. This suggests that the endothelium has now acquired the functional properties associated with arterial endothelium. These findings also suggest a possible temporary palliation of stenoses that threaten the patency of the graft. The response of grafts to glyceryl trinitrate indicates that the medial smooth muscle responds to nitric oxide normally, with relaxation. We have used local application of glyceryl trinitrate (with patches) to improve the velocity gradient through vein graft stenoses (Fig. 5) [13]. In the case of a stenosis equal or superior to 90%, this could *buy time* to permit treatment of the stenosis on an elective basis rather than an emergency basis. This is likely to be of particular benefit for frail patients.

ability of cells to activate protein C [8]. These are changes which are unaffected by using an external stent to abolish the circumferential deformation on the vein.

The effect of arterial flow to attenuate the anticoagulant properties of the endothelium may be partially offset by the increase in endothelial nitric oxide synthase and nitric oxide production with increased shear stress. However, these changes are

Early changes in smooth muscle function in vein grafts

Unless the vein graft is vasodilated, saphenous vein responds to the increased hemodynamic stress of the arterial circulation with vasoconstriction, i.e., with the generation of increased contractile force. This is an immediate response and occurs within 5 minutes of the vein being implanted into an arterial circulation [14]. The increased contractility of the vein is in response to circumferential deformation in the arterial circulation, since the increased contractility is abolished if the vein is externally stented [14]. There are several possible reasons to indicate that the venous smooth muscle becomes hypoxic early after implantation of the vein graft. For in-situ grafts the vasa vasorum are likely to be obliterated by the increased pressure, whilst in reverse grafts the vasa vasorum lose their feeder vessels. In addition the vein must work much harder to conduct the pulse pressure of the arterial circulation in comparison to its non-pulsatile functions in the venous system. The vein dilates and this places stress upon the molecular interactions between smooth muscle cells and these cells and their underlying connective tissue matrix. The reflex response to this dilatation, is to thicken and strengthen the muscular media and remodel to reduce the lumen size. Intimal hyperplasia, the migration of synthetic smooth muscle cells into the intima, is one of the reflex responses to this injury and could be considered as a healing mechanism. While there are reasons to suppose that the medial smooth muscle cells of a newly implanted vein graft become hypoxic, this may be counteracted by the greatly increased oxygen tension of the arterial circulation. The anti-oxidant defenses of the smooth muscle may be insufficient to cope with this oxida-

tive stress and the generation of oxygen radicals is another possible mechanism underlying the development of vein graft pathology. There is evidence to support this latter hypothesis from experiments with cultured smooth muscle cells exposed to cyclic strain, when after several hours there is increased production of hydrogen peroxide and oxygen radicals with increased lipid peroxidation [15]. Cyclic strain also increases the production of platelet-derived growth factor by smooth muscle cells [16] and this is likely to stimulate the development of intimal hyperplasia. We have suggested that potassium channel opening drugs may be useful in this situation. This class of drugs is used for conditioning ischemic myocardium and in some countries is used for the treatment of hypertension. The potassium channel openers act as vasodilators and act by opening adenosine triphosphate (ATP) dependent potassium channels. The function of these channels is related to intracellular ATP concentration; reduction of ATP by metabolic stress leads to channel activation, reduced cell excitability and hence a reduction in workload. The channels are regulated directly by intracellular ATP concentration. As the concentration of ATP falls, the channels open resulting in K+ efflux from cells and cellular hyperpolarization. These changes oppose the opening of other channels leading to calcium influx and hence promote vasorelaxation. Thus ATP-dependent potassium channels represent an elegant physiological mechanism through which the contractile ability of a cell is coupled directly to its metabolic status. It is possible that potassium channel opening drugs could be used at very low concentrations to avoid hypotensive effects, since saphenous vein exposed to arterial flow conditions in-vitro rapidly becomes very sensitive to the benzopyran class of potassium channel opening drugs [14].

The adaptation of the venous smooth muscle, with medial muscle hypertrophy and limitation of lumen diameter with intimal hyperplasia is almost complete within 1 month following implantation of saphenous vein in the arterial circulation. This covers the period when the graft is most susceptible to complications. When the normal remodeling is interrupted, excessive localized intimal hyperplasia with development of graft stenosis may occur. One possibility is that this results from the clonal expansion of a single intimal smooth muscle cell, which escapes growth control by having abnormal interactions with heparan sulphates and other extracellular matrix components [16].

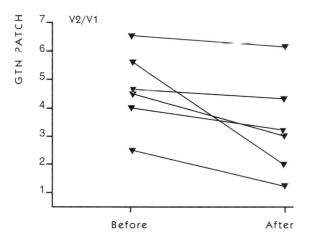

FIG. 5 The influence of a glyceryl trinitrate (GTN) patch on the velocity gradient through vein graft stenoses. The GTN patch had been applied for 24 hours.

The influence of plasma components on maturation of the vein graft

Interactions between the flowing blood and the vessel wall also influence the maturation of vein grafts in the arterial circulation. In coronary artery vein grafts, there is considerable evidence to suggest that hypercholesterolemia is associated with accelerated proximal and distal atherosclerosis as well as new atherosclerotic changes which may cause the vein graft to fail. Aggressive reduction of plasma cholesterol concentrations improves the patency of coronary artery vein grafts [17]. In contrast, hypercholesterolemia has not been well documented as a risk factor for early vein graft pathology in the lower limb [18]. In the lower limb other factors assume greater importance in predicting the outcome of femorodistal vein grafts. These factors relate to matters already discussed. First, smoking alters platelet behavior and increases plasma fibrinogen concentration to increase the pro-thrombotic tendency. Smoking also is associated with excessive production of free radicals, and nicotine causes an increase in catecholamine release, with resultant increase in sympathetic tone and vasoconstriction. It is not surprising that continuing smokers have double the risk of femoropopliteal vein graft occlusion compared with ex-smokers or non-smokers [18]. Both smoking and the acute phase response triggered by major surgery cause an increase in circulating concentrations of fibrinogen, associated with an increased thrombotic tendency. Increased concentrations of plasma fibrinogen are associated with the development of vein graft stenosis and vein graft occlusion [18,19]. The mechanisms underlying these very strong associations are likely to be the direct interaction of fibrinogen and its derivatives with the cells of the vessel wall. Fibrinogen at physiological concentrations stimulates the proliferation of smooth muscle cells cultured from human saphenous vein [20]. Fibrin monomer is an even more potent mitogen for cultured smooth muscle cells and has additive effects with the fibrinopeptide B released from fibrinogen by either thrombin or urokinase. The concentration of plasma fibrinogen has a very important effect on the maturation of lower limb vein grafts.

There may be other circulating factors that have influence on the maturation of vein grafts. Clearly platelet activation and deposition, with release of platelet derived growth factor, could stimulate the proliferation of intimal smooth muscle cells to exacerbate the development of intimal hyperplasia. The clinical observations that antiplatelet drugs are less effective than coumadin derivatives in preventing vein graft attrition, indicate that platelet activation is less important than thrombosis in provoking vein graft pathology. Hypertriglyceridemia and hyperhomocysteinemia are other potential factors likely to provoke vein graft pathology. In particular, elevated plasma concentrations of homocysteine are known to cause endothelial cell dysfunction.

Graft flow: an important regulator of vein graft maturation

Clinicians have long recognized that a minimum blood flow through the graft (more than 45 mL/min) is critical to vein graft maturation and patency. Graft blood flow directly alters endothelial function, the interaction of circulating blood cells with the graft wall and vascular remodeling. If sufficient flow is achieved through a newly implanted vein graft, will the graft remain patent? Unfortunately, although good flow through the newly implanted vein graft is an essential prerequisite for graft performance and patency, thrombosis at the vessel wall and the adverse effects of circumferential deformation on smooth muscle cell behavior must be considered. The evidence to support a new policy of external stenting of vein grafts is growing, but as yet is insufficient to alter clinical practice. There is strong evidence to support the use of anticoagulation in newly implanted vein grafts [9]. So at least one step forward has been taken in methods to reduce the failure rate of lower limb vein grafts. Adjunct methods such as graft surveillance may help improve secondary graft patency.

Conclusion

The vascular surgeon is a perfectionist. The vascular surgeon will have to be patient while evidence accrues to further improve the results of femorodistal vein bypass surgery. The new methods being investigated include external vein graft stenting, genetic manipulation of the vein graft and vein graft preconditioning.

ACKNOWLEDGEMENTS
All the original work reported here was supported by the British Heart Foundation and I thank my many colleagues, particularly Rob Hicks, Jon Golledge, Martin Gosling, David Beattie, Alun Davies and Roger Greenhalgh for their contributions.

REFERENCES

1 Dobrin PB, Littooy FN, Endean ED. Mechanical factors predisposing to intimal hyperplasia and medial thickening in autogenous vein grafts. *Surgery* 1989 ; 105 : 393-400.

2 Resnick N, Gimbrone MA Jr. Hemodynamic forces are complex regulators of endothelial gene expression. *FASEB J* 1995 ; 9 : 874-882.

3 Izzat MB, Mehta D, Bryan AJ et al. Influence of external stent size on early medial and neointimal thickening in a pig model of saphenous vein bypass grafting. *Circulation* 1996 ; 94 : 1741-1745.

4 Angelini GD, Izzat MB, Bryan AJ, Newby AC. External stenting reduces early medial and neointimal thickening in a pig model of arteriovenous bypass grafting. *J Thorac Cardiovasc Surg* 1996 ; 112 : 79-84.

5 Bambang L, Moczar M, Lecerf L, Loisance D. External biodegradable supporting conduit protects endothelium in vein graft in arterial interposition. *Int J Artif Organs* 1997 ; 20 : 397-406.

6 Szentivanyi M Jr, Berczi V, Huttl T et al. Venous myogenic tone and its regulation through K+ channels depends on chronic intravascular pressure. *Circ Res* 1997 ; 81 : 988-995.

7 Golledge J, Turner RJ, Harley SL et al. Circumferential deformation and shear stress induce differential responses in saphenous vein endothelium exposed to arterial flow. *J Clin Invest* 1997 ; 99 : 2719-2726

8 Gosling M, Golledge J, Turner RJ, Powell JT. Arterial flow conditions downregulate thrombomodulin on saphenous vein endothelium. *Circulation* 1999 ; 99 : 1047-1053.

9 Anonymous. Efficacy of oral anticoagulants compared with aspirin after infrainguinal bypass surgery (The Dutch bypass oral anticoagulants or Asprin study) : a randomised trial. *Lancet* 2000 ; 355 : 346-351.

10 Hirokawa K, Aoki N. Regulatory mechanisms for thrombomodulin expression in human umbilical vein endothelial cells in vitro. *J Cell Physiol* 1991 ; 147 : 157-165.

11 Cook JM, Cook CD, Marlar R et al. Thrombomodulin activity on human saphenous vein grafts prepared for coronary artery bypass. *J Vasc Surg* 1991 ; 14 : 147-151.

12 Celermajer DS, Sorensen KE, Gooch VM et al. Non-invasive detection of endothelial dysfunction in children and adults at risk of atherosclerosis. *Lancet* 1992 ; 340 : 1111-1115.

13 Golledge J, Hicks RC, Ellis M et al. Dilatation of saphenous vein grafts by nitric oxide. *Eur J Vasc Endovasc Surg* 1997 ; 14 : 41-47.

14 Beattie DK, Gosling M, Davies AH, Powell JT. The effects of potassium channel openers on saphenous vein exposed to arterial flow. *Eur J Vasc Endovasc Surg* 1998 ; 15 : 244-249.

15 Howard AB, Alexander RW, Nerem RM et al. Cyclic strain induces oxidative stress in endothelial cells. *Am J Physiol* 1997 ; 272 : C 421-427.

16 Refson JS, Schachter M, Patel MK et al. Vein graft stenosis and the heparin responsiveness of human vascular smooth muscle cells. *Circulation* 1998 ; 97 : 2506-2510.

17 Campeau L, Hunninghake DB, Knatterud GL et al. Aggressive cholesterol lowering delays saphenous vein graft atherosclerosis in women, the elderly, and patients with associated risk factors. NHLBI post coronary artery bypass graft clinical trial. Post CABG Trial Investigators *Circulation* 1999 ; 99 : 3241-3247.

18 Wiseman S, Kenchington G, Dain R et al. Influence of smoking and plasma factors on patency of femoropopliteal vein grafts. *Br Med J* 1989 ; 299 : 643-646.

19 Hicks RCJ, Ellis M, Mir-Hasseine R et al. The influence of fibrinogen concentration on the development of vein graft stenoses. *Eur J Vasc Endovasc Surg* 1997 ; 9 : 115-420.

20 Sturge J, Carey N, Davies AH, Powell JT. Fibrin monomer and fibrinopeptide B act additively to increase DNA synthesis in smooth muscle cells cultured from human saphenous vein. *J Vasc Surg* 2000 (in press).

7

MECHANISMS AND PREVENTION
OF MYOINTIMAL HYPERPLASIA

JONATHAN S REESON, JOHN H N WOLFE

Arterial stenosis (or restenosis) is one of the most important barriers to long-term patency following arterial interventions such as coronary [1,2] and peripheral [3] angioplasty, percutaneous atherectomy [4], and coronary [5] grafting. It is responsible for approximately 80% of all peripheral arterial bypass graft failures [6], resulting in the loss of about 30% of all arterial bypass grafts. Myointimal hyperplasia [MIH] comprising vascular smooth muscle cell (VSMC) proliferation and migration with deposition of extra-cellular matrix is one major cause of stenoses that develop between six weeks and one year following vessel injury [7]. However, it should also be appreciated that in about one-half of the affected vessels, remodeling without hyperplasia appears to be the cause of stenosis [8-10].

53

The process of myointimal hyperplasia

Ultrastructural analysis of the MIH lesion reveals it to have a cellular basis. The predominant cell type is the VSMC, while cells with an appearance similar to fibroblasts are also seen, as are cells of indeterminate appearance. However, in the uninjured artery there are no fibroblasts present in the media or intima, VSMCs making up virtually all of the media, with the occasional representation in the intima [11,12]. There is believed to be a continuum of histological appearances between the fibroblast and the VSMC, implying that these are not distinct cell types, but can differentiate from a common origin in both directions (both are mesodermal in origin) [13]. There is support for this from cell culture studies in which cells have been made to differentiate into either a contractile (VSMC-like) phenotype or a synthetic (fibroblast-like) phenotype [14]. It is likely that these observations could account for the historic confusion that has arisen around the term graft *fibrosis* and the appearances of MIH. The proliferating VSMCs in the developing MIH lesion adopt a synthetic phenotype similar to the fibroblast and secretes collagen and extracellular matrix, which ultimately form the bulk of the mature lesion;

the graft stenosis represents the mature MIH lesion. The source of the proliferating VSMCs is from the media underlying the lesion. These VSMCs initially migrate into the intima and proliferate [15,16]. The stimulus for the process is arterial trauma resulting in endothelial denudation and exposure of the basement membrane and media to platelets. The platelets degranulate, resulting in the release of peptide growth factors that are both chemotactic [17,18] and mitogenic [7] for VSMCs, thus stimulating the VSMCs to migrate and proliferate in the intima. There is evidence of autocrine and paracrine stimulation of VSMCs, allowing the process to continue well beyond the resolution of the original platelet stimulation [19,20].

Only 30% of the medial VSMCs respond to the injurious agent by proliferation and migration [21,22] as assessed by labeled thymidine uptake by the VSMC in the balloon-injured rat carotid model, though this is not necessarily applicable to humans. The relative importance of the contribution of the various peptide growth factors in the development of the MIH lesion in humans is not yet clear. However, platelet derived growth factor (PDGF) transcripts have been found by in situ hybridization in atherosclerotic plaque [23], and PDGF-like mitogen is secreted by cultured VSMC derived from anastomotic hyperplastic lesions [24]. PDGF is also expressed by cultured human venous endothelial cells [25] and intimal cells, around the anastomosis, after placement of PTFE grafts into the circulation [20]. This all lends weight to the concept that endothelial injury and exposure of the media to platelets with subsequent growth factor release is the precursor to MIH. There is, however, evidence to the contrary from the rat model, demonstrating that, following induced thrombocytopenia, the injured vessel will still develop a MIH lesion, due to VSMC proliferation, although it will be attenuated. This fact prompted these authors to propose that platelets may be more involved in stimulating VSMC migration than proliferation [26]. More recent work suggests that the human VSMC undergoes a biphasic response to PDGF, particularly the BB moiety, which is concentration-dependent: low concentrations of PDGF-BB stimulate VSMC migration and high concentrations of PDGF-BB inhibit migration, but stimulate VSMC proliferation. The authors of the work have suggested a mechanism to tie these two observations together: consider a distant source of PDGF-BB and its effect. A concentration gradient would be produced by the growth factor, so that dis-

tant VSMCs would be exposed to a small concentration of PDGF-BB sufficient to induce chemotaxis but not proliferation. The cells would migrate towards the source of PDGF-BB and, in doing so, ascend the concentration gradient. At higher concentrations, they would receive a signal to stop migrating and receive a signal to start proliferating (Fig. 1) [27].

It is fairly certain that peptide growth factors cause cellular proliferation and migration and hence MIH. However, it is not clear why some individuals and not others develop vein graft stenosis, or why stenosis occurs at one particular site in the graft. It therefore seems logical to assume that other factors are influencing the development of MIH.

Mechanical factors: shear stress and compliance

Mechanical factors, in particular those related to blood flow, have been implicated in the etiology of MIH in animal models. The normal laminar flow pattern in arteries produces a slow-moving boundary layer, and the force this exerts on the vessel wall is known as shear stress. In conditions of slow flow or turbulence, flow in the boundary layer may be static or even reversed, causing boundary layer separation, as blood constituents and platelets are in prolonged contact with the artery wall. This has been proposed as a possible trigger for arterial wall damage.

The phenomenon of low flow causing low shear stress and being associated with the development of MIH was demonstrated initially using the dog femorofemoral crossover bypass [28]. Using a plexiglass model of an end-to-side 45 degree anastomosis, a complex helical flow pattern at normal arterial pressure with pulsatile flow has been demonstrated [29]. The areas of localized low shear stress roughly corresponded to the sites of predilection for MIH. Bassiouny et al. modeled casts derived from rabbit arteries and identified flow patterns by passing microbeads through these models. A relationship between low shear stress and turbulent flow was demonstrated, with the location of these forces corresponding to sites of known predilection for MIH: the floor of the recipient vessel and the suture line [30]. Sottiurai et al. looked at adult human carotid bifurcations obtained at autopsy and also demonstrated that intimal thickening and atherosclerosis develop largely in regions of low wall shear stress [31]. It appears that the endothelial cell is responsible for sensing the change in shear stress [32] and then either releases or stimulates the release of peptide growth factors [33].

Conversely, high shear stress has also been proposed as a causative factor in the production of MIH, with the vein graft adapting to this higher shear by wall thickening, probably a different process to focal thickening [34].

Ideally, vein is the first choice for bypass conduit with graft patency for vein being far superior to PTFE alone (62% vs. 30% at three years) [35]. The reason for this is thought to be compliance mismatch [40] predominantly at the distal anastomosis.

However, the advent of the distal anastomotic interposition Miller collar [36], Taylor patch [37] and St. Mary's boot [38], have all improved the patency of PTFE femorocrural bypass to approximately 50% at 3 years. This is of crucial importance, especially in patients undergoing reconstruction who have had vein used for previous reconstructions in the leg or coronary circulation. Vein interposition techniques optimize the mechanical properties of saphenous vein and protect small arteries from anastomotic distortion; hence MIH develops in the venous interposition graft where the vessel is more capacious and so protects the recipient vessel. These benefits do not occur with direct PTFE-artery anastomosis [39].

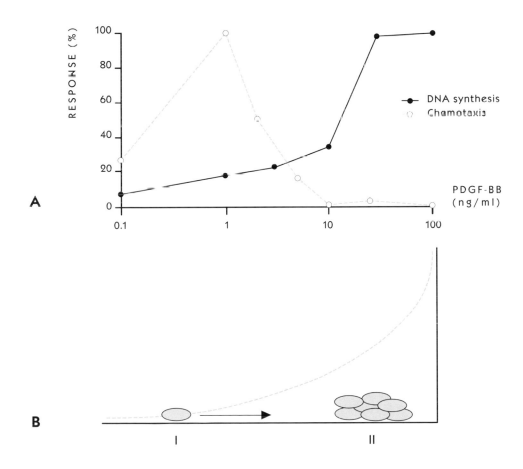

FIG. 1 A - Superimposed plots of the typical chemotaxis and [^{3}H]-thymidine incorporation dose-response relationships in response to platelet-derived growth factor (PDGF)-BB in human saphenous vein smooth muscle cells. Data are expressed as the percentage of the maximum response for both DNA synthesis and chemotaxis. B - Schematic drawing of a model system aligned with the chemotaxis and DNA synthesis profile described in A. A source of PDGF-BB, located at the vertical bar, gives rise to a concentration gradient of PDGF-BB (dotted line) declining with increasing distance away from the source. A smooth muscle cell (position I) is exposed to a small concentration of PDGF-BB sufficient to induce chemotaxis towards the source, depicted by the arrow. As the cell ascends the concentration gradient the signal for chemotaxis is switched off (refer to A), but the signal to proliferate is switched on. The result is the location of proliferating cells at position II.

The hemodynamic forces discussed above make a strong case for anastomotic MIH, but do not explain the occurrence or location of intra-graft stenosis.

Vein graft factors: intrinsic and extrinsic

INTRINSIC
To further answer the question of graft body stenosis it is important to consider pre-existing venous disease. Several workers have observed that pre-existing morphological changes seen in the intimal layer in long saphenous veins were very similar to MIH [41,42]. These damaged veins have a reduced vein-wall compliance, as a result of thickened vein, and are associated with an increased rate of stenosis [43]. Some of these histological findings have, however, been refuted [44].

EXTRINSIC
The *response to injury* is widely accepted as the explanation for MIH and atherosclerosis. Local mechanical injury must be considered as an etiological factor in the development of the discrete intrabody-vein graft stenosis. In an elegant study by Moody et al., all sites where vein graft trauma had occurred were marked with surgical clips: clamp injury, venotomies, valve division, tributaries and residual valve cusps. There was no relationship between the development of subsequent vein graft stenosis and the site of the clips [45]. It also contrasts with work from Mills et al., who demonstrated that vein grafts with normal early duplex doppler scans exhibited a low incidence of subsequent stenosis development, whereas, early focal flow abnormalities developed into a high grade stenosis in 50% of patients [46].

In an attempt to understand the development of MIH stenosis, much work has focused on various animal models, seeking treatments that prevent its progression. The problems with this approach are manifold; for example the biological responses of animal VSMC to growth factors differ from that of humans, and some animal models do not produce the progressive stenotic type of MIH lesion seen in humans [47]. Additionally, the pharmacology and pharmacokinetics of most therapeutic agents differ substantially between species, and a therapeutic response in an animal model cannot be assumed to translate into a favorable response in patients.

This may go some way to explain why the battery of cardiovascular drugs that have been used successfully in animal models to prevent the development of stenosis, have been almost universally unsuccessful when piloted in the human [48,49]. There are some exceptions to this statement, but there are as yet no therapeutic agents available that have consistently demonstrated an ability to prevent MIH in humans (Table). It is important to mention a recent randomized study comparing radiotherapy delivered via a coronary angiography catheter versus placebo: in a group of patients who developed restenosis following angioplasty there was a significant reduction in the incidence of restenosis in the radiotherapy treated group (17% vs. 54%) [50]. This is an interesting result, but the incidence of restenosis in the untreated group was higher than might normally be expected, at 54%, so these results must be treated with some caution.

The many animal models described probably demonstrate a normal response to injury in a normal vessel. MIH in humans is almost certainly a maladaptive response of diseased vessels. As the small mammal model does not do justice to this human problem, some of us have turned to a human cell culture system to further investigate the biology of MIH. Angelini et al. have popularized a human saphenous vein organ culture model developed by Pederson and Bowyer, and have demonstrated tissue

Table	TREATMENTS FOR (RE)STENOSIS
Effective in animals - Ineffective in man	
➤ Heparin/LMW heparin	
➤ Aspirin/antiplatelet drugs	
➤ Fish oils	
➤ ACE inhibitors/Ang II antagonists	
➤ Calcium channel blockers	
➤ Steroids	
➤ Lipid-lowering agents	
➤ Angiopeptin	
➤ Trapidil	

viability throughout 14 days in culture [51, 52]. They have demonstrated an intimal hyperplastic response composed largely of extracellular matrix, which is only sparsely cellular. This is in contrast to the in-vivo lesion, which is densely cellular during the first 14 days. Saphenous vein can only be cultured for 14 days because there is subsequent deterioration. Also, very high concentrations (30%) of fetal calf serum are required to maintain the endothelial cells. At this concentration VSMC do not proliferate. This is supported by their own experiments that show that by removing the intima, the hyperplastic response can be abolished. This contrasts with the in vivo model, where endothelial denudation promotes the MIH response [53].

Over 20 years ago it was found that heparin inhibited VSMC proliferation, both in-vivo [54, 55] and in vitro [56] a phenomenon that has also been exploited in the human VSMC culture model developed by Chan et al. [57]. In our experiments on the effect of heparin on VSMC proliferation, we demonstrated a pronounced heterogencity of responses between VSMCs derived from different individuals. This was the first time that human VSMCs, from a single individual, had been repeatedly cultured. Of particular interest was the finding that VSMCs from

patients who had already developed graft stenosis were predominantly resistant to the antiproliferative effects of heparin, in culture. Even more striking was the finding that this resistance was consistent within an individual and did not depend on the cell being taken from the affected vessel [58]. We then showed these properties were consistent from passage to passage in the same cell line [59], and that within an individual, VSMCs taken from different sites along the same segment of saphenous vein (proximal, middle and distal) behave in a consistent fashion, in response to heparin, as do VSMCs from paired vein and artery [59]. These data raise fundamental issues: since the VSMCs derived from patients who have developed stenosis are resistant to the inhibition of the proliferative response due to heparin in culture, and since these findings are consistent in an individual, can we predict the fate of their graft?

In an attempt to answer this question, we prospectively correlated cultured VSMC responses to heparin with subsequent graft behavior. This demonstrated, at a minimum of one year of follow up, that there was a significant correlation between VSMC culture response and subsequent graft stenosis (Fig. 2). These prospective data strongly support

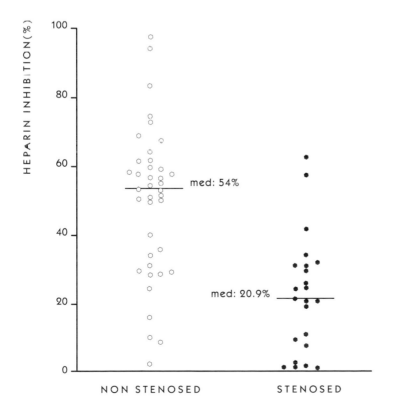

FIG. 2 Inhibition of proliferation by heparin (7mM) of vascular smooth muscle cells derived prospectively from saphenous vein of patients with and without stenosis of infra-inguinal vein grafts, between six weeks and one year of surgery. Percentage inhibition along vertical axis. Each symbol represents a patient. (p < 0.001: *Mann Whitney*).

the hypothesis that VSMC heparin resistance is a marker for excessive MIH and hence graft stenosis [60]. Furthermore, it might explain why heparin is so effective at preventing MIH in animal models, but does not prevent graft stenosis in humans.

Heparin inhibits VSMC proliferation and migration, but the mechanism of its antiproliferative action remains unclear. Heparin has been reported to bind to high affinity cell surface sites on animal VSMC before undergoing receptor mediated endocytosis, resulting in signal transduction into the cytoplasm and modulation of genes involved in proliferation [61]. Heparin binding to human VSMC occurs in a specific manner, on the cell surface and is both saturable and reversible. Kinetic and steady state data suggest a single class of binding sites. Our group has also demonstrated a correlation between the density of binding sites on the cell surface and the cell responsiveness to heparin [62]. These studies seem to demonstrate a cellular marker in vascular smooth muscle which is predictive of subsequent stenosis in vein graft recipients; they also hint at a

possible mechanism (i.e., a deficiency of heparin binding sites on the VSMC surface) that prevents the normal *damping down* of VSMC proliferation in the vein graft, thus allowing an excessive response to a trivial injury.

The role of extracellular matrix proteins as regulators of cell growth and differentiation is a possible mechanism that needs further investigation. Altered responsiveness to heparin may itself be a marker for a more fundamental disturbance of growth regulation in the vascular wall, though this does not preclude the possibility that a failure to interact appropriately with glycosaminoglycans in the vessel wall has in itself an important role in the disease process. Understanding these mechanisms and how they could be modulated will contribute to better understanding of the biology of the vascular wall, and may also lead to more rational and effective management of an important clinical problem, with the intriguing prospect of identifying individuals at increased risk of graft failure and ultimately reducing the likelihood of an unfavorable outcome.

REFERENCES

1 McBride W, Lange RA, Hillis LD. Restenosis after successful coronary angioplasty. *N Engl J Med* 1988; 318: 1734-1737.

2 Popma JJ, Califf RM, Topol EJ. Clinical trials of restenosis after coronary angioplasty. *Circulation* 1991; 84: 1426-1436.

3 Anonymous. Second European consensus document on critical leg ischaemia. European working group on critical leg ischaemia. *Eur J Vasc Surg* 1992; 6 (suppl A): 15-16.

4 Snyder SO, Wheeler JR, Gregory RT et al. Peripheral vascular experience with the trac-weight atherectomy device. In: Greenhalgh R, Hollier L (eds.). *The maintenance of arterial reconstruction*. London: WB Saunders, London, 1991 pp; 231-243.

5 Bourassa MG, Fischer LD, Campeau L et al. Long term fate of bypass grafts the CASS and Montreal Heart Institute experiences. *Circulation* 1985; 72: V71-78.

6 Taylor PR, Wolfe JH, Tyrell MR et al. Graft stenosis: justification for one year surveillance. *Br J Surg* 1990; 77: 1125-1128.

7 Ross R. The pathogenesis of atherosclerosis: a perspective for the 1990s. *Nature* 1993; 362: 801-809.

8 Waller BF, Pinkerton CA, Orr CM et al. Morphological observations late (greater than 30 days) after clinically successful balloon angioplasty. *Circulation* 1991; 83 (suppl 2): I 28-41.

9 Mintz GS, Douek PC, Bonner RF et al. Intravascular ultrasound comparison of de novo and restenotic coronary artery lesions. *J Am Coll Cardiol* 1993; 21: 118A.

10 Strauss BH, Chisholm RJ, Keeley FW et al. Extracellular matrix remodeling after balloon angioplasty injury in a rabbit model of restenosis. *Circ Res* 1994; 75: 650-658.

11 Woolf N. The origins of atherosclerosis. *Postgrad Med J* 1978; 54: 156-162.

12 Chamley-Campbell J, Campbell GR, Ross R. The smooth muscle cell in culture. *Physiol Rev* 1979; 59 (1): 1-61.

13 Sottiurai VS, Yao JS, Flinn WR, Batson RC. Intimal hyperplasia and neointima: an ultrastructural analysis of thrombosed grafts in humans. *Surgery* 1983; 93: 809-817.

14 Chamley-Campbell JH, Campbell GR. What controls smooth muscle phenotype? *Atherosclerosis* 1981; 40: 347-357.

15 Dilley RJ, McGeachie JK, Prendergast FJ. A review of the histologic changes in vein-to-artery grafts, with particular reference to intimal hyperplasia. *Arch Surg* 1988; 123: 691-696.

16 Forrester JS, Fishbein M, Helfant R, Fagin J. A paradigm for restenosis based on cell biology: clues for the development of new preventive therapies. *J Am Coll Cardiol* 1991; 17: 758-769.

17 Bell L, Madri JA. Effect of platelet factors on migration of cultured bovine aortic endothelial and smooth muscle cells. *Circ Res* 1989; 65: 1057-1065.

18 Madri JA, Kocher O, Merwin JR et al. The interactions of vascular cells with solid phase (matrix) and soluble factors. *J Cardiovasc Pharmacol* 1989; 14 (Suppl 6): S70-75.

19 Fritze LM, Reilly CF, Rosenberg RD. An antiproliferative heparan sulfate species produced by postconfluent smooth muscle cells. *J Cell Biol* 1985; 100: 1041-1049.

20 Golden MA, Au YP, Kenagy RD, Clowes AW. Growth factor gene expression by intimal cells in healing polytetrafluoroethylene grafts. *J Vasc Surg* 1990; 11: 580-585.

21 Clowes AW, Schwartz SM. Significance of quiescent smooth muscle migration in the injured rat carotid artery. *Circ Res* 1985; 56: 139-145.

22 Clowes AW, Clowes MM, Fingerle J et al. Kinetics of cellular proliferation after arterial injury. V. Role of acute distention in the induction of smooth muscle proliferation. *Lab Invest* 1989; 60: 360-364.

23 Wilcox JN, Smith KM, Williams LT et al. Platelet-derived growth factor mRNA detection in human atherosclerotic plaques by in situ hybridization. *J Clin Invest* 1988; 82: 1134-1143.

24 Birinyi LK, Warner SJ, Salomon RN et al. Observations on human smooth muscle cell cultures from hyperplastic lesions of prosthetic bypass grafts: production of a platelet-derived growth factor-like mitogen and expression of a gene for a platelet-derived growth factor receptor - a preliminary study. *J Vasc Surg* 1989; 10: 157-165.

25 Limanni A, Fleming T, Molina R et al. Expression of genes for platelet-derived growth factor in adult human venous endothelium. A possible non-platelet-dependent cause of intimal hyperplasia in vein grafts and peri-anastomotic areas of vascular prostheses. *J Vasc Surg* 1988; 7: 10-20.

26 Fingerle J, Johnson R, Clowes AW et al. Role of platelets in smooth muscle cell proliferation and migration after vascular injury in rat carotid artery. *Proc Natl Acad Sci* USA 1989; 86: 8412-8416.

27 Clunn GF, Refson JS, Lymn JS et al. Platelet-derived growth factor beta-receptors can both promote and inhibit chemotaxis in human vascular smooth muscle cells. *Arterioscler Thromb Vasc Biol* 1997; 17: 2622-2629.

28 Rittgers SE, Karayannacos PE, Guy JF et al. Velocity distribution and intimal proliferation in autologous vein grafts in dogs. *Circ Res* 1978; 42: 792-801.

29 Ojha M, Cobbold RS, Johnston KW et al. Detailed visualization of pulsatile flow fields produced by modelled arterial stenoses. *J Biomed Eng* 1990; 12: 463-469.

30 Bassiouny HS, White S, Glagov S et al. Anastomotic intimal hyperplasia: mechanical injury or flow induced. *J Vasc Surg* 1992; 15: 708-717.

31 Sottiurai VS, Batson RC. Role of myofibroblasts in pseudo-intima formation. *Surgery* 1983; 94: 792-801.

32 Kraiss LW, Kirkman TR, Kohler TR et al. Shear stress regulates smooth muscle proliferation and neointimal thickening in porous polytetrafluoroethylene grafts. *Arterioscler Thromb* 1991; 11: 1844-1852.

33 Hsieh HJ, Li NQ, Frangos JA. Shear stress increases endothelial platelet-derived growth factor mRNA levels. *Am J Physiol* 1991; 260: H642-646.

34 Kohler TR, Kirkman TR, Clowes AW. The effect of rigid external support on vein graft adaptation to the arterial circulation. *J Vasc Surg* 1989; 9: 277-285.

35 Wolfe JH, Tyrrell MR. Justifying arterial reconstruction to crural vessels - even with a prosthetic graft. *Br J Surg* 1991; 78: 897-899.

36 Miller JH, Foreman RK, Ferguson L et al. Interposition vein cuff for anastomosis of prosthesis to small artery. *Aust N Z J Surg* 1984; 54: 283-285.

37 Taylor RS, Loh A, McFarland RJ et al. Improved technique for polytetrafluoroethylene bypass grafting: long-term results using anastomotic vein patches. *Br J Surg* 1992; 79: 348-354.

38 Tyrrell MR, Wolfe JH. New prosthetic venous collar anastomotic technique: combining the best of other procedures. *Br J Surg* 1991; 78: 1016-1017.

39 Tyrrell MR, Chester JF, Vipond MN et al. Experimental evidence to support the use of interposition vein collars/patches in distal PTFE anastomoses. *Eur J Vasc Surg* 1990; 4: 95-101.

40 LoGerfo FW, Soncrant T, Teel T et al. Boundary layer separation in models of side-to-end arterial anastomoses. *Arch Surg* 1979; 114: 1369-1373.

41 Sanchez LA, Gupta SK, Veith FJ et al. A ten-year experience with one hundred fifty failing or threatened vein and polytetrafluoroethylene arterial bypass grafts. *J Vasc Surg* 1991; 14: 729-738.

42 Marin ML, Gordon RE, Veith FJ et al. Human greater saphenous vein: histologic and ultrastructural variation. *Cardiovasc Surg* 1994; 2: 56-62.

43 Davies AH, Magee TR, Sheffield E et al. The aetiology of vein graft stenoses. *Eur J Vasc Surg* 1994; 8: 389-394.

44 Varty K, Porter K, Bell PR et al. Vein morphology and bypass graft stenosis. *Br J Surg* 1996; 83: 1375-1379.

45 Moody AP, Edwards PR, Harris PL. The aetiology of vein graft strictures: a prospective marker study. *Eur J Vasc Surg* 1992; 6: 509-511.

46 Mills JL, Bandyk DF, Gahtan V et al. The origin of infrainguinal vein graft stenosis: a prospective study based on duplex surveillance. *J Vasc Surg* 1995; 21: 16-25.

47 Muller DW, Ellis SG, Topol EJ. Experimental models of coronary artery restenosis. *J Am Coll Cardiol* 1992; 19: 418-432.

48 Chan P. Cell biology of human vascular smooth muscle. *Ann R Coll Surg Engl* 1994; 76: 298-303.

49 Ferrell M, Fuster V, Gold HK et al. A dilemma for the 1990s. Choosing appropriate experimental animal model for the prevention of restenosis. *Circulation* 1992; 85: 1630-1631.

50 Teirstein PS, Massullo V, Jani S et al. Catheter-based radiotherapy to inhibit restenosis after coronary stenting. *N Engl J Med* 1997; 336: 1697-1703.

51 Angelini GD, Soyombo AA, Newby AC. Smooth muscle cell proliferation in response to injury in an organ culture of human saphenous vein. *Eur J Vasc Surg* 1991; 5: 5-12.

52 Pederson DC, Bowyer DE. Endothelial injury and healing in vitro: studies using an organ culture system. *Am J Pathol* 1985; 119: 264-272.

53 Clowes AW, Clowes MM, Reidy MA. Kinetics of cellular proliferation after arterial injury. III. Endothelial and smooth muscle growth in chronically denuded vessels *Lab Invest* 1986; 54: 295-303.

54 Clowes AW, Karnowsky MJ. Suppression by heparin of smooth muscle cell proliferation in injured arteries. *Nature* 1977; 265: 625-626.

55 Guyton JR, Rosenberg RD, Clowes AW et al. Inhibition of rat arterial smooth muscle cell proliferation by heparin. *Circ Res* 1980; 46: 625-633.

56 Hoover RL, Rosenberg R, Haering W et al. Inhibition of rat arterial smooth muscle cell proliferation by heparin. *Circ Res* 1980; 47: 578-583.

57 Chan P, Munro E, Patel M et al. Cellular biology of human intimal hyperplastic stenosis. *Eur J Vasc Surg* 1993; 7: 129-135.

58 Chan P, Patel M, Munro E et al. Abnormal growth regulation of vascular smooth muscle cells by heparin in patients with restenosis. *Lancet* 1993; 341: 341-342.

59 Munro E, Chan P, Patel M et al. Consistent responses of the human vascular smooth muscle cell in culture: implications for restenosis. *J Vasc Surg* 1994; 20: 482-487.

60 Refson JS, Schachter M, Patel MK et al. Vein graft stenosis and the heparin responsiveness of human vascular smooth muscle cells. *Circulation* 1998; 97: 2506-2510.

61 Castellot JJ Jr, Wong K, Herman B et al. Binding and internalization of heparin by vascular smooth muscle cells. *J Cell Physiol* 1985; 124: 13-20.

62 Patel MK, Refson JS, Schachter M et al. Characterisation of [3H]- heparin binding in human vascular smooth muscle cells and its relationship to the inhibition of DNA synthesis. *Br J Pharmacol* 1999; 127: 361-368.

7

8

POSTOPERATIVE ARTERIAL INFECTION: EPIDEMIOLOGY, BACTERIOLOGY AND PATHOGENESIS

ROBERTO CHIESA, GERMANO MELISSANO
RENATA CASTELLANO, DOMENICO ASTORE, SILLIA FRIGERIO
LUCA GARRIBOLI, GIAN PIETRO GESU, ANGELO ANZUINI
GIUSEPPE PICCOLO, GIROLAMO SIRCHIA, MARIO SCALAMOGNA

Reconstructive vascular surgery was first reported in the early 1950s; homografts have been the only means of vascular grafting until the introduction of prosthetic grafts. Vascular reconstruction with prosthetic grafts provided acceptable results, however, prosthetic infection soon appeared as an infrequent but severe complication. A large variety of treatments have been proposed in the management of this complication, with poor results due to high mortality and amputation rate. Successful treatment requires an understanding of bacteriology, pathogenesis, and prevention of risk factors to eradicate vascular prosthesis infection.

Epidemiology

Overall rates for major graft infection average around 2%, ranging from less than 1% to 6% in published series [1]. The reported incidence of graft infection varies with the indication for implantation and the site of the graft. Graft infection is more common after emergency procedures and when an anastomosis in the groin is performed. The incidence is well below 2% after primary operations but in case of redo surgery it may increase to 3%-4% [2]. The actual incidence of prosthetic graft infection may be higher than the level reported in these studies because of the variable time interval between the primary procedure and the recognition of graft infection, and because of the management of this complication at a hospital different from the original one.

Prosthetic graft infection can occur in the perioperative period, largely due to contamination, despite routine antimicrobial prophylaxis. A second peak of incidence occurs later. The mean time interval from primary procedure to onset of clinical manifestations has been reported in the range of 25 to 41 months [3]. Clinical recognition of vascular prosthesis infection is commonly associated with anastomotic pseudo-aneurysms or graft-enteric fistula formation.

An anastomotic pseudo-aneurysm occurs with an incidence between 1% and 5% and is most frequently located at the femoral anastomosis of an aortofemoral graft [3]. Although several factors may lead to anastomotic aneurysm formation, infection may be a contributing event. In this case it is very important to inspect the anastomosis in an effort to determine the cause of the suture line disruption and particularly to evaluate the possibility of infection, as this dictates a radically different therapeutic approach. Indeed, positive cultures are found in 90% of anastomotic pseudo-aneurysms [3]. Development of an aorto-enteric fistula with associated gastro-intestinal hemorrhage is an infrequent (0.4%-2.4%) but devastating late complication of aortic vascular procedures, and it is often associated with graft infection [3].

Despite aggressive antibiotic administration and surgical treatment, the mortality and amputation rates associated with prosthetic infections remain high, with the highest morbidity occurring when sepsis or anastomotic bleeding is involved. Infection of an aortic bypass graft induces mortality rates ranging between 40% and 75% [4,5]. In contrast, infection involving femoropopliteal grafts has an associated mortality of only about 10%, although the rate of limb loss is substantially higher [4,5].

In order to better understand epidemiology, Szilagy et al. [4] divided infections into three grades according to the depth of involvement. Grade I and II involve skin and subcutaneous tissue, and grade III is reserved for infection involving the prosthesis itself. This is the oldest classification, but still the most useful because of its simplicity. Newer classifications have been proposed: Bunt et al. [6] classified the aortic graft infection according to presence or absence of aorto-enteric fistula, while Bandyk [7] classified according to the micro-organisms, having noticed different types of micro-organisms in an early and late graft infection. Another classification by Goëau-Brissonnière (see chapter 9) classified the graft infection according to the time of presentation (before 3 months or after 3 months) in four stages:
- stage 0, no manifestations of infection,
- stage I, local signs like inflammatory perigraft mass, cellulitis, hematoma, seroma, and skin necrosis,
- stage II, positive local culture but without graft infection, and prosthesis infection.

However, in order to accurately classify graft infection, it is important to further specify the type of graft material, graft site and the time of early or late presentation. Despite the availability of different antibiotics and a large variety of surgical treatments, prosthetic graft infection remains one of the most dramatic complications in vascular surgery.

Bacteriology

In general, any organism can infect a graft in the postoperative period, however, *Staphylococcus aureus* has been the most frequently indentified. In the last decade there has been an increase of infections caused by *Staphylococcus epidermidis*, Gram-negative bacteria (*Escherichia* [E] *Coli, Pseudomonas, Klebsiella, Enterobacter* and *Proteus*) which are found in 40%, and mixed Gram-positive and Gram-negative infections occurring in 10%-15% of cases [3]. Graft infections with negative cultures are, however, no exception and are cited in 5%-20% [3].

Negative cultures can occur with late infection, and are generally caused by *Staphylococcus epidermidis* and other coagulase-negative staphylococci with low virulence. The infections caused by Gram-negative bacteria (*E. Coli, Pseudomonas, Klebsiella, Enterobacter* and *Proteus*) are frequently associated with a high incidence of rupture and anastomotic failure: those manifestations could be caused by the production of endotoxins, elastase, and alkaline protease which can subsequently decrease the integrity of the graft material. Graft infections caused by fungi (*Candida, Micobacterium, Aspergillus*) are rare and may be associated with the altered immune function in case of malignancy, lymphoproliferative disorders, or drug administration (steroids or chemotherapy), which can predispose to this kind of graft infection. These different characteristics of graft infection can be better understood when studying the different phases of graft adhesion and colonization by micro-organisms. The process of infection involves several steps:
1 - bacteria adhesion to biomaterial surfaces,
2 - microcolony formation within a bacterial bio-film, which is a complex structure composed of an

extracellular nutrient glycocalyx produced by the microorganism,

3 - activation of host defense,

4 - an inflammatory response involving perigraft tissue and the anastomosis. Bacterial adherence to the prosthesis depends on cell wall and growth characteristics of the bacteria species and physical and chemical properties of the vascular material.

The cell wall structures of gram-positive and gram-negative bacteria differ, thereby influencing their adherence to biomaterials. *Staphylococcus aureus* has been demonstrated to adhere better to suture material than *E. Coli* [8]. *Staphylococcus epidermidis* has been implicated as the prevalent pathogen causing late graft infection [9] by the production of an extracellular mucinoid substance. Although specific virulence factors are not as clearly established as they are in *Staphylococcus aureus*, it seems clear that factors such as bacterial polysaccharide components are involved in the attachment and persistence of *Staphylococcus epidermidis* on foreign materials. Clinical culture isolates of *Staphylococcus epidermidis* are frequently referred to produce a biofilm, known as slime, involved in adherence to medical devices [10]. Bandyk et al. [11] found that the latest graft infections might be caused by coagulase-negative staphylococci, which harbor and survive within a biofilm on biomaterial surfaces.

The adhesion of bacteria to the surface of prosthetic implants is recognized as an important initial step of an infectious process and has been shown to depend on many factors, including physical properties and chemical composition of the material, the duration of exposure, and the protein biolayer that forms on all prosthetic surfaces after graft implantation.

Vascular graft composition and construction can influence bacterial adherence. Graft fiber surface characteristics, the relative degree of material hydrophobicity, and the presence of anionic versus cationic surface charge all affect initial bacterial adherence [12]. Dacron vascular grafts have been shown to have a greater propensity for bacterial adherence than expanded polytetrafluoroethylene (ePTFE) grafts [13].

Irreversible changes to the structure of the prosthesis are induced by colonization of the biomaterial by micro-organisms, which in most cases necessitates total replacement of the prosthesis. Macroscopic and microscopic examination of experimental and clinical implants revealed alterations to the ePTFE structure, such as areas of fragmentation, fracture lines, and detachment of fine layers of ePTFE that harbored numerous *Staphylococcus* colonies [14]. PTFE prostheses may reduce tissue reaction which causes local ischemia and low pH. These alterations inhibit phagocytosis and lysosome enzymes activity, facilitating the development of infection.

Graft infections can become clinically evident at different times after the implant. If graft infection occurs within 4 months, the infection is generally caused by bacteria with high virulence like *Staphylococcus aureus*. These coagulase-positive micro-organisms are able to induce autolysis and generate a very important inflammatory process. Late graft infection can occur months or years following the original implant. They are caused by low-virulence bacteria like *Staphylococcus epidermidis* and other coagulase-negative bacteria. These micro-organisms are saprophytes of the skin and in some case can become opportunistic. They are able to produce bacteria biofilms which protect bacteria against antibiotics and can inhibit host defense. In these cases, infection can be very difficult to treat, and management might be complicated by negative cultures.

Pathogenesis

The exact pathogenesis of vascular graft infections is not completely established and is likely to be multifactorial. The type of graft material, method of graft fabrication, implant site, extended operating time, use of antibiotic prophylaxis, host defense and nutritional state of the patient, presence of remote infection, and pathogenicity of contaminating organisms are all factors that influence the risk of graft infection [7]. All prosthetic vascular grafts are susceptible to infection via direct contamination during implantation or bacteremia after operation. Exposure of vascular grafts to micro-organisms and successive colonization can occur at different times. Incorrect sterilization of the graft or surgical instruments or a nonsterile operative field are obvious sources of direct, immediate contamination. Emergency procedures are at greater risk for contamination due to inadequate preparation of the patient, and in fact are associated with a higher incidence of graft infection. Grafts may also be contaminated by direct contact with the patient's skin. Concomitant biliary, bowel, and urologic procedures also increase the risk of graft colonization by bacteria. Infected lymph nodes or vessels can also lead to direct graft contamination. This is of particular concern when a bypass is performed in the presence of ischemic ulcers of the lower extremities.

Patients requiring graft revision for failed vascular reconstruction commonly harbor bacteria within scar tissue, lymphoceles and on the surfaces of previously implanted prosthetic vascular grafts and suture material. The development of a wound infection adjacent to a vascular graft can lead to graft infection by direct spreading of the infection, explaining the high incidence of infections of grafts in the groin region.

Porous fabric prostheses develop a thin layer of luminal fibrin which is gradually replaced by mature collagen growing in from the outer surface of the prosthesis, resulting in a stable and relatively non-thrombogenic luminal surface and increased resistance to late hematogeneous infections. Bacteremia may contaminate all the non-endothelialized prostheses. Although the infection has no significant adverse effect upon the prosthesis itself, it inevitably spreads to the host tissue with incorporated graft, ultimately weakening and disrupting the anastomosis between the graft and the host artery. This disruption of the anastomosis can lead to the formation of a false aneurysm, sepsis, graft enteric fistula, or hemorrhage, with potential limb loss or death. The prosthesis becomes less susceptible to colonization as the luminal pseudo-intimal lining develops and matures over time, but vulnerability to infection from bacteremia has been documented one year after implantation. Late graft infection due to bacteremia caused by dental extraction, urinary tract manipulations or endovascular invasive procedures, also occur.

In an attempt to offer local protection and overcome the risk of infection at the time of surgery, methods of incorporating antibiotics or protein carrier molecules into grafts have been developed [15]. Rifampicin is a hydrophobic semi-synthetic substance with a high affinity for gelatin-coated grafts and is active against the commonly causative microorganisms involved in graft infection. Gentamicin beads have been used to treat infections in vascular surgery, offering the advantage of providing very high concentrations of gentamicin locally [16].

The concern about the development of drug-resistant micro-organisms and drug sensitivity has limited the widespread adoption of this approach.

There is considerable interest in the development of a vascular prosthetic graft which is resistant to infection. Several methods have been evaluated, including the recent introduction of a vascular graft that incorporates silver as an antimicrobial agent. Silver has a long history of medical use and exerts its antimicrobial effect by interacting with bacteria at multiple levels. Based upon its low cellular toxicity and minimal local tissue response, silver is deemed highly biocompatible and suitable for incorporation into implantable medical devices. The use of an antimicrobial vascular graft for in-situ replacement is a promising treatment alternative which warrants additional clinical investigation and longer term follow-up. The use of metals such as silver in the bonding process increases retention of the surrounding tissue.

Future remedies will likely involve utilization of new biomaterial designs and application of either highly potent antimicrobials or agents which penetrate biofilms and eradicate the organisms.

Endovascular treatment

Percutaneous transluminal angioplasty (PTA) and stent implantation are considered to be safe and effective modalities to treat selective cases of peripheral arterial occlusive disease [17-19]. However, both PTA [20] and stent implantation [21] may lead to acute thrombosis, aneurysm formation, vessel rupture, embolization, long-term restenosis, and septic complications.

Although stent infection is uncommon, this complication is severe and may result in the death of the patient. Because strict longitudinal follow-up of patients undergoing stenting is lacking, the true incidence of such complications remains obscure. So far, only five cases of infection that occurred after stent implantation were reported [22-26]. Fatal outcome was observed in two of the five patients [25,26] and serious morbidity occurred in three. The bacterial organism implicated in all patients was *Staphylococcus aureus*, which was isolated from the false aneurysm [22], or excised stents [22-26] and was grown in blood cultures [25-27]. The reason of infection remains uncertain, although the culprit organism and the early presentation of infection (1 to 2 weeks after procedure) suggest that periprocedural contamination is likely. Another possibility could be bacteremia at the time of the procedure. In both situations, a balloon angioplasty and stent deployment determine intimal disruption with predisposition of arterial infection, necrotizing angiitis with subsequent weakening of vessel wall, aneurysm formation, and arterial rupture. The necrotizing angiitis may be widespread, and the renal failure often observed in these cases is thought to be a consequence of this vasculitis. The cause of death is related to multi-organ failure as a result of septic or hemorrhagic shock, disseminated intravascular coagulopathy, or diffuse necrotizing angiitis. In addition, surgical and cardiologic experience have identified factors associated with an increased likelihood of bacteremia after stenting. Prolonged procedure times, repeated use of indwelling sheaths within 24 hours, repeated femoral access within 7 days, and puncture side hematomas have been implicated as contributing factors for infection [28]. So far, no guidelines regarding antibiotic prophylaxis exist for patients undergoing endovascular therapies. We recommend antibiotic prophylaxis for all endovascular procedures, particularly in the presence of an indwelling catheter.

Despite appropriate precautions, vascular specialists will be confronted with this complex problem. Endovascular infections after PTA and stenting have rarely been reported, however, the increasingly liberal application of endovascular procedures will probably augment these complications. It thus becomes imperative for the interventionalists performing these procedures to be aware of this potential complication. Strict sterile technique, antibiotic prophylaxis, and elimination of potential sources of periprocedural bacteremia may limit the occurrence of such arterial infections. When this uncommon complication is identified, it is important to expeditiously treat these patients to prevent uncontrolled sepsis and death [27].

Personal experience

We reviewed the records of 33 consecutive patients treated for graft infection at our institution between January 1994 and October 2000. The diagnosis of aortic infection was made on the basis of clinical presentation (fever, leukocytosis, blood cultures, draining wounds, and gastro-intestinal hemorrhage) and computed tomographic scanning.

Fifty-two percent of the patients underwent the original reconstructive procedure at our institution, while the others had their reconstructive procedure done elsewhere. Thirty were males, three were females, and their mean age was 65.6 ± 12.4 years. Twenty patients had an infected aortobifemoral (ABF) graft, 5 had infected aortic tube grafts (AO), 1 had an infected aortobiliac (ABI) graft, 1 had an infected iliofemoral graft, 2 had iliopopliteal grafts, and 5 had infected femoropopliteal grafts. The original indication for aortic and peripheral reconstruction was aneurysmal disease in 13 patients, and occlusive disease in 20 patients. Eleven patients presented with clinical evidence of infection: groin infection in 3, pseudo-aneurysm in 4, cutaneous graft fistula in 2; systemic evidence of sepsis in 2. Eleven patients presented with gastro-intestinal bleeding due to secondary aorto-enteric fistulas. Seven patients presented with acute limb ischemia due to occlusion of one limb of an ABF graft or complete graft occlusion; three patients presented with abdominal abscess, and one with *chylothorax* (Table I). The average time interval between primary reconstruction and presentation of graft infection was 19.3 months (range 0.5 to 144 months).

Cultures were taken from graft material and perigraft fluid. The bacterial organisms that were

8
65

Table I	CLINICAL PRESENTATION OF 33 PATIENTS WITH VASCULAR GRAFT INFECTION *		
Clinical presentation		*Number*	*%*
Aorto-enteric fistula		11	34
Graft occlusion		7	21
Sepsis		2	6
Pseudo-aneurysm		4	12
Abdominal abscess		3	9
Groin abscess		3	9
Cutaneus fistula		2	6
Chylotorax		1	3
Total		**33**	**100**

* Patients treated at our center between January 1994 and October 2000

cultured are listed in Table II. There were 24 dacron grafts, and 9 PTFE grafts (Table III).

TREATMENT

Local therapy with iodine and antibiotic irrigation was used to treat the infected aortic graft in two patients. One patient was treated with complete excision of the infected aortic graft combined with endarterectomy of the native aorto-iliac artery segment and reconstruction with interposition of bovine pericardium. One patient was treated with complete excision of the infected peripheral graft with revascularization with autologous graft. Ten patients were treated with in-situ reconstruction with cryopreserved homografts after complete aortic graft excision (Figs. 1-6). In seven patients, revascularization was performed by in-situ prosthetic graft replacement: four with PTFE grafts and three

Table III	PRIMARY RECONSTRUCTION IN 33 PATIENTS WITH VASCULAR GRAFT INFECTION		
Primary reconstruction	Dacron (%)	PTFE (%)	Total (%)
Aorto-aortic bypass	5 (15)	0 (0)	5 (15)
Aortobi-iliac bypass	1 (3)	0 (0)	1 (3)
Aortobifemoral bypass	14 (43)	6 (18)	20 (61)
Iliacofemoral bypass	0 (0)	1 (3)	1 (3)
Iliacopopliteal bypass	0 (0)	1 (3)	1 (3)
Femoropopliteal bypass	4 (12)	1 (3)	5 (15)
Total	**24 (73)**	**9 (27)**	**33 (100)**

Table II	DIFFERENT MICRO-ORGANISMS CULTURED FROM THE EXPLANTED GRAFT AND THE PROSTHETIC FLUID *	
Organism	Number graft	%
Staphylococcus aureus	15	20
Candida albicans	9	12
Staphylococcus epidermidis	6	8
Coagulase-negative Staphylococcus	5	6
Pseudomonas aeruginosa	5	6
Enterococcus faecalis	5	6
Enterococcus species	4	5
Lactobacillus species	3	4
Escherichia Coli	2	3
Streptococcus intermedius	2	3
Klebsiella pneumoniae	2	3
Topulopsis glabrata	2	3
Enterobacter cloacae	2	3
Enterococcus faecium	2	3
Others	12	15

* *Staphylococci* are the most commonly involved in graft infection

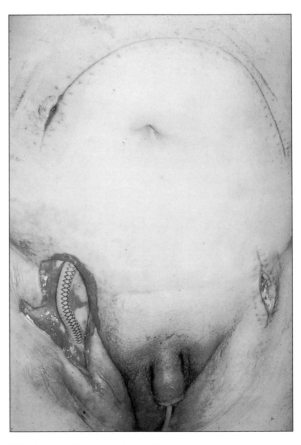

FIG. 1 A 51-year-old patient, one month after aortobifemoral bypass with dacron graft, presents with visible graft exposed in an open bilateral groin wound. The bacterial organism that was cultured is *Staphylococcus aureus*.

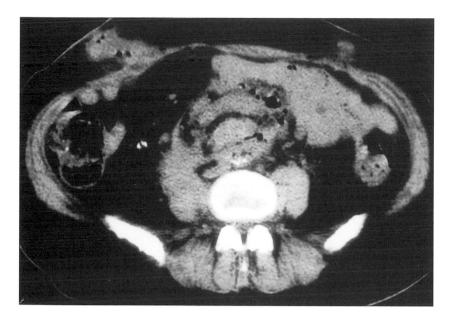

FIG. 2 Computed tomograms of the inflammatory perigraft mass and air in aortobifemoral bypass.

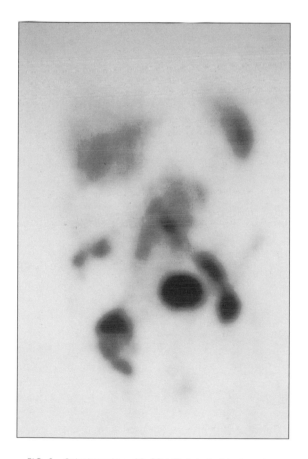

FIG. 3 Scintigraphy with 99 MTc labeled leukocytes.

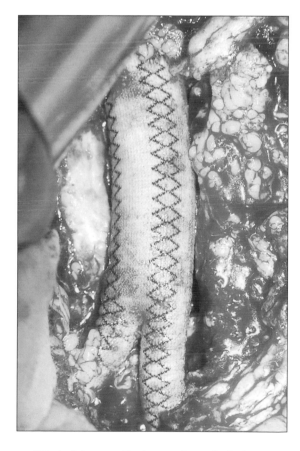

FIG. 4 Intra-operative image of prosthetic tissue.

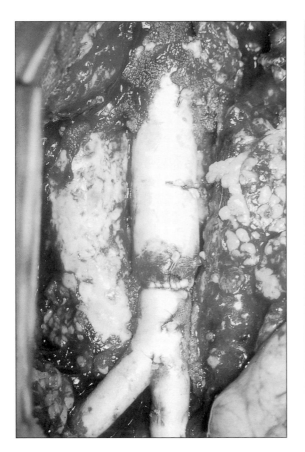

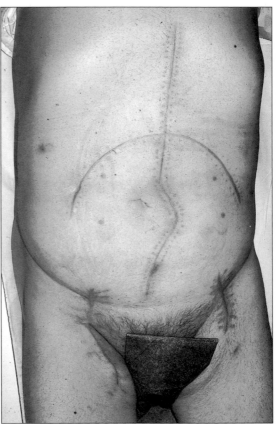

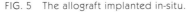

FIG. 5 The allograft implanted in-situ.

FIG. 6 One month after secondary surgery, the groin wounds healed.

with rifampin impregnated dacron grafts. In 11 patients, extra-anatomic bypass grafting and subsequent excision of the infected aortic graft was performed: axillobifemoral bypass with PTFE graft in 6 patients, axillobifemoral bypass with PTFE and homograft graft in 2 patients. Three patients were treated with partial prosthetic excision and reconstruction with interposition of homograft segment (Table IV).

Systemic antibiotics were continued for two weeks postoperatively. Thereafter, therapy was changed to an appropriate oral or intramuscular antibiotic regimen for six more weeks. The decision to stop antibiotic therapy at six weeks was based on microbiological advice or CT scanning, provided there was no evidence of ongoing infection.

RESULTS

The perioperative mortality rate was 18%. Perioperative death was caused by sepsis (4 patients), hemorrhagic shock as a result of aorto-enteric fistula (1 patient), and multi-organ failure (1 patient). Postoperative mortality was highest in patients who presented with aorto-enteric fistula (37%), and in those who presented with sepsis (100%). Postoperative mortality was lowest in patients who presented with a groin infection, without involving the prosthesis, or infection of the distal segment of the graft (14%). No amputation was required in our patients. Patients were evaluated at one month and at three months after operation, then at intervals of six months.

The mean follow-up period was 18 months (range 1-71 months): in this period 9 patients died within 2 years after surgical treatment (rate 27%). Total mortality was 45 % (Table IV). Postoperative death was caused by sepsis (3 patients), hemorrhagic shock for aortic stump rupture (1 patient), stroke (1 patient), malignancy (2 patients), and unknown causes (1 patient). One patient died of sepsis 5 years after surgical treatment (Table V). The cumulative mortality rate was highest in patients presenting with aorto-enteric fistula (60%), in those treated with homograft in-situ replacement (50%), and in those treated with simultaneous aortic graft excision and extra-anatomic bypass (50%).

Of the 18 survivors, 17 remained alive and clinically free of infection; one patient recently presented with a recurrent groin infection one year later.

Experience of the North Italian Transplant Programme (NITP)

INTRODUCTION

Following the experience of cardiac surgeons with homografts in the treatment of infective aortic valve endocarditis, cardiovascular surgeons have investigated in-situ revascularization using homografts in the management of vascular prosthetic infections. Preliminary results are encouraging, but long-term results and influence of preservation techniques are still under investigation. We report the experience of the *Italian Collaborative Vascular Homograft Group* [30], with the use of fresh and cryopreserved arterial homografts for the treatment of aortic graft infections.

MATERIALS AND METHODS

This program, named *Collaborative Vascular Homograft Group* (CVHG) is organized in close cooperation with the Reference Center (RC) of the *North Italian Transplant Programme* (NITP), 10 departments of vascular surgery (Table VI), and a homograft bank *(Banca Italiana Omoinnesti)*. Homograft procurement, allocation, and transplantation activity were coordinated by NITP's RC.

The NITP is a transplant organization which has coordinated organ procurement and transplantation activity since 1976 and actually serves an area of about 20 million inhabitants. The tasks of the Reference Center include: managing the waiting list; performing immunological evaluation of recipients and donors; allocating organs and tissues; organizing transports; collecting data from recipients; donors, grafted patients; setting up protocols together with the operative units; planning information campaigns; supporting donor families; and finally, promoting research in the field of transplantation.

Table IV	OVERALL MORTALITY ACCORDING TO THE TYPE OF SECONDARY RECONSTRUCTION RECEIVED	
Secondary reconstruction	*Patients (%)*	*Deaths (%)*
Excision + homograft in-situ	10	5
Excision + PTFE in-situ	4	1
Excision + dacron in-situ	3	1
Excision + axillobifemoral PTFE	6	3
Partial excision + homograft	3	1
Excision + PTFE + homograft	2	1
Local therapy	2	2
Other	2	0
No therapy (intra-operative death)	1	1
Total	**33 (100)**	**15 (45)**

Table V	COMPARISON OF CLINICAL PRESENTATION AND FOLLOW-UP OF THE PATIENTS *	
Clinical presentation	*Survivals (%)*	*Deaths (%)*
Aorto-enteric fistula	4 (12)	7 (21)
Graft occlusion	6 (18)	1 (3)
Sepsis	0	2 (6)
Pseudo-aneurysm	3 (9)	1 (3)
Abdominal abscess	1 (3)	2 (6)
Groin abscess	2 (6)	1 (3)
Cutaneus fistula	2 (6)	0
Chylothorax	0	1 (3)
Total	**18 (55)**	**15 (45)**

* Aorto-enteric fistula is associated with the worst prognosis

Table VI	DEPARTMENTS OF VASCULAR SURGERY OF THE *ITALIAN COLLABORATIVE VASCULAR HOMOGRAFT GROUP*

H. Ancona (Prof. G. Alò)

H. Bassini, Cinisello Balsamo (Prof. G. Biasi)

H. Busto Arsizio (Prof. A. Costantini)

IRCCS Centro Cardiologico Fondazione Monzino, Milano (Prof. P. Biglioli)

H. Fatebenefratelli, Milano (Prof. G.P. Spina)

I.C.P., Milano (Prof. G. Agrifoglio)

Istituto ortopedico Gaetano Pini, Milano (Prof. A.M. Sironi)

IRCCS Policlinico, Pad. Zonda, Milano (Prof. U. Ruberti)

IRCCS H.S. Matteo, Pavia (A. Odero)

IRCCS H.S. Raffaele, Milano (R. Chiesa)

The operative protocol included the following criteria.
1 - Only patients suffering from infections of an infrarenal aortic prosthesis could be proposed as potential recipient for an aortic allograft.
2 - NITP multi-organ donors were chosen as a source of vascular allografts at the Procuring Centers (PC);
3 - An *ad hoc* authorization from the Ministry of Health (mandatory in the Italian legislation), was required to the Transplant Center (TC) to perform vessel harvesting and transplantation.
4 - Before the homograft bank was activated, the TC were allowed to use fresh homografts.

For each operative unit of the CVHG we defined the following tasks.
- *Procuring Center:* report and evaluate all potential organ/tissue donors and perform vessel harvesting.

- *Homograft Bank:* perform tissue processing and cryopreservation, quality certification according to standard operating procedures.
- *Transplant Centers:* perform recipient evaluations, aortic transplantation, post-transplant follow-up.
- *Reference Center:* perform data registration, tissue and organ procurement coordination, graft allocation, post-transplant data collection.

For our program we adopted a *3 level organizational model:*
1 - reference Center coordinates all steps from potential donor to the transplantation;
2 - homograft Bank is responsible for tissue quality and safety;
3 - procuring Center are responsible for donor quality and safety, and Transplant Centers for recipient evaluation and transplantation.

Between March 1994 and December 1999, 512 arterial segments were harvested from multi-organ donors, 444 were cryopreserved at the bank, and 68 were preserved at 4°C (fresh) in antibiotic solution. Eighteen per cent of arterial segments was discarded because of anatomical alteration or bacterial-fungal contamination. The homografts were used in 70 patients with aortic graft infections. The analysis was performed on 60 cases whose data were sufficient and reliable.

Eleven patients were treated with homografts preserved at 4°C and 49 patients were treated with cryopreserved homografts. The mean age of the patients was 66 years (range 40-78 years). Emergency surgical procedures were performed in 12 patients (20%). Aorto-enteric fistula was diagnosed in 19 patients. The mean interval between the first procedure and the insertion of a homograft implantation for patients with an infected aortic graft was 3 years (range 1-15 years). *Staphylococcus* was the main cause of infection identified at intraoperative culture in 50% of causes. The vascular infections were due to more than one micro-organism in 37% of the cases. The types of vascular reconstruction were: 40 aortobifemoral, 9 aorto-aortic, 6 aortobiiliac, and 5 aortofemoral grafts. Antibody and human lymphocyte antigen (HLA) compatibility between donor and recipient were not respected. All patients started broad-spectrum antibiotics when vascular infection was diagnosed, and were replaced by selective antibiotics on the basis of microbiological findings. The duration of antibiotic therapy was influenced by the type of micro-organisms and the extension of the infection.

The mean duration of follow-up was 33 months (range 1-68 months). Clinical and duplex scanning evaluation were routinely performed. Computed tomography (CT), magnetic resonance (MR), scanning, or arteriography were performed on the basis of duplex scanning results.

HARVESTING

Arteries were not removed from donors over 60 years of age, donors with the presence of risk factors for HIV, hepatitis, signs or symptoms of transmittable disease (including malignancies), or with donor serology positive for anti-HIV, HbsAg, anti-HCV, or syphilis. Descending thoracic aorta, aortic bifurcation, and iliac and femoral arteries were harvested on a peri-adventitial plain. Hypogastric and deep femoral arteries were transected 4-5 centimeters towards their origin. Small collateral branches were transected a few millimeters distal to their origin to facilitate ligation or suture. Finally, after being flushed with heparinized saline solution to eliminate residual blood, homografts were placed in ice-cold sterile Eurocollins solution and transported to the bank.

BANKING

The arterial segments were prepared, measured, and evaluated at the bank in a first-grade laminar flow room. Arteries were discarded in case of aneurysms, wall calcifications, intimal ulcerations, or when sample cultures were positive for bacterial or fungal contaminations. Homografts used as fresh tissue were stored at 4°C for a period ranging from 48 hours, to decrease cellular antigenicity, to 30 days, to avoid later degenerative changes. The preservation medium is Eurocollins 1000 ml, heparin 10 000 IU, netilmicin 80 mg, ceftriaxone 1 g, amphotericin B 50 mg.

Cryopreservation was carried out after antibiotic decontamination with an antibiotic solution (see above) and kept at 4°C for 48-96 hours. The cryoprotective solution was composed of RPMI 1640, 10% dimethylsulfoxide (DMSO), and 10% fetal cow serum (FCS). Starting temperature was 4°C and the cooling rate was -1°C/minute until temperatures reached -100°C. Arterial grafts were stored in a vapor phase of liquid nitrogen (-150°C) and quarantined for at least 50 days before distribution in order to complete cultures for mycobacterium. Before the transplant procedure, rapid thawing was carried out by submersion of the graft in a 40°C water bath; the DMSO was quickly removed by progressive dilution of the medium to avoid cellular membrane damage. Arterial samples and solution were cultured for bacterial and fungal contamination after each operational step, and grafts were discarded if necessary.

HOMOGRAFT IMPLANTATION

The side branches of the homograft were ligated or sutured. In case of inadequate dimensions the homografts were obtained by anastomoses of more arterial segments. In all cases the infected prosthetic graft was removed and the periprosthetic tissue carefully debrided. The periprosthetic fluid and fragment of the infected graft were cultured for aerobes, anaerobes, and fungi. The homografts were implanted with most of the side branches (i.e., intercostal arteries) anteriorly, in order to detect bleeding and to facilitate hemostasis.

RESULTS

Thirty-day mortality was 15% (nine patients). In four cases the mortality was homograft-related because death was caused by peri-anastomotic rupture. In five cases the mortality was non-homograft-related; cause of death was multi-organ failure in three cases and congestive heart failure in two cases.

The mean follow-up was 33 months (range 1-68 months). There were 15 late deaths with a mortality rate of 25%. In seven cases mortality was homograft-related; the cause of death was peri-anastomotic rupture in five patients and homograft rupture in two patients. In eight cases the mortality was non homograft-related; congestive heart failure in two cases, myocardial infarction in four cases, pulmonary neoplasm in one case and unknown in one patient.

Eleven patients had graft occlusion; six cases were successfully treated with thrombectomy, five patients received a femoropopliteal bypass with autologous vein. In three cases leg amputation was necessary (one case for irreversible ischemia beginning before the homograft reconstruction).

The results of fresh and cryopreserved homografts were compared. No significant differences in early postoperative mortality, late mortality, homograft-related mortality, and graft failure were observed. Thirty-six months after surgery the actuarial survival rate was 57% and the actuarial patency was 41% (Fig. 7-8).

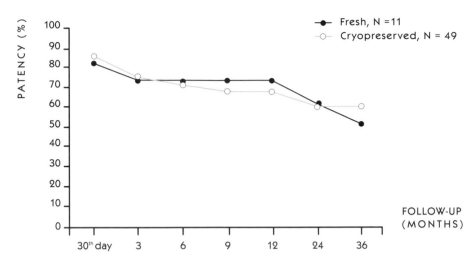

FIG. 7   Actuarial patency of fresh and cryopreserved homografts.

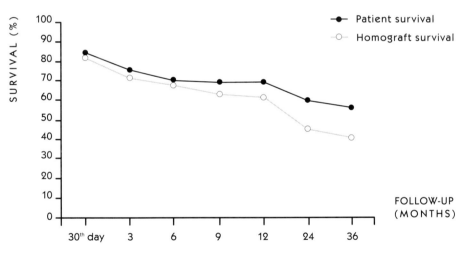

FIG. 8   Actuarial survival patency rates.

Conclusion

Vascular graft infection, despite low incidence, remains a significant problem and a challenge to all vascular surgeons. Even though several techniques have been proposed for the treatment of this complication such as in-situ repair with vascular prostheses or extra-anatomic prosthetic bypass, mortality and amputation rates remain high. Homografts are less vulnerable to infection than prosthetic grafts, allowing in-situ replacement with lower risk of reinfection, thereby reducing complications like aortic stump rupture, infection, or occlusion of the extra-anatomic prosthetic bypass. However, occlusion and late degeneration of the homograft may be expected due to preservation techniques and chronic rejection.

REFERENCES

1 Hayes PD, Nasim A, London NJ et al. in-situ replacement of infected aortic grafts with rifampicin-bonded prostheses: the Leicester experience (1992 to 1998). *J Vasc Surg* 1999; 30: 92-98.

2 Johnson G, Kempczinski RF, Moore WS et al. In: Rutherford RB, ed. *Vascular Surgery*. Saunders, Philadelphia 1998 pp; 588-604.

3 Bandyk DF. Vascular graft infections: epidemiology, microbiology, pathogenesis, and prevention. In: Bernhard VM, Towne JB (eds). *Complications in Vascular Surgery*. Quality Medical Publishing, St. Louis 1991; pp 223-234.

4 Szilagyi DE, Smith RF, Elliott JP et al. Infection in arterial reconstruction with synthetic grafts. *Ann Surg* 1972; 176: 321-333.

5 Goldstone J, Moore WS. Infection in vascular prostheses. Clinical manifestations and surgical management. *Am J Surg* 1974; 128: 225-233.

6 Bunt TJ. Synthetic vascular graft infections I. Graft infections. *Surgery* 1983; 93: 733-746.

7 Bandyk DF. Aortic graft infection. *Sem Vasc Surg* 1990; 3:122.

8 Chu CC, Williams DF. Effects of physical configuration and chemical structure of materials on bacterial adhesion. A possible link to wound infection. *Am J Surg* 1984; 147: 197-204.

9 Bandyk DF, Berni GA, Thiele BL et al. Aortofemoral graft infection due to *Staphylococcus epidermidis*. *Arch Surg* 1984; 119: 102-108.

10 Arciola CR, Montanaro L, Baldassarri L et al. Slime production by *Staphylococci* isolated from prosthesis-associated infections. *New Microbiol* 1999; 22: 337-341.

11 Bandyk DF, Bergamini TM, Kinney EV et al. in-situ replacement of vascular prostheses infected by bacterial microfilms. *J Vasc Surg* 1991; 13: 575-583.

12 Sugarman B. In vitro adherence of bacteria to prosthetic grafts. *Infection* 1982; 10: 9-14.

13 Boyce B. Physical Characteristics of expanded polytetrafluorethylene grafts. In: James Stanley, ed. *Biological and synthetic vascular prostheses*. Grune and Stratton Inc., New York 1996; pp 554-561.

14 Bellon JM, Contreras LA, Bujan J. Ultrastructural alterations of polytetrafluoroethylene prostheses implanted in abdominal wall provoked by infection: clinical and experimental study. *World J Surg* 2000; 24: 528-532.

15 Vicaretti M, Hawthorne W, Ao PY et al. Does in-situ replacement of a staphylococcal infected vascular graft with a rifampicin impregnated gelatin sealed dacron graft reduce the incidence of subsequent infection? *Int Angiol* 1999; 18: 225-232.

16 Benaerts PJ, Ridler BM, Vercaeren P et al. Gentamicin beads in vascular surgery: long-term results of implantation. *Cardiovasc Surg* 1999; 7: 447-450.

17 Tetteroo E, Van der Graaf Y, Bosch LJ et al. Randomized comparison of primary stent placement versus primary angioplasty followed by selective stent placement in patients with iliac-artery occlusive disease. Dutch Iliac Stent Trial Study Group. *Lancet* 1998; 351: 1153-1159.

18 Dorros G, Jaff M, Mathiak L et al. Four-year follow-up of Palmaz-Shatz stent revascularization as treatment for atherosclerotic renal artery stenosis. *Circulation* 1998; 98: 642-647.

19 Dorros G. Stent-supported carotid angioplasty: should it be done, and, if so, by whom? A 1998 perspective. *Circulation* 1998; 98: 927-930.

20 Samson H, Sprayegen S, Veith F. Management of angioplasty complications, unsuccessful procedures and early and late failures. *Ann Surg* 1984; 199: 234-240.

21 Palmaz J, Laborde J, Rivera F. Stenting of the iliac arteries with the Palmaz stent: experience from a multicenter trial. *Cardiovasc Intervent Radiol* 1992; 15: 291-297.

22 Chalmers N, Eadington D, Gandanhamo D. Case report: infected false aneurysm at the site of an iliac stent. *Br J Rad* 1993; 66: 946-948.

23 Cooper JC, Woods DA, Spencer P et al. The development of an infected false aneurysm following iliac angioplasty. *Br J Radiol* 1991; 64: 759-760.

24 Deiparine MK, Ballard JL, Taylor FC et al. Endovascular stent infection. *J Vasc Surg* 1996; 23: 529-533.

25 Thérasse E, Soulez G, Cartier P et al. Infection with fatal outcome after endovascular metallic stent placement. *Radiology* 1994; 192: 363-395.

26 Schachtrupp A, Chalabi K, Fischer U et al. Septic endarteritis and fatal iliac wall rupture after endovascular stenting of the common iliac artery. *Cardiovasc Surg* 1999; 7: 183-186.

27 Gordon GI, Vogelzang RL, Curry RH et al. Endovascular infection after renal artery placement. *J Vasc Intervent Radiol* 1996; 7: 669-672.

28 Chiesa R, Astore D, Piccolo G et al. Fresh and cryopreserved arterial homograft in the treatment of prosthetic graft infections: experience of the Italian Collaborative Vascular Homograft Group. *Ann Vasc Surg* 1998; 12: 457-462.

8

73

9

PREVENTION AND TREATMENT
OF ARTERIAL GRAFT INFECTIONS

OLIVIER GOËAU-BRISSONNIÈRE, MARC COGGIA

The development of synthetic arterial prostheses was a major advance in vascular surgery, allowing complex revascularizations with very good mid- and long-term clinical results. However, arterial graft infection is the most feared complication in vascular surgery, and remains a challenging problem despite numerous refinements in graft fabrication, implantation techniques and routine antibiotic prophylaxis. Graft infection is always difficult to eradicate, and if not recognized or adequately treated, eventually causes prosthesis failure, life-threatening hemorrhage, or sepsis. Even in very experienced centers and in recent series, mortality and amputation rates associated with infected grafts remain significant [1-4].

During the past decade, experimental works allowed a better understanding of the pathogenesis of vascular graft infections. Diagnostic advances due to new imaging techniques and the improvement of microbiological techniques contributed to the elaboration of better therapeutic strategies, adapted to the anatomic lesions and the clinical presentation. The encouraging results obtained with in-situ replacement with arterial homografts, autologous veins, or rifampin-bonded grafts have also led to the reappraisal of the role of conventional treatment of vascular graft infections, i.e., total prosthetic graft excision and extra-anatomic bypass [1,2,5,6].

Epidemiology

CLASSIFICATION

Several classifications of wound and graft infections have been proposed. Szilagyi et al. [7] divided postoperative incisional infections into three grades, according to the depth of wound involvement. Grade I infections are superficial infections which only involve the skin, grade II are subcutaneous infections, and grade III involve the arterial prosthesis. This very simple classification probably lacks clinical detail, but it is still widely used. Bunt [8] further classified grade III infections to specify the anatomic extension of the lesions and the associated complications, i.e., graft infection, graft-enteric erosion, graft-enteric fistula and aortic stump sepsis. Because these two classifications did not classify the infections according to the results of bacteriological cultures and histological sampling, we recently proposed a new classification. In this classification, early postoperative wound and graft infection are classified as shown in Table I. After the third postoperative month, vascular graft infections are defined using the criteria of grade III.

INCIDENCE

The overall incidence of prosthetic graft infection is difficult to determine because most reported series were retrospective. In the literature, the incidence of graft infection varies with the institution, the operative indication and the site of graft implantation. From most series, the incidence of graft infection appears to be lower after purely abdominal aortoiliac and cervical arterial prosthetic surgery. It increases notably after aortofemoral, femoropopliteal, femorofemoral, or axillofemoral prosthetic replacement, and after the operations replacing the descending thoracic aorta or the thoracoabdominal aorta. In two reviews of the literature done in 1983 [8] and 1998 [9], the overall incidence of graft infection was estimated to be about 2%. Nevertheless, the epidemiology of arterial graft infection has undergone an evolution over the past two decades, with coagulase-negative staphylococci (CNS) emerging as important pathogens responsible for late graft infections, which may present several years after the initial operation. The cumulative incidence

of graft infection may then be underestimated because of the long delay that often occurs between the initial operation and the first clinical manifestation of infection. However, the true incidence of graft infection may be estimated as high as 5%, if both early and late infections are included.

DELAY OF ONSET

In old series, most vascular graft infections were early infections, occurring within four months after graft implantation. Sixty-five percent of the cases reported by Szilagyi et al. in 1972 [7] were early graft infections. However, over the two past decades, the number of late infections increased, and, at present, in some series, most infections are late infections. In a recent series of 24 graft infections reported by Henke et al. [10], the average interval from graft implantation to presentation of infection was 29 months. Three reasons can explain this change:
1 - antibiotic prophylaxis reduces the number of early infections through the decreased number of wound infections,
2 - the change in microbial ecology, with the emergence of *Staphylococcus epidermidis (S. epidermidis)*,
3 - the advances made in the diagnosis, leading to the inclusion of several late postoperative complications that were previously not considered as infectious, such as false aneurysms or periprosthetic seromas.

MICROBIOLOGY

Graft infection is mostly bacterial, although a wide range of microorganisms have been implicated, including fungi or mycoplasmas. In early series of

Table I	CLASSIFICATION OF WOUND AND GRAFT INFECTION
Grade 0	Normal healing.
Grade I	Infection unlikely, but presence of one of the following criteria associated with a negative culture: inflammation, hematoma, lymphocele, skin necrosis.
Grade II	Confirmed wound infection, prosthesis probably free of infection; presence of one of the following criteria: grade I and also positive wound culture, pus discharge; none of the grade III criteria.
Grade III	Graft infection; presence of at least one of the following criteria: pus contiguous to the prosthesis, positive prosthetic or periprosthetic microbiological examination (Gram stain or culture), prosthetic or periprosthetic histological signs of infection.

graft infections, *Staphylococcus aureus (S. aureus)* was the leading pathogen, involved in up to 50% of cases. Other bacteria isolated were mainly enterobacteriaceae, and *S. epidermidis* was rarely cultured. Since the early 1970s, this microbiological pattern has progressively changed, and infections due to *S. epidermidis* have increased in frequency. The analysis of recent series clearly shows a new repartition of the bacteria involved in arterial graft infections. The incidences of *S. aureus* and *S. epidermidis* are now similar, about 20% in most series, and Gram-negative bacteria are often isolated in about 50% of cases [9]. The most frequently cultured Gram-negative bacteria are *Escherichia coli (E. coli)*, *Pseudomonas sp.* and *Klebsiella sp.* Polymicrobial infections have also been reported with an increased incidence. In a prospective study we evaluated early postoperative wound and graft infection in 633 patients undergoing aortofemoral reconstruction, 39 bacterial strains were isolated in 27 of 30 patients having a grade II or III infection. Isolated bacteria were 14 *S. aureus*, 9 CNS, 9 enterobacteriaceae, 4 streptococci, 2 acinetobacters, and one Hafnia alvei.

The increased incidence of Gram-negative bacteria may be related to the widespread use of prophylactic antibiotics which are very active against *S. aureus*, and the increasing prevalence of these microorganisms in the hospital environment. The increased number of *S. epidermidis* may also relate to improved culture techniques and a better report of positive cultures, *S. epidermidis* being considered as a true pathogen.

When looking at the distribution of microorganisms according to the site of graft implantation, three points deserve mention. First, intestinal microorganisms (enterobacteriaceae, anaerobes) appear responsible for most aortoiliac infections when no groin incision has been done. Second, *S. epidermidis* is now the leading pathogen after aortofemoral reconstruction. Third, *S. aureus* remains the principal pathogen in most series after infrainguinal reconstructions. In these distal reconstructions, an increased incidence of *Pseudomonas sp.* has also been observed. No matter the site of graft implantation, about 6% of bacteriological cultures are negative despite clinical evidence of infection. This was the case in our own experience, in which two from 27 cultures (6%) were reported as negative. These negative cultures are often observed in late infections and may be due to inadequate sampling, inadequacy of laboratory techniques to recover CNS, or the previous administration of broad spectrum antibiotics when a graft infection is suspected. The adjunct of histological criteria of infection may contribute to the diagnosis of infection.

Pathogenesis

Infection of a prosthetic vascular graft is always the consequence of a bacterial colonization of the graft material. Following bacterial adhesion to the biomaterial surface, the pathogenesis of graft infection involves several steps in which biomaterials and bacteria act together:
1 - microcolony formation within a bacterial biofilm,
2 - activation of host defenses,
3 - an inflammatory response involving perigraft tissues and the graft-artery anastomoses.

Neutrophil chemotaxis, decreased phagocytosis, complement activation, secretion of cytokines and an intense immune foreign body reaction creates an acidic ischemic microenvironment which contributes to bacterial proliferation and biofilm formation. This intense inflammatory reaction leads to the autolysis of perigraft tissues creating a perigraft cavity or abscess, and the spread of the infection along the graft and adjacent organs. The involvement of graft-artery anastomoses is associated with an arteritis which decreases the tensile strength of sutures and contributes to the formation of anastomotic pseudoaneurysm and anastomotic disruption. Infections due to Gram-negative bacteria such as *E. coli*, *Pseudomonas*, *Klebsiella*, *Enterobacter*, and *Proteus* species are particularly virulent. These bacteria produce toxins that contribute to the autolysis of perigraft tissues and anastomotic dehiscence. Alternatively, low-virulence bacteria such as CNS are mostly responsible for late infections. The slime produced by these bacteria contributes to their adhesion to vascular grafts within a biofilm made of microcolonies surrounded with glycocalyx.

Microorganisms can colonize the biomaterial during the implantation procedure or through the wound when a healing complication occurs. Hematogenous or lymphatic seeding of a prosthesis may also happen in the presence of remote sites of infection, such as urinary tract infection, venous catheter sepsis, ischemic foot ulcer. A perioperative contamination remains the most frequent modality of graft colonization, and several predisposing factors have been identified (Table II). Besides lapses in aseptic technique by the surgical team or very unusual sterilization accidents, the higher incidence of graft infection observed when at least one of the anastomoses is below the inguinal ligament [7,11] suggests that contaminating bacteria more often belong to the patient's endogenous flora than to the environment. Despite preoperative cutaneous preparation, many bacteria remain over the skin and in the dermis. The skin of operated patients is often colonized with CNS which produce a slime, and hospitalization is enough to increase the resistance of these microorganisms from 15% to 50% [12]. Inguinal cutaneous flora is then the origin of the sepsis, and microorganisms can colonize the prosthesis by migrating in the groin incision or through a direct contact between the skin and the graft. Disruption of inguinal lymphatics may also contribute to graft colonization, especially in the presence of infected skin ulcers or gangrenous toes. An infected wound can also lead to the development of graft infection by direct extension.

Other potential sources of graft contamination are the arterial wall, the periarterial tissues or an aneurysmal thrombus [13], but the significance of positive arterial cultures remains debated. In some series, a relationship was established between the positivity of aneurysmal content cultures and the occurrence of a postoperative graft infection. This was not confirmed in other studies, and, for some groups, routine bacterial cultures are probably not necessary during elective primary arterial recon-structions. However, the follow-up of these studies was always limited. Since *S. epidermidis* is the leading pathogen isolated from arterial wall cultures, a longer follow-up should be obtained to get a definitive opinion regarding the true infectious risk of these cultures.

In abdominal aortic surgery, concomitant operation on other organs may contaminate the graft, and most authors advise against the performance of a second surgical procedure. An exception should be made for this admonition regarding cholecystectomy for asymptomatic cholelithiasis, since a significant incidence of postoperative acute cholecystitis has been reported in patients with cholelithiasis undergoing aortic replacement, with a risk of bacteremia, and in the absence of an increased risk of infection after concomitant cholecystectomy. Nevertheless, cholecystectomy should be performed only after the retroperitoneum has been closed over the aortic graft. Bacteremia or bacterial transudation may also result from a colic ischemia and contaminate a vascular prosthesis [11], and residual intraperitoneal microabscesses may contaminate a prosthesis several months after surgery for peritonitis. During graft implantation, the graft must be isolated from the intestine in order to avoid intestinal erosions leading to graft infection and/or graft-enteric fistula.

The risk of graft infection is also increased following reoperation, especially after a repeated groin incision, due to an increased number of postoperative wound complications. In patients undergoing

Table II	Factors predisposing to graft infection	
Preoperative factors	*Postoperative factors*	*Altered host defenses*
Inguinal incision	Postoperative wound infection	Age grater than 80 years
Reoperative surgery	Colic ischemia	Malnutrition
Emergency procedure	Intestinal erosion	Diabetes
Asepsis breaks	Graft puncture	Malignancy
Simultaneous gastrointestinal procedure	Bacteremia	Corticosteroid treatment
Non sterile graft		Leukopenia
Prolonged preoperative stay		Immunodeficiency
Operating time more than 4 hours		
Remote infection		
Diseased artery walls		

an iterative vascular reconstruction, the predictive value of positive arterial wall cultures has clearly been demonstrated, as well as the frequent bacterial colonization of occluded grafts or false aneurysms, even in the absence of overt signs of infection.

Several other factors increase the risk of peroperative graft colonization, such as a prolonged preoperative in-hospital stay with skin colonization by more resistant bacteria, an operating time longer than 4 hours [14], emergency surgery [15], or early reoperation for hematoma, graft thrombosis, or hemorrhage [12].

Graft puncture in the groin to perform an arteriography is a logical cause of prosthetic infection. However, despite the report of local infectious complications, the risk of graft infection appears low, and most authors recommend graft puncture rather a trans-humeral angiogram [16].

Early or late bacteremia may also lead to vascular graft infection. The hematogenous infectability of arterial prostheses has been experimentally demonstrated and was confirmed in the clinical setting by the similarity of bacteria isolated from infected grafts and a remote site of infection. The susceptibility of vascular prostheses to bacteremic seeding progressively decreases as the pseudointimal lining develops, but a risk persists, even years after graft implantation.

Several host-related factors have been noted to increase the incidence of graft infection, including age greater than 80 years, diabetes, obesity, malnutrition, corticosteroid administration, malignancy, or immunodeficiency. The physical and the chemical properties of the graft material also influence bacterial adhesion and graft infectability. Experimental studies demonstrated that the affinity of some bacterial strains was 10 to 100 times higher for polyester than for expanded polytetrafluoroethylene (ePTFE), and that the adherence of *S. epidermidis* to polyester was decreased when the graft material was precoagulated or albumin-coated [17, 18]. Bacterial adherence to vascular biomaterials also depends on the bacteria species and the ability of bacteria to produce slime. *S. aureus* was demonstrated to adhere 10 to 1000 times more on graft material than *E. coli* did. Slime-producing CNS adhere in greater numbers to polyester and ePTFE than do nonproducing strains [17]. The increased adherence of staphylococci is due to specific capsular adhesins that mediate bacterial attachment and graft colonization [19]. Antibodies to these glycoproteins can be developed, which can inhibit the adherence of adhesin-producing staphylococci to the graft material. Moreover, the infective threshold of bacteria required to cause an invasive graft infection, i.e., the minimum number of bacteria necessary to cause graft infection in more than 50% of grafts contaminated, varies with bacterial species. As demonstrated by White et al. [20] it is 1 x 107 for *S. aureus* and 1 x 109 for *S. epidermidis*, but similar graft infections can be induced with as few as 1 x 102 *Pseudomonas aeruginosa* organisms.

Techniques of prevention

The infectious risk of graft implantation justifies preventive strategies before, during, and after operation. Whenever possible, the re-establishment of satisfactory immune defenses and of an acceptable nutritional status should be obtained. In some debilitated patients, prosthetic grafting should be avoided other than for limb salvage. The timing of arteriography in relation to surgery has been debated. Even if some authors consider that the infectious risk of angiography is limited [21], we agree with Landreneau that surgery should be performed within 24 hours of angiography or delayed beyond one week [22]. Preoperative hospital stay should be reduced to the strict minimum in order to limit skin colonization by a nosocomial flora resistant to commonly used prophylactic antibiotics. Preoperative skin preparation is also crucial. It must be performed as close as possible from the operation, at best immediately before the surgical procedure. Clipping the skin or using a depilatory cream decreases the rate of infection compared with shaving. Preoperative shower using a bactericidal soap also contributes to reduce the risk of infection. Preparation of the skin for incision should be thorough, using povidone-iodine or chlorhexidine. During the operation, surgical technique, handling of tissues, and hemostasis must be very careful, and the graft should be protected from any contact with the skin. The incisions should be closed in layers to eliminate dead space and reduce the incidence of wound complications. The use of double gloving is probably wise, but the advantage of ultraclean air systems has not been demonstrated in vascular surgery. In the postoperative period, intravenous lines and urinary catheter should be removed as soon as possible and dressings should not be changed unnecessarily.

ANTIBIOTIC PROPHYLAXIS

Perioperative antibiotic prophylaxis has been shown in prospective clinical trials to significantly reduce the incidence of wound infections that can lead to vascular graft infection, and its use in prosthetic vascular surgery is mandatory [23,24]. The antibiotic used should be bactericidal against most of the bacterial species involved in graft infections, and administered systemically at the time of anesthetic induction and at regular intervals during the surgical procedure to maintain serum and tissue levels above the minimal inhibitory concentration for the expected pathogens. Local antibiotic irrigation plays little role in addition to intravenous antibiotics [24]. Most groups recommend a 24-hour prophylaxis, and there are no solid data to support a longer administration. Since most graft infections are caused by staphylococci, *E. coli*, and streptococci, first and second generation cephalosporins such as cefazolin or cefamandole are still widely used

(Table III). Recent peroperative pharmacokinetic studies contributed to optimize the modalities of administration of these prophylactic antibiotics, suggesting to use closer injections and higher doses during the surgical procedure. In patients with allergies to penicillin or cephalosporins, the association of vancomycin or teicoplanin and an aminoglycoside is an appropriate alternative.

Several points remain debated regarding the modalities of antibiotic prophylaxis in vascular surgery. In the presence of a distal tissue loss, it appears logical to continue the prophylaxis during 5 to 7 days, but there is no study justifying this widely adopted attitude. The higher risk of postoperative infection reported after vascular reoperations or a prolonged preoperative hospital stay may also justify to prefer the association of vancomycin or teicoplanin and an aminoglycoside, and a longer duration of antibiotic administration, e.g., 48 hours. Finally, the occurrence of *true* failures of a correctly

Table III PROPOSALS FOR PERIOPERATIVE ANTIBIOTIC PROPHYLAXIS IN VASCULAR SURGERY

Standard regimen	- Cefazolin, 1 g IV* 1 hour before surgery, then every 2 or 3 hours during surgery and every 6 hours until the 24th hour. *Or* - Cefamandole, 1.5 g IV 1 hour before surgery, then every 2 or 3 hours during surgery and every 6 hours until the 24th hour.
Allergy to penicillin or cephalosporins, reoperation or prolonged preoperative stay (> 48 h)	- Vancomycin, 1 g IV over 1 hour, 1 or 2 hours before surgery, then 12 hours later. *Or* - Teicoplanin, 6 mg/kg IV over 30 minutes, 1 or 2 hours before surgery, then 12 hours later. *AND* - Netilmicin, 3 mg/kg IV over 1 hour, 1 hour before surgery, then 12 hours later. *Or* - Amikacin, 7.5 mg/kg IV over 1 hour, 1 hour before surgery, then 12 hours later.
Leg or remote site infection	- Culture adapted prophylaxis, 5 to 7 days.

* Intravenous

administered prophylaxis reported with cephalosporins, i.e., the occurrence of an infection due to microorganisms sensitive to the administered antibiotic, and the increased role of Gram-negative bacteria bring the choice of prophylactic antibiotics to discussion [25]. However, this discussion is difficult because many questions remain unanswered about the pathophysiology of vascular graft infection and the mechanisms of the prophylactic activity of antibiotics. In order to limit the emergence of resistant strains, it appears mandatory to avoid the use of molecules very active against multiresistant strains. Apart from this rule, other antimicrobial agents could turn out to be a better choice. Antibiotics reducing the adhesion of bacteria or acting against slowly growing bacteria or demonstrating a postantibiotic effect [26] and molecules with a very long half-life time should deserve attention. Fluoroquinolones meet these criteria, with a spectrum of activity adapted to most of the pathogens responsible for vascular graft infections. We recently performed a multicenter prospective randomized trial in 633 patients and compared the efficacy of pefloxacin and cefamandole to prevent postoperative wound and graft infection after aortofemoral prosthetic surgery. In this trial, true failures of prophylaxis were more frequent with cefamandole, but initial resistances, i.e., the occurrence of a grade II or III infection due to microorganisms sensitive to the administered antibiotic, were more frequent with pefloxacin. Nevertheless, a single dose of pefloxacin was as efficient as five doses of cefamandole to prevent wound and graft infections, with 4.1% and 5.5% of grade II and grade III infections, respectively. Fluoroquinolones might then represent an interesting alternative.

The low but persistent risk of late graft colonization probably justifies a short duration antibiotic prophylaxis in patients bearing a vascular prosthesis immediately before procedures which carry a risk of bacteremia, such as dental extraction, manipulation of the urinary tract and, particularly, angiographic examinations.

ANTIBIOTIC-BONDED VASCULAR PROSTHESES

Since the appropriate use of antibiotic prophylaxis in conjunction with other preventive measures did not totally eradicate graft sepsis, the development of prostheses that are intrinsically resistant to infection was a very appealing concept. Many experimental studies have demonstrated the efficacy of antibiotic-bonded grafts to reduce the incidence of graft infection. The advent of protein-sealed polyester grafts has raised the possibility of using the sealant as vehicle for antibiotic delivery. However, an infection-resistant prosthesis should comply with several prerequisites. The antimicrobial agent bonded to the prosthesis should have a bactericidal effect against the bacteria involved in graft infections. It should be nonallergenic and have a minimal risk of toxicity. The duration of the antibacterial activity of the bonded graft should be as long as possible to allow a satisfactory graft healing without infection. Finally, the technique used to bind the antimicrobial agent should be easy to accomplish in the usual clinical setting.

From these prerequisites, rifampin was a good candidate for bonding, with a strong affinity for gelatin-sealed polyester grafts. Rifampin demonstrates a wide antibacterial activity against most aerobic Gram-positive cocci, notably with remarkable anti-staphylococcal potency, and against many aerobic Gram-negative organisms that cause vascular graft infection. It is, overall, a well tolerated drug, especially after the parenteral administration of a single dose slowly released in the bloodstream. Using a dog model of bacteremic graft infection, we demonstrated the resistance of rifampin-bonded grafts to an early postoperative methicillin-resistant *S. aureus* bacteremia [27]. We also demonstrated that rifampin-bonded gelatin-sealed grafts were resistant to infection when used for in-situ replacement of a graft by *S. epidermidis* [5]. These experimental results were the rationale for a prospective randomized study evaluating the efficacy of rifampin bonding to prevent early wound and graft infection after prosthetic aortoiliofemoral reconstruction. In this study conducted in 2610 patients in 90 centers, the incidence of wound infection was significantly reduced in patients receiving a rifampin-bonded graft in association with perioperative systemic antibiotic prophylaxis [28]. Since wound infection is a factor predisposing to graft infection, the results of this trial justify the use of rifampin-bonded grafts, especially in patients at risk of infection.

Treatment

The management of prosthetic vascular graft infection remains a formidable challenge. The two main objectives are to eradicate the infection and to maintain an adequate limb perfusion. Systemic antibiotic therapy is mandatory and should always begin before any reoperation, as soon as the diagnosis of graft infection is made. If the pathogen or the pathogens have been identified in a preoperative microbiological sample, bactericidal antibiotics should be administered preoperatively and perioperatively. If the responsible organisms have not been identified before operation, broad spectrum antibiotics should be administered. The intravenous association of vancomycin, an aminoglycoside and a third generation cephalosporin would then be appropriate. Once operative cultures have grown bacteria, the antibiotic treatment should be adapted to the results of antibiotic susceptibility testing of the isolated strains. The optimal duration of antibiotic therapy after surgical treatment of vascular graft infection remains under debate. However, the incidence of graft reinfection and complications such as aortic stump rupture may be reduced with long-term antibiotic administration. Four to 6 weeks of parenteral administration, followed by oral antibiotics for 6 months are often advocated, but some authors have recommended lifetime administration of oral antibiotics in high-risk situations [29].

The surgical part of the treatment depends upon the site of graft implantation, the severity and the extension of the sepsis, the virulence of the pathogen, and the vascular anatomy. Familiarity with multiple treatments, experience with complex surgical reconstructions, and careful long-term follow-up are crucial to achieve optimal results. Graft excision can rarely be done alone, without revascularization. The most common surgical option is total graft removal preceded or followed by an ex-situ prosthetic bypass. In many series dealing with aortoiliac prosthetic infections, such a major procedure has been associated with mortality and amputation rates as high as 40% and 30%, respectively [30-32]. However, some recent series of staged extra-anatomic bypass grafting and aortic graft removal showed improved early and long-term outcomes with an overall treatment related mortality between 12% and 19%, and lower amputation rates between 7% and 11% [3,4]. Very good early and long-term results have also been reported by Darling et al. with the use of a retroperitoneal in line aortic bypass through clean tissue planes [33]. At the aortoiliac level, some authors have also proposed to combine graft excision with an autogenous revascularization associating endarterectomy and in-situ replacement

with autologous veins or arteries [34]. However, this procedure is also very difficult to perform, with few indications. in-situ prosthetic replacement has also been explored as an alternative method, with variable results. This technique should be applied primarily to treat low grade, late appearing infections with the microbiological characteristics of a CNS infection (bacterial biofilm, negative cultures) and without anastomotic hemorrhage [35]. Selective graft preservation should also be used very cautiously in carefully selected patients, only when the infection appears strictly limited to a non anastomotic segment of a patent peripheral graft, and in the absence of systemic sepsis [36]. This technique is more likely to be successful in early than in late extracavitary graft infections [37].

Facing these poor results, Kieffer et al. recently proposed to treat graft infection by in-situ replacement with arterial allografts, with very interesting early results, particularly in terms of limb salvage [1]. This new technique was an important advance in the management of graft infection, and the antibiotics used to decontaminate and preserve the allografts probably play a role in their resistance to infection [38]. However, despite these gratifying early clinical results, the procurement of arterial allografts is often difficult to organize and preservation techniques are still debated. An alternative technique for in-situ replacement has been proposed by Clagett et al. [39] and Nevelsteen et al. [2], using the lower extremity deep veins to create autogenous conduits for in-situ replacement of an excised infected graft. The early results of this therapeutic option using an autogenous material are also very satisfactory in terms of limb salvage, but the long-term behavior of these venous conduits should be studied.

Among ongoing developments, using antibiotic-bonded grafts for in-situ replacement of infected grafts may also be a promising alternative. Using a dog model, we were able to demonstrate that rifampin-bonded gelatin-sealed grafts resisted to reinfection after in-situ replacement of an infrarenal aortic prosthesis infected with *S. epidermidis* RP62, a strain susceptible to rifampin [5]. In the same animal model, rifampin-bonded grafts were also resistant to reinfection with a rifampin-resistant isogenic mutant of *S. epidermidis* RP62 [40]. Early clinical results with rifampin-bonded prostheses appear to be favorable [6,41], but more studies are warranted to investigate these antibiotic-conduits further.

In all the cases, a wide debridement of all devitalized and infected tissues must be associated to the removal of an infected graft to provide a suitable environment in which healing may occur. Since the artery wall adjacent to the infected graft may contaminate a new conduit, the arterial wall should also be debrided back to normal-appearing tissues.

Future directions and emerging problems

A better understanding of the interaction between bacteria and biomaterials and of the mechanisms of action of antibiotics will help in the prevention of arterial graft infections.

The continuous amelioration of the resistance of arterial substitutes also warrants further research. In particular, the use of antibiotic-bonded grafts will probably significantly be very useful in patients at high risk for infection, and for treatment of vascular graft infection by in-situ replacement.

Finally, well designed and conducted clinical trials should be carried out to determine which group of patients should benefit from a specific therapeutic alternative, according to the severity and the extent of the sepsis.

Besides these advances in the management of arterial graft infections, physicians who care for patients with vascular disease must be aware of the seriousness of infectious complications after stent or endovascular prosthesis deployment [42,43]. The true incidence of these infections is currently unknown, but an increasing number of cases are reported, and *S. aureus* is the leading pathogen. Radical surgical therapy is always needed and will be a major procedure in most cases, with arterial and stent resection in addition to antibiotic treatment. In light of the potentially devastating nature of this complication, the administration of prophylactic antibiotics should be considered before any procedure in which placement of an arterial stent or an endovascular prosthesis is considered possible.

9

83

REFERENCES

1 Kieffer E, Bahnini A, Koskas F et al. in-situ allograft replacement of infected infrarenal prosthetic grafts: results in forty-three patients. *J Vasc Surg* 1993; 17: 349-356.

2 Nevelsteen A, Lacroix H, Suy R. Autogenous reconstruction with the lower extremity deep veins: an alternative treatment of prosthetic graft infection after reconstructive surgery for aortoiliac disease. *J Vasc Surg* 1995; 22: 129-134.

3 Yeager RA, Taylor LM Jr, Moneta GL et al. Improved results with conventional management of infrarenal aortic infection. *J Vasc Surg* 1999; 30: 76-83.

4 Seeger JM, Pretus HA, Welborn MB et al. Long-term outcome after treatment of aortic graft infection with staged extra-anatomic bypass grafting and aortic graft removal. *J Vasc Surg* 2000; 32: 151-161.

5 Goëau-Brissonnière O, Mercier F, Nicolas MH et al. Treatment of vascular graft infection by in-situ replacement with a rifampin-bonded gelatin-sealed dacron graft. *J Vasc Surg* 1994; 19: 739-744.

6 Hayes PD, Nasim A, London NJ et al. in-situ replacement of infected aortic grafts with rifampicin-bonded prostheses: the Leicester experience (1992 to 1998). *J Vasc Surg* 1999; 30: 92-98.

7 Szilagyi DE, Smith DF, Elliott JP, Vrandecic MP. Infection in arterial reconstruction with synthetic grafts. *Ann Surg* 1972; 176: 321-333.

8 Bunt TJ. Synthetic vascular graft infections. I. Graft infections. *Surgery* 1983; 93: 733-746.

9 Leschi JP, Goëau-Brissonnière O, Coggia M. Epidémiologie des infections de prothèse artérielle. In: Kieffer E, Goëau-Brissonnière O, Pechère JC, (eds). *Infections artérielles*, Paris: AERCV, 1998, pp 55-71.

10 Henke PK, Bergamini TM, Rose SM, Richardson JD. Current options in prosthetic vascular graft infection. *Am Surg* 1998; 64: 39-45.

11 Sharp WJ, Hoballah JJ, Mohan CR et al. The management of the infected arterial prosthesis: a current decade of experience. *J Vasc Surg* 1994; 19: 844-850.

12 Levy MF, Schmitt DD, Edmiston DE et al. Sequential analysis of staphylococcal colonization of body surfaces of patients undergoing vascular surgery. *J Clin Microbiol* 1990; 28: 664-669.

13 Wakefield TW, Pierson CL, Schaberg DR et al. Artery, periarterial adipose tissue, and blood microbiology during vascular reconstructive surgery: perioperative and early postoperative observations. *J Vasc Surg* 1990; 11: 624-628.

14 Rebollo MH, Bernal JM, Llorca J et al. Nosocomial infections in patients having cardiovascular operations: a multivariate analysis of risk factors. *J Thorac Cardiovasc Surg* 1996; 112: 908-913.

15 Koskas F, Kieffer E. Chirurgie pour rupture d'anévrysme de l'aorte abdominale: résultats à court et long terme d'une étude prospective de l'AURC. *Ann Chir Vasc* 1997; 11: 90-99.

16 AbuRahma AF, Robinson PA, Boland JP et al. Facteurs de complications dans une série récente de 707 artériographies. *Ann Chir Vasc* 1993; 7: 122-129.

17 Schmitt DD, Bandyk DF, Pequet AJ et al. Mucin production by *Staphylococcus epidermidis*: a virulence factor promoting adherence to vascular grafts. *Arch Surg* 1986; 121: 89-95.

18 Siverhus DJ, Schmitt DD, Edmiston CE et al. Adherence of mucin and non-mucin producing staphylococci to preclotted and albumin-coated velour knitted vascular grafts. *Surgery* 1990; 107: 613-619.

19 Tojo M, Yamashita N, Goldman DA et al. Isolation and characterization of a capsular polysaccharide adhesion of *Staphylococcus epidermidis*. *J Infect Dis* 1988; 157: 713-722.

20 White JV, Nessel CC, Wang K. Differential effect of type of bacteria on peripheral graft infections. In: Calligaro KD, Veith FJ, (eds). *Management of infected vascular grafts*. Quality Medical Publishing St. Louis, 1994, pp 25-42.

21 Ameli FM, Knackstedt J, Provan JL et al. Influence des artériographies par ponction fémorale sur l'incidence des contaminations et des infections inguinales postopératoires. *Ann Chir Vasc* 1990; 4: 328-332.

22 Landreneau MD, Raju S. Infections after elective bypass surgery for lower limb ischemia: the influence of preoperative transcutaneous arteriography. *Surgery* 1981; 90: 956-962.

23 Kaiser AB, Clayson KR, Mulherin JL Jr et al. Antibiotic prophylaxis in vascular surgery. *Ann Surg* 1978; 188: 283-289.

24 Pitt HA, Postier RG, McGowan AW et al. Prophylactic antibiotics in vascular surgery. Topical, systemic or both? *Ann Surg* 1980; 192: 356-364.

25 Kernodle DS, Classen DC, Burke JP et al. Failure of cephalosporins to prevent *Staphylococcus aureus* surgical wound infections. *JAMA* 1990; 263: 961-966.

26 Davidson RJ, Zhanel GG, Phillips R et al. Human serum enhances the postantibiotic effect of fluoroquinolones against *Staphylococcus aureus*. *Antimicrob Agents Chemother* 1991; 35: 1261-1263.

27 Goëau-Brissonnière O, Leport C, Bacourt F et al. Prevention of vascular graft infection by rifampin bonding to a gelatin-sealed dacron graft. *Ann Vasc Surg* 1991; 5: 408-412.

28 Goëau-Brissonnière O, Koskas F, Pechère JC, and the participants in the Rifampin Bonded Grafts European Trial. Prevention of early wound and graft infection with rifampin-bonded polyester grafts. *Ann Vasc Surg*, in press.

29 Chan FY, Crawford ES, Coselli JS et al. in-situ prosthetic graft replacement for mycotic aneurysm of the aorta. *Ann Thorac Surg* 1989; 47: 193-303.

30 O'Hara JP, Hertzer NR, Beven EG et al. Surgical management of infected abdominal aortic grafts: review of a 25-year experience. *J Vasc Surg* 1986; 3: 725-731.

31 Reilly LM, Stoney RJ, Goldstone J et al. Improved management of aortic graft infection: the influence of operation sequence and staging. *J Vasc Surg* 1987; 5: 421-431.

32 Ricotta JJ, Faggioli GL, Stella A et al. Total excision and extra-anatomic bypass for aortic graft infection. *Am J Surg* 1991; 162: 145-149.

33 Darling RC 3rd, Resnikoff M, Kreisenberg PB et al. Alternative approach for management of infected aortic grafts. *J Vasc Surg* 1997; 25: 106-112.

34 Ehrenfeld WK, Wilbur BG, Olcot CN et al. Autogenous tissue reconstruction in the management of infected prosthetic grafts. *Surgery* 1979; 85: 85-92.

35 Bandyk DF, Bergamini TM, Kinney EV et al. in-situ replacement of vascular prostheses infected by bacterial biofilms. *J Vasc Surg* 1991; 13: 575-583.

36 Calligaro KD, Veith FJ, Schwartz ML et al. Selective preservation of infected prosthetic arterial grafts. Analysis of a 20-year experience with 120 extracavitary-infected grafts. *Ann Surg* 1994; 220: 461-471.

37 Calligaro KD, Veith FJ, Schwartz ML et al. Differences in early versus late extracavitary arterial graft infections. *J Vasc Surg* 1995; 22: 680-688.

38 Knosalla C, Goëau-Brissonnière O, Leflon V et al. Treatment of vascular graft infection by in-situ replacement with cryopreserved aortic allografts: an experimental study. *J Vasc Surg* 1998; 27: 689-698.

39 Clagett GP, Bowers BL, Lopez-Viego MA et al. Creation of a neo-aortoiliac system from lower extremity deep and superficial veins. *Ann Surg* 1993; 218: 239-249.

40 Coggia M, Goëau-Brissonnière O, Leflon V et al. Traitement expérimental d'une infection de prothèse à *Staphylococcus epidermidis* résistant par remplacement in situ avec une prothèse en polyester enduite de gélatine et imprégnée de rifampicine. *Ann Chir Vasc*, in press.

41 Torsello G, Sandmann W, Gehrt A et al. in-situ replacement of infected vascular prostheses with rifampin-soaked vascular grafts: early results. *J Vasc Surg* 1993; 17: 768-773.

42 DeMaioribus CA, Anderson CA, Popham SS et al. Mycotic renal artery degeneration and systemic sepsis caused by infected renal artery stent. *J Vasc Surg* 1998; 28: 547-550.

43 Tiesenhausen K, Amann W, Koch G et al. Endovascular stentgraft infection: a life threatening complication. *Vasa* 2000; 29: 147-150.

10

RENAL COMPLICATIONS
AFTER ENHANCED
CONTRAST MEDIA INJECTION

HENRIK S THOMSEN, SAMEH K MORCOS

Contrast media nephrotoxicity refers to a condition in which impairment of renal function occurs following intravascular administration of contrast media in the absence of an alternative etiology. The literature is conflicting with regard to the level of renal dysfunction that must be present to diagnose contrast media nephropathy. Some are in favor of a high sensitivity, but a low specificity (e.g. an increase in S-creatinine by more than 25% or 44 μmol/L) whereas opt for a lower sensitivity, but a high specificity (e.g. an increase in S-creatinine by more 50% or 90 μmol/L). The most important features of contrast medium nephrotoxicity are a) a decrease in creatinine clearance, b) a reduction in renal function which often resolves within 1-2 weeks, c) an increase in serum creatinine that peaks within 3-4 days after the administration of the contrast medium, and d) oliguria. A persistent nephrogram is not always associated with a reduction in renal function. The patients at highest risk for developing contrast-induced acute renal failure are those with pre-existing renal impairment particularly when the reduction in renal function is secondary to diabetic nephropathy.

In most cases no specific treatment is required. Several measures have been recommended in preventing contrast medium-induced nephropathy. Extracellular volume expansion and use of low-osmolar contrast media were found to be the most effective. The European Society of Urogenital Radiology has recently forwarded guidelines for diminishing the risk of contrast medium-induced nephropathy. A specific problem occurs in patients with noninsulin dependent diabetes mellitus receiving metformin. The combination of metformin, diabetic nephropathy, and contrast media may cause fatal lactic acidosis. Guidelines on the use of metformin and contrast media have recently been proposed.

Definition of contrast media nephrotoxicity

The term contrast media nephrotoxicity is widely used to refer to the reduction in renal function induced by contrast media. It implies impairment in renal function (an increase in serum creatinine by more than 25% or 44μmol/L) that has occurred within 3 days following the intravascular administration of contrast media and the absence of alternative etiology [1].

Contrast medium nephrotoxicity is considered an important cause of hospital-acquired renal failure. This is not surprising, since diagnostic and interventional procedures using contrast media are performed with increasing frequency. In addition, the patient population subjected to these procedures is progressively older with more co-morbid conditions [2]. Prevention of this iatrogenic condition is important to avoid the substantial morbidity and even mortality that can be sometime associated with contrast medium nephrotoxicity. It was recognized that even a small decrease in renal function may greatly exacerbate the morbidity and mortality caused by coexisting conditions. Acquired sepsis, bleeding, coma, and respiratory failure are more frequent in patients with acute renal failure.

The renal handling of contrast media

When the contrast media molecules reach the systemic circulation, the molecules quickly equilibrate across capillary membranes (except an intact blood-brain barrier). During the first phase of distribution, the increase in intravascular osmolality for hypertonic agents as well as the low-osmolar contrast media causes a rapid fluid shift across capillary membranes toward the intravascular compartment. At the same time, the contrast medium molecules move rapidly through capillary pores into the interstitial, extracellular space, as well as glomerular filtration into the renal tubules. Less than 1% is excreted through extra renal routes [3]. The elimination half-life following intravascular administration in patients with normal renal function is about 2 hours and 75% of the administered dose is excreted in urine within 4 hours [4].

The plasma concentration of iodine follows a bi-exponential decay curve, like drugs which are freely distributed in the extracellular phase and excreted by pure glomerular filtration (e.g. Tc99m-DTPA). The first exponential term represents the mixing of the contrast media in the plasma volume and then its distribution into the interstitial space. After approximately 150 minutes the concentration of contrast medium decreases in a monoexponential way in patients with normal renal function; in patients with severely reduced renal function this phase is delayed [5]. Iodinated contrast media are useful for determination of glomerular filtration rate both in relation to an X-ray examination and as an alternative to the methods using radionuclides [6]. For pure determination of either the plasma clearance or the renal clearance a low dose (e.g. 10 mL of a 300 mg I/mL solution) of contrast medium can be used. A low dose does not seem to be nephrotoxic [7].

The kidneys are just 0.4% of the total body mass, but receive approximately 1.2-1.3 L blood each minute (20%-25% of total cardiac output). The normal glomerular filtration rate (GFR) for human beings is 125 mL or 180 L/d (60 times plasma volume). Since more than 99% of the filtrate is reabsorbed, the normal urine volume is approximately 1 L/day. The glomerular membrane allows passage of substances of up to around 4 nm in diameter and excludes substances larger than 8 nm in diameter. The threshold for filtration is a molecular weight of around 40 000. Albumin has a molecular weight of 43 500 and a diameter of 3 nm, and approximately 22% pass through the glomerular filtration threshold. Subsequently it is reabsorbed in the proximal tubules of normal kidneys. Since the molecular weight of currently used iodinated intravascular media are below 2 000, and since protein binding of modern urographic contrast media is negligible, the contrast media molecules are freely filtered without hindrance through the glomerular basement membrane [4].

The concentration of contrast medium within the tubule depends on the concentration in the glomerular filtrate and on the amount of water reabsorbed as the filtrate passes down the tubule. The concentration in the initial filtrate is the same as that in plasma. However, the concentration in mature urine is 50 to 100 times that in the plasma, since 75% of the filtered water is reabsorbed in proximal tubule, 5% in the loop of Henle, 15% in the distal tubule, and nearly 5% in the collecting ducts [3].

Because molecules of contrast material, like those of mannitol, are not reabsorbed, they continue to exert an osmotic force, markedly reducing reabsorption of water from the tubules. This increases pressure in the Bowman capsule and creates an acute internal hydronephrosis associated with individual nephron dilatation; this leads to global renal enlargement. The main resistance to urine flow in the kidney is at the level of the collecting ducts, which have a total cross-sectional intraluminal area that is smaller than the total cross-sectional intraluminal area of the tubules of the nephrons. The contrast-induced reductions in glomerular filtration rate, filtration fraction, and renal perfusion are explainable on the basis of these intratubular and intracapsular pressure changes caused by the hypertonic solution. On the basis of Sterling's law, the increase in proximal tubular hydrostatic pressure decreases the gradient for filtration from the glomerular capillary. These effects are markedly attenuated when low osmolar contrast media and isotonic contrast media are used.

Within minutes after an intravascular osmotic diuretic is injected, the water and sodium excretion from the kidney increases markedly. Much of the diuretic action can be accounted for on the basis of inhibition of sodium and water reabsorption in the proximal tubule, along with inhibition of sodium and water transport in the loop of Henle. During brisk osmotic diuresis, the distal tubule and collecting duct fail to recapture any notable portion of the increased sodium and water load delivered into the early distal tubule. Increases in the rate of perfusion of the distal portion of the loop lead to decreases in whole kidney glomerular filtration rate, which is a function of the so-called tubuloglomerular feedback (TGF) mechanism. This is, in part, related to the marked increase in proximal tubular pressure with increased flow rates within the nephron.

Results of micropuncture studies in rats after slow intravenous infusions of large doses of contrast medium have been useful in our understanding of the tubular handling of contrast media. Monomers decrease single nephron glomerular filtration rate during the infusion phase. A marked pressure drop between the distal tubules and the renal pelvis has been noted and provides supporting evidence that the most distal part of the nephron, including the collecting ducts, is the main site of resistance to outflow of urine after the injection of contrast medium.

The depression of single nephron glomerular filtration rate is attributed to the intratubular concentration, which is higher when the osmolality is lower. The higher the concentration is, the higher the tubular urine viscosity of the medium is. Increased tubular urine viscosity causes a prolonged increase in tubular hydrostatic pressure and a more prolonged depression of single nephron glomerular filtration rate. The higher concentrations of isoosmotic nonionic dimers, iotrolan and iodixanol, especially in the proximal tubules, where the contrast agents have a decreased osmotic force, might be due to a combination of the isoosmotic nature and the dimeric configuration, which result in higher urine viscosity. Thus the nonionic isoosmolar dimers produce a more prolonged depression of single nephron glomerular filtration rate than the nonionic low osmolar monomers do, which again cause longer depression of single nephron glomerular filtration rate than the ionic high osmolar contrast media do. Whether the drop in the single nephron glomerular filtration rate is of clinical importance remains to be solved. All literature indicates that those monomers, which cause the shortest drop in single nephron glomerular filtration rate, are the most nephrotoxic.

Renal susceptibility to toxic challenge

Since the kidney is the main route of elimination of contrast media, their effects on this organ require careful examination. Ideally, the molecules of contrast media should be filtered without inducing functional or structural changes in the kidney. Unfortunately, this is far from the truth and these agents induce alteration in renal function as well as structural changes in the renal tubules. These effects are usually of no clinical significance in patients with normal kidneys. However, in the presence of renal impairment a further significant deterioration in renal function may develop which can lead to significant morbidity and even mortality in some cases [8].

There are several reasons for the renal susceptibility to a toxic challenge in general.

1 - The kidneys represent 0.4% of body mass and receive 20%-25% of resting cardiac output per minute, so that all blood-borne solutes are rapidly delivered to the renal parenchyma.

2 - High renal oxygen consumption produces sensitivity to agents causing impaired cellular uptake or utilization of oxygen.

3 - Solutes are reabsorbed from luminal fluid increasing the concentration in parenchymal cells.

4 - Other solutes are secreted into luminal fluid increasing the concentration near luminal cell membranes.

5 - The counter-current mechanism and the action of antidiuretic hormone (ADH) further increase luminal fluid concentrations of solutes.

6 - Certain compounds taken up by renal cells are retained for long periods of time, so that both solute concentration and duration of toxic exposure are increased.

7 - Patients with reduced nephron population excrete all solutes through fewer nephrons, thereby increasing the *dose* per nephron.

8 - Volume depletion, or obstruction to flow of urine, may lead to greater reabsorption of a solute or to prolonged exposure of susceptible tissue to a toxic solute.

Not all points have the same importance with regard to contrast media.

Features of contrast medium nephrotoxicity (CMN)

An increase in serum creatinine and a decrease in creatinine clearance reflecting a decrease in the glomerular filtration rate characterize the clinical features. The increase in serum creatinine often peaks within 3 to 4 days after the administration of contrast media [8]. Mild proteinuria and oliguria may also be observed. The majority of patients with contrast medium nephrotoxicity tend to be non-oliguric except those with pre-existing advanced chronic renal failure. Heavy proteinuria is an unusual feature of contrast medium nephrotoxicity. Fortunately, most episodes of contrast medium nephrotoxicity are self-limited and resolve within 1-2 weeks. Permanent renal damage is rare and occurs only in a very few instances. However, contrast medium nephrotoxicity can increase the risk of developing severe nonrenal complications and prolong the hospital stay [2].

Contrast media nephrotoxicity can be confused with the syndrome of atheroembolism that may develop post angiographic examinations. This condition is not caused by contrast media but results from trauma to the atherosclerotic blood vessels precipitating cholesterol microemboli. The clinical picture is characterized by acute renal failure associated with distal digital infarction and skin mottling. Renal histology demonstrates the pathognomonic microvascular cholesterol emboli.

Parameters used to detect the presence of CMN

Serum Creatinine

This measurement can be used to monitor renal function in patients with pre-existing renal impairment before the administration of contrast media [9].

Glomerular Filtration Rate

Measurement of glomerular filtration rate (GFR) is the best sensitive test to assess renal function but is not easy to obtain. Creatinine clearance is often used as a measurement of the GFR. However, creatinine is not a perfect marker for measuring glomerular filtration rate as it is both filtered by the glomeruli and secreted by the tubules.

Recently, it was suggested that intravascular contrast medium enhanced computed tomography examinations can be used to measure renal function and glomerular filtration rate. However, the usefulness of contrast media as a marker to measure glomerular filtration rate in the clinical context of contrast medium nephrotoxicity is not known.

Enzymuria

Urinary enzymes are often raised following the administration of contrast media. However, no relationship has been established between a reduction in GFR and the presence of enzymuria following the administration of contrast media [9]. Therefore, the detection of urinary enzymes is thought to be of little importance to the clinical assessment and management of contrast medium nephrotoxicity.

Proteinuria

Transient proteinuria is a common feature after contrast media injection [8]. This is most likely, secondary only to increased leakage through the glomeruli, although reduced reabsorption by the renal tubules has also been suggested. Contrast media in urine may interfere with some of the protein assay techniques leading to false-positive results. This is probably a pH effect and care must be exercised in interpreting tests for proteinuria in the presence of any contrast agent in the urine.

PERSISTENT NEPHROGRAM

Persistent nephrogram on plain radiography or CT of the abdomen for 24-48 hours post contrast media injection has been described as a feature of CMN [8-10]. However, this sign is now considered nonspecific and can be observed in a number of cases without nephrotoxicity [9]. However, the presence of this sign may discourage the administration of further doses of contrast media [1].

Incidence of CMN

There are wide variations in the reported incidence of CMN because of differences in patient selection, the type of the radiological procedures and the definition of renal impairment [9]. It is now evident that the development of CMN is low in people with normal renal function varying from 0% to 10% [1,9]. Pre-existing renal impairment increases the frequency of this complication (10). An incidence of CMN ranging from 12% to 27% was reported in several prospective controlled studies. In one study, an incidence as high as 50% was reported in patients with diabetic nephropathy undergoing coronary angiography in spite of the use of low osmolar contrast media (LOCM) and adequate hydration. Dialysis was necessary in 15% of these patients [11].

Predisposing factors to CMN

The patients at highest risk for developing contrast-induced acute renal failure are those with pre-existing renal impairment particularly when the reduction in renal function is secondary to diabetic nephropathy. Diabetes mellitus per se without renal impairment is not a risk factor. The degree of renal insufficiency present before the administration of contrast media determines to a great extent the severity of contrast media nephrotoxicity. Large doses of contrast media and multiple injections within 72 hours increase the risk of developing CMN. The route of administration is also important and contrast media are less nephrotoxic when

administered intravenously than when given intra-arterially in the renal arteries or in the aorta proximal to the origin of the renal blood vessels. The acute intrarenal concentration of contrast media is much higher after intra-arterial injection than after an intravenous administration. Dehydration and congestive cardiac failure are risk factors as they are associated with a reduction in renal perfusion, which enhances the ischemic insult of contrast media. Multiple myeloma has been considered in the past as a risk factor for CMN. However, if dehydration is avoided contrast media administration rarely leads to acute renal failure in patients with myeloma.

Old age (over 60 years) is a risk factor because of the reduction in renal mass, function and perfusion, which occurs with age and predisposes the elderly patients to CMN. The concurrent use of nephrotoxic drugs such as nonsteriodal anti-inflammatory drugs (NSAID) and aminoglycosides increase the potential nephrotoxic effects of contrast media. The importance of hypertension, hyperuricemia or proteinuria per se as risk factors for CMN is not clear.

The type of contrast media is also an important predisposing factor for CMN. Recent reports have shown that high osmolar contrast media (HOCM) are more nephrotoxic in comparison to LOCM particularly in patients with pre-existing renal impairment. Whether the newly developed non-ionic dimers, which are iso-osmolar and highly hydrophilic are less nephrotoxic is not yet clear. Clinical experience has so far demonstrated no difference in the renal tolerance of non-ionic monomeric LOCM and the iso-osmolar dimers.

Pathophysiology of CMN

A reduction in renal perfusion caused by a direct effect of contrast media on the kidney and toxic effects on the tubular cells is generally accepted as the main factors in the pathophysiology of contrast medium nephropathy. However, the importance of direct effects of contrast media on tubular cells is contentious. The mechanisms responsible for reduction in renal perfusion involve tubular and vascular events. High osmolality contrast media produce marked natriuresis and diuresis that can activate the tubuloglomerular feedback (TGF) response. This leads to vasoconstriction of the glomerular afferent arterioles causing a decrease in glomerular filtration rate and an increase in renal vascular resistance (RVR). The tubuloglomerular feedback may be responsible for almost 50% of the increase in renal vascular resistance induced by high-osmolar ionic contrast media. In contrast, iso-osmolar dimers which induce only a mild diuresis and natriuresis do not activate this mechanism. The activation of the tubuloglomeular feedback is osmolality dependent and low osmolar contrast media, which are still hypertonic solutions compared to blood, may also stimulate this mechanism. Possible other tubular events in the pathogenesis of contrast medium induced nephropathy include an increase in the intratubular pressure, and tubular obstruction by Tamm-Horsfall protein and abnormal proteins. However, there is no strong evidence to support the importance of these tubular effects in the pathophysiology of contrast medium induced nephropathy.

The structural effects of contrast media on the renal tubules include vacuolization of the epithelial cells of the proximal tubules, DNA fragmentation (abnormal activation of apoptosis or *programmed* cell death), and necrosis of the cells of the thick ascending limbs of loops of Henle in the renal medulla. Active engulfing of contrast media in tubular cells causes the vacuolar responses in the tubular cells, which cause lysosomal changes. The vacuolization is reversible and resolves within a few days of contrast medium administration. There is no correlation between the degree of vacuolization in the tubular cells and the reduction in renal function. The structural effect of contrast medium in the renal medulla is due to ischemia and is less with low-osmolar contrast media. Activation of apoptosis may play an important role in the nephron injury and renal failure induced by contrast media.

The vascular events following contrast media administration are mainly secondary to the direct renal effects of contrast media, which modulate the synthesis and release of vasoactive mediators within the kidney. The endogenous vasodilators prostaglandins and nitric oxide are not directly involved in the renal hemodynamic effects of contrast media. Nevertheless, the intrarenal production of these vasodilators is important in maintaining the perfusion and oxygen supply of the medulla, a tissue that is poorly perfused and inadequately supplied with oxygen. In situations where the synthesis of these mediators is hampered, the renal insult produced by contrast media is enhanced.

The vasoactive substances endothelin and adenosine are important in the mediation of the renal hemodynamic effects of contrast media. Contrast agents stimulate the release of endothelin by endothelial cells in culture and increase both the plasma endothelin concentration and the urinary endothelin excretion following intravascular administration. Endothelin receptor antagonists may prevent the fall in glomerular filtration rate and the reduction in renal perfusion induced by contrast media. In addition, following contrast media administration, the increase in plasma endothelin is greater in patients whose renal function declines when compared to those whose renal function remains unchanged.

Adenosine is an important mediator of the reduction in glomerular filtration rate and renal blood flow induced by contrast media. The biological interaction between adenosine and endothelin is unknown.

Long-term renal effects of contrast media

High-osmolar contrast media can enhance the progression of glomerulosclerosis and renal failure in old spontaneously hypertensive male rats [13]. However, the long-term effects of contrast media on renal function in man are not known.

PREVENTION OF
CONTRAST MEDIUM NEPHROTOXICITY

Several measures have been recommended to prevent contrast medium-induced nephropathy [14], which include:

1 - volume expansion;
2 - hydration with intravenous administration of normal saline (NaCl 0.9%) or half-strength saline (NaCl 0.45%);
3 - infusion of mannitol;
4 - administration of atrial natriuretic peptide, loop diuretics, calcium antagonists, theophylline, or dopamine;
5 - use of low-osmolar non-ionic contrast media instead of high-osmolar ionic contrast media;
6 - hemodialysis rapidly after contrast administration;
7 - injection of small volume of contrast medium;
8 - avoiding short intervals (less than 48 hours) between procedures requiring intravascular administration of contrast media.

Of all these measures, extracellular volume expansion and use of low osmolar contrast media were found to be the most effective [1,15]. Patients with pre-existing renal impairment or multiple myeloma should be adequately hydrated prior to contrast medium administration. This can be achieved with the intravenous injection of 100 mL/hour of 0.9% saline starting 4 hours prior to contrast medium administration and continued for 24 hours afterwards [14]. This regime is suitable for patients who are not in congestive heart failure and are not allowed to drink or eat prior to undergoing an interventional or surgical procedure. If there is no contraindication to oral administration, free fluid intake should be encouraged. At least 500 mL of water or soft drinks before and 2500 mL during the following 24 hours should be offered orally. This fluid intake should secure a diuresis of at least 1 mL/minute. In addition to the use of nonionic low-osmolar contrast media, concurrent administration of nephrotoxic drugs such as gentamicin and NSAID should be avoided. Guidelines on how to diminish the risk of contrast medium-induced nephropathy has recently been proposed by the *Contrast Media Safety Committee* of *the European Society of Urogenital Radiology* (Table I).

The efficacy of the use of renal vasodilators, theophylline and calcium antagonists in the prevention of contrast medium nephrotoxicity remains contentious but the administration of furosemide and mannitol is no longer recommended [1, 14, 15].

Treatment of CMN

The treatment of contrast induced nephropathy begins with recognition of the condition. For high risk patients measurement of serum creatinine between the 2nd and 4th postprocedural day will identify the nonoliguric form of contrast medium induced nephropathy, for oliguric patients a

Table I		ESUR* SIMPLE GUIDELINES TO AVOID CONTRAST MEDIUM NEPHROTOXICITY
Definition		Contrast medium nephrotoxicity is a condition in which an impairment in renal function *(an increase in serum creatinine by more than 25% or 44μmol/L)* occurs within 3 days following the intravascular administration of a contrast medium (CM) in the absence of an alternative etiology.
Risk factors	**Look for**	- S-creatinine levels, particularly secondary to diabetic nephropathy. - Dehydration. - Congestive heart failure. - Age over 70 years old. - Concurrent administration of nephrotoxic drugs, e.g. non-steroid anti-inflammatory drugs.
In patients with risk factor(s)	**Do**	- Make sure that the patient is well hydrated. Give at least 100 mL - oral (e.g. soft drinks) or intravenous (normal saline) depending on the clinical situation - per hour starting 4 hours before to 24 hours after contrast administration. In warm areas increase the fluid volume. - Use low- or iso-osmolar contrast media. - Stop administration of nephrotoxic drugs for at least 24 hours. - Consider alternative imaging techniques, which do not require the administration of iodinated contrast media.
	Do not	- Give high osmolar contrast media. - Administer large doses of contrast media. - Administer mannitol and diuretics, particularly loop-diuretics. - Perform multiple studies with contrast media within a short period of time.

* ESUR = European Society of Urogenital Radiology

24-hours urine volume less than 400 mL will trigger the diagnosis. There is no specific treatment. Hemodialysis has been tried, but this should only be done on clinical need. Some patients with contrast medium nephrotoxicity may require temporary dialysis support, while for those with oliguria such dialysis support often becomes permanent. The acute management of such patients is the same as for other patients with acute renal failure and should include careful monitoring of serum electrolytes to detect hyperpotassiemia, meticulous attention to fluid intake and output to prevent hypovolemia or hypervolemia, daily serum creatinine measurements, daily weights, plus adequate nutritional intake. Attempts to convert oliguric renal failure to the nonoliguric form using mannitol

and furosemide have been unsuccessful. The patient should not be re-exposed to contrast media before the kidney function has returned to its previous function. If contrast is to be given again, the patient must be adequately hydrated.

Metformin-induced lactic acidosis and the intravascular administration of contrast media

The biguanide metformin (dimethylbiguanide) are used in noninsulin dependent diabetes mellitus and was introduced into clinical practice in 1957.

TABLE II	ESUR* GUIDELINES FOR THE ADMINISTRATION OF CONTRAST MEDIA TO DIABETICS TAKING METFORMIN
	Serum creatinine level should be measured in every diabetic patient treated with biguanides prior to intravascular administration of contrast media. Low-osmolar contrast media should always be used in these patients.
Elective studies	A. *If the serum creatinine is normal,* the radiological examination should be performed and intake of metformin stopped from the time of the study. The use of metformin should not be resumed for 48 hours and should only be restarted if renal function/serum creatinine remains within the normal range. B. *If renal function is abnormal,* the metformin should be stopped and the contrast study should be delayed for 48 hours. Metformin should only be restarted 48 hours later, if renal function/serum creatinine is unchanged.
Emergency cases	A. *If the serum creatinine is normal,* the study may proceed as suggested for elective patients. B. *If the renal function is abnormal (or unknown),* the physician should weigh the risks and benefits of contrast administration. Alternative imaging techniques should be considered. If contrast media administration is deemed necessary and the following precautions should be implemented. - Metformin therapy should be stopped. - The patient should be hydrated (e.g. at least 100 mL per hour of soft drinks or intravenous saline up to 24 hours after contrast medium administration. - In hot areas more fluid should be given). - Monitor renal function (serum creatinine), serum lactic acid and pH of blood. - Look for symptoms of lactic acidosis (vomiting, somnolence, nausea, epigastric pain, anorexia, hyperpnea, lethargy, diarrhea and thirst). Blood test results indicative of lactic acidosis: pH less than 7.25 and lactic acid more than 5 mmol.

ESUR = European Society of Urogenital Radiology

Approximately 90% of metformin are eliminated via the kidneys in 24 hours. Renal insufficiency (GFR less than 70 mL/min, or serum creatinine more than 140 μmol/L) will lead to retention of these biguanides in the tissues and the potential for the development of fatal lactic acidosis [16].

The use of contrast media in patients receiving metformin should be carried out with care. Contrast media can induce a reduction in renal function leading to retention of metformin that may induce lactic acidosis. However, no conclusive evidence was found to indicate that the intravascular use of contrast media precipitated the development of metformin induced lactic acidosis in patients with normal S-creatinine (less than 130 μmol/L). The complication was almost always observed in noninsulin dependent diabetic patients with abnormal renal function before injection of contrast media.

In Europe it is currently advised that metformin should be stopped 48 hours before and 48 hours subsequent to the administration of contrast media. Serum creatinine should be monitored to check that it has remained at the precontrast level before metformin is resumed. The contrast media safety committee of the *European Society of Urogenital Radiology* (opposite Table II) has recently produced a new guideline on the use of metformin and contrast media.

REFERENCES

1 Morcos SK, Thomsen HS, Webb JAW. Contrast media induced nephrotoxicity: a consensus report. Contrast Media Safety Committee of the European Society of Urogenital Radiology (ESUR). *Eur Radiol* 1999; 9: 1602-1613.

2 Solomon R. Contrast-medium-induced acute renal failure. *Kidney Int.* 1998; 53: 230-242.

3 Thomsen HS, Golman K, Hemmingsen L et al. Contrast medium induced nephropathy: animal experiments. *Frontiers Eur Radiol* 1993; 9: 83-108.

4 Katzberg RW, Urography into the 21st century: new contrast media, renal handling, imaging characteristics, and nephrotoxicity. *Radiology* 1997; 204: 297-312.

5 Almén T, Frennby B, Sterner G. Determination of glomerular filtration rate (GFR) with contrast media. In: Thomsen HS, Muller RN, Mattrey RF (eds) *Trends in contrast media.* 1999, Berlin, Springer Verlag, pp 81-94.

6 Thomsen HS, Vestergaard A, Nielsen SL et al. Renal clearance of an ionic high-osmolar and a non-ionic low-osmolar contrast medium. *Invest Radiol* 1991; 26: 564-568.

7 Frennby B. Use of iohexol clearance to determine the glomerular filtration rate. A comparison between different clearance techniques in man and animal. *Scand J Urol Nephrol Suppl* 1997; 182: 1-63.

8 Berns AS. Nephrotoxicity of contrast media. *Kidney Int* 1989; 36: 730-740.

9 Morcos SK. Contrast media-induced nephrotoxicity- questions and answers. *Brit J Radiol* 1998; 71: 357-365.

10 Love L, Johnson MS, Bresler ME et al. The persistent computed tomography nephrogram: its significance in the diagnosis of contrast-associated nephrotoxicity. *Br J Radiol* 1994; 67: 951-957.

11 Rudnick MR, Goldfarb S, Wexler L et al. Nephrotoxicity of ionic and nonionic contrast media in 1196 patients: a randomized trial. *Kidney Int* 1995; 47: 254-261.

12 Morcos SK, El Nahas AM. Advances in the understanding of the nephrotoxicity of radiocontrast media *Nephron* 1998; 78: 249-252.

13 Duarte CG, Zhang J, Ellis S (1997). The SHR as a small animal model for radiocontrast renal failure. Relation of nephrotoxicity to animal's age, gender, strain, and dose of radiocontrast. *Renal Fail.* 19: 723-743.

14 Thomsen HS. Contrast nephropathy. In: Thomsen HS, Muller RN, Mattrey RF (eds) *Trends in contrast media.* 1999, Berlin, Springer Verlag, pp 103-116.

15 Solomon R, Werner C, Mann D et al. Effects of saline, mannitol and furosemide to prevent acute decreases in renal function induced by radiocontrast agents. *N Engl J Med* 1994; 331: 1416-1420.

16 Thomsen HS, Morcos SK. Contrast media and metformin. Guidelines to diminish the risk of lactic acidosis in non-insulin dependent diabetics after administration of contrast media. *Eur Radiol* 1999; 9: 738-740.

10

11

RENAL FAILURE FOLLOWING RECONSTRUCTIVE VASCULAR SURGERY

GEORGE HAMILTON

Renal failure remains a frequent complication of major vascular interventions of all kinds but in particular after aortic procedures. This is despite the major advances that have been made in recent years in peri-operative and postoperative management of vascular hemodynamics. At this present time the onset of renal failure or acute tubular necrosis after a vascular procedure, endovascular or open, heralds significant morbidity and increased probability of death in the afflicted patient. High prevalence of associated renal artery disease in patients undergoing arterial interventions further increases the risk of renal failure in our group of patients.

Pathophysiology of renal failure in arterial disease

In addition to its other important hemostatic mechanisms, the healthy kidney regulates the intravascular and extravascular fluid compartments, electrolyte concentration and blood pressure. Thus acute renal failure complicating vascular surgery results in profound hemodynamic effects commonly associated with multi organ failure and high mortality rates. For example a recent review of patients undergoing cardiac surgery found an incidence in the postoperative period of acute renal failure requiring renal replacement therapy of only 1.1%. Mortality in this group, however, was 64%

compared to only 4.3% in patients who did not develop acute renal failure; subsequent analysis of this group revealed a corrected odds ratio for death of 7.9 [1,2]. This major increase in mortality holds true also for renal failure following vascular surgery.

MECHANISMS OF ACUTE RENAL FAILURE IN THE VASCULAR PATIENT

In the greatest majority, acute renal failure develops as a result of ischemia of the tubular cells of the nephron. More specifically the anatomical region of the kidney most susceptible is the outer medulla. Here there is a high metabolic demand combined with relatively low blood flow, indeed this region has a *water shed* blood supply with the medulla typically having half the partial oxygen pressure of the cortex [3]. Thus renal ischemia affects primarily the tubules at the outer medulla where cellular death will occur. This process involves not only necrosis but also apoptosis or programmed cell death, which is probably triggered by ischemia. Necrosis occurs as a result of profound decrease in intracellular ATP with activation of phospholipases which act on the cellular membrane. These release arachidonic acid by degrading its constituent phospholipids. In addition to this destabilization of the cell membrane, loss of the epithelial brush border, destruction of cellular tight junctions and activation of cytokines occurs causing an acute inflammatory response. Subsequently, tubular cells in this area swell and die, slough into the tubular lumen and obstruct filtrate flow. This progression explains the common pattern of onset of renal failure with the initial loss of concentrating ability in the urine followed by oliguria and anuria, as massive tubular cell death, denudation then obstruction of the tubules by sloughed cells occurs. Apoptosis occurs at this time secondary to ischemia but this event is not associated with an inflammatory response. It is also seen in the recovery phase when there is tubular epithelial proliferation and presumably is involved in the modulation of the proliferative process to restore normal tubular architecture [4].

Blood flow within the kidneys is also regulated by the interplay of vasoactive substances on renal blood vessel tone. This interaction between vasodilatory substances such as nitric oxide and prostaglandin E_2, and vasoconstricting substances such as endothelin, catecholamines and angiotensin II has significant effects on perfusion. A commonly encountered clinical example of the importance of microvascular renal blood flow is the renal failure which will complicate ACE inhibitor therapy in the presence of severe renal artery stenosis. This results from the decreased glomerular perfusion pressure resulting from decreased tone of the efferent arteriolar vessels. Renal ischemia will result in ATP breakdown and release of adenosine and also reduce nitric oxide production, both causing parenchymal vasoconstriction. The use of non steroidal anti-inflammatory drugs (NSAIDS) will inhibit PGE_2 production, and also X-ray contrast media in themselves can cause intense vasoconstriction [5].

Renal failure can result from mechanical obstruction at the level of the tubular system. Rhabdomyolysis can complicate reperfusion of an acutely ischemic muscle bed. This results in release of myoglobin which will concentrate in the kidneys and particularly in conjunction with hypovolemia will produce acute renal failure. Typically, acute renal failure will result from the presence of more than one predisposing factor with preoperative renal dysfunction recognized in many studies as the single most important predictor of the likelihood of the development of this complication.

There are therefore many mechanisms which can adversely affect the nephron but the most common pathway for acute renal failure development in vascular patients is ischemia with reperfusion. Vascular patients have a high prevalence of underlying renal disease particularly renal artery stenosis and diabetes. When parenchymal disease is added to recent exposure to angiographic contrast agents, intraoperative hypovolemia from blood and fluid loss, and particularly the major effects of aortic cross clamping, the relatively high predisposition to renal failure seen in vascular patients can be readily understood (Table I) [6].

EFFECTS OF AORTIC CROSS CLAMPING

Cross clamping of the aorta provokes major changes affecting primarily cardiac function. These changes depend on the level of aortic cross clamping. Suprarenal clamping causes dramatic increases in mean arterial pressure, filling pressures and ventricular wall motion abnormalities with an up to 40% decrease in ejection fraction [7]. Increasing duration of cross clamping also causes increased systemic vascular resistance and decreased cardiac output. The details of these effects are beyond the scope of this chapter but central to these phenomena are the effects of major blood volume redistribution dictated by the level of aortic cross clamping.

Direct renal ischemia occurs in suprarenal clamping, but major hemodynamic effects on the kidney occur even with infrarenal clamping. The hypervolemia, vasodilatation and increased blood flow in tissue proximal to the clamp can result in significant microcirculatory disturbance which can adversely affect oxygen exchange in these tissues. Associated with aortic cross clamping is substantial arteriovenous shunting through the upper body tissues and also there is increased discharge of noradrenaline and adrenaline. These factors result in arteriolar constriction and decreased capillary flow in the kidney [7]. Thus infrarenal aortic cross clamping results in increased vascular resistance in the renal parenchyma and a 30% decrease in renal blood flow. Furthermore this effect may persist for some time after unclamping of the aorta. In infrarenal aortic clamping intuitively the renal blood flow would not be expected to be compromized, but these deleterious effects on the kidney circulation help to explain the up to 5% incidence of renal failure requiring renal replacement therapy which has been described following infrarenal aortic procedures. Ischemia and reperfusion injury which occurs with suprarenal aortic clamping compounds these effects and results in the much higher rate of renal complications seen when the clamp is placed across the thoracic aorta.

Clinical features

Renal failure after vascular reconstructive surgery can vary from minor serum electrolyte and creatinine disturbance to full blown acute tubular necrosis. Diagnosis mostly is made on the basis of oliguria and elevated serum creatinine levels. Thorough physical examination in particular to assess for the presence of hypovolemia, hypotension, sepsis or congestive cardiac failure is vitally important in the management of these patients. Early postoperative renal failure may be due to fluid depletion and hypovolemia or less commonly where there is compromized cardiac function. Indeed in the elderly vascular patient there may be a combination of both conditions present. The classification of causes of renal failure into prerenal, renal or parenchymal and postrenal is useful in the management of these patients (Table II).

Most patients who develop renal failure after vascular surgery fall into the prerenal group of causes. The major clinical decision that must be made in

Table I	RISK FACTORS FOR POSTOPERATIVE RENAL FAILURE
➤ Preoperative renal dysfunction	➤ Renal artery stenosis
➤ Aortic procedures	➤ Recent X-ray contrast
➤ Hypovolemic shock	➤ NSAIDS
➤ ACE inhibitors, furesemide	➤ Diabetes
➤ Sepsis, endotoxemia	➤ Jaundice, cirrhosis
➤ Congestive cardiac failure	➤ Athero-embolism
➤ Reperfusion injury, rhabdomyolysis	➤ Cyclosporin, tacrolimus
➤ Multiple myeloma	➤ Aminoglycosides, amphotericin B

Table II	CLASSIFICATION OF RENAL FAILURE	
Prerenal	*Renal*	*Postrenal*
Hypovolemia Blood and fluid loss Dehydration, third space sequestration, ascites, edema	**Acute renal failure** Acute tubular necrosis, myoglobinuria, contrast nephropathy, drug nephropathy	**Obstruction** Catheter: clot, kink
Cardiogenic Poor left ventricular function Decreased cardiac output	**Chronic** Amyloidosis, diabetic nephropathy,	Bladder: clot, tumour
Sepsis Endotoxic shock	renal artery stenosis, atheroembolic disease, glomerulonephritis	Ureter: extrinsic compression (e.g. graft limb, suture), clot, tumour

these patients is in distinguishing between hypovolemia and cardiogenic shock. Renal or parenchymal causes such as nephrotoxicity from drugs or
contrast media may also be an important and common aggravating feature of the development of
renal failure. Severe renal artery stenosis causing
ischemic nephropathy can also present in up to 40%
of this group of patients. Preoperative detection and
treatment of these disorders is vitally important in
reduction of the incidence of postoperative renal
failure.

Technical considerations in avoidance of post-reconstructive renal failure

Technical problems arising during surgery can
contribute significantly to the development of renal
failure. The importance of the anesthetist's role in
management of cardiovascular hemodynamics in
these procedures has already been emphasized.
Technical prowess of the surgeon is a further obvious but relatively overlooked factor. Adequate preoperative investigation, assessment and patient
selection are clinical skills of paramount importance. The presence of severe aortic disease around
the renal artery origins raises quite significantly the
risk of atheroembolism into the renal circulation.
A further clamp associated injury is that of renal
osteal occlusion occurring from displacement of calcified aortic plaque. These problems can be avoided
by identification of such high risk aortic necks and
the use of supraceliac rather than juxta or suprarenal clamping [8].

Prolonged aortic clamping, particularly above the
renal artery origins, will increase renal failure. This
can result from technical difficulties in bypass anastomoses, difficult renal endarterectomy particularly
using the lumenal approach and from previously
unrecognized renal accessory arteries arising from
the infrarenal aorta. These are technical problems
which in most cases can be avoided by careful preoperative assessment, imaging and planning of the
details of the reconstruction. If, for example, preoperative angiography indicates that renal ischemia
is likely to be longer than 40 minutes, surgical techniques such as presutured separate renal bypass
grafts on the main aortic graft, renal perfusion
either warm or cooled, extra-anatomical bypass, or
bench surgery can be planned and employed.

A rushed repair of a thoracoabdominal aneurysm,
particularly in type IV were renal perfusion is not
commonly used, can result in inadvertent compromise of the renal artery orifice by the suture line.
Similarly repair of a juxtarenal aneurysm without
careful identification of the renal osteal orifices can
result in suture compromise of the renal artery origin. Technical detail to the identification of the
renal and visceral artery origins, meticulous clearing of thrombus and atheroma as required will
reduce these complications. Inadvertent suturing or
ligation of the ureters is, of course, rare in the hands
of vascular surgeons but does occur and must be
avoided. Finally postoperative bleeding of significance can cause dramatically raised intra-abdominal
pressure. When this pressure becomes greater than
that in the inferior vena cava and renal vein, renal
engorgement and edema will result and eventually
give renal shutdown. Prompt relief of this situation
by laparotomy and evacuation of clot with hemostasis will guarantee avoidance of renal failure.

Renal failure following thoracoabdominal aneurysm repair

Renal failure in patients having thoracoabdominal aneurysm repair is reported in major series over
the last decade to occur on average in 18% (ranges
0%-40%), with an average of 8% (range 0%-27%)
requiring dialysis (Table III). All series report
significantly increased postoperative mortality in
patients requiring hemodialysis; reported mortality
rates in this group can be as high as 70% representing an up to ten fold increase in comparison
to those who do not require renal replacement
therapy.

Several independent predicting factors of renal
failure have been identified in the major series presented over this last decade. Consistently present is
preoperative renal dysfunction with increasing risk
present with serum creatinine levels greater than
1.5 - 2.0 mg/dl or 132 - 166 mm/l (Table IV) [24].
Other predictors include prolonged aortic clamp
times (greater than 100 minutes) and increased age.
Different series have identified further predictors
such as type I and II thoracoabdominal aneurysms,
male gender, the presence of renal occlusive disease, the need for visceral perfusion and left renal
artery reattachment. There is little concordance

Table III REVIEW OF LITERATURE ON RENAL FAILURE AFTER THORACOABDOMINAL PROCEDURES

1sr author [ref.]	Year	Number of cases	Renal failure (%)	Dialysis (%)
Schmidt [9]	1990	40	7 (17)	2 (5)
Fox [10]	1991	51	NR	2 (4)
Golden [11]	1991	57	23 (40)	NR
Cox [12]	1992	120	35 (29)	33 (27)
Hollier [13]	1992	150	14 (9)	6 (4)
Svensson [14]	1993	1 509	269 (18)	136 (9)
Schepens [15]	1994	85	NR	12 (14)
Coselli [16]	1994	372	54 (14.5)	NR
Acher [17]	1994	110	NR	3 (2.7)
Gilling-Smith [18]	1995	110	NR	20 (18)
Grabitz [19]	1996	260	NR	27 (10.4)
Kashyap [20]	1997	183	21 (11.5)	5 (2.7)
Jacobs [21]	1999	52	0	0
Cooley [22]	2000	132	9 (6.8)	9 (6.8)
Martin [23]	2000	165	55 (34)	23 (14)
			(76 TAA, type III & IV : rest suprarenal)	9 (12)

NR.: not recorded

Table IV ACUTE RENAL FAILURE AFTER THORACOABDOMINAL AORTIC ANEURYSM REPAIR: RESULTS OF UNIVARIATE ANALYSIS (SAFI ET AL. [24])

Preoperative creatinine *	Number of patients (%)	Number renal failures (%)
All patients	234 (100)	41 (17.5)
0.4 - 0.9	47 (20.1)	3 (6.4)
0.9 - 1.0	57 (24.4)	8 (14.1)
1.1 - 1.3	59 (25.2)	3 (5.1)
1.4 - 1.7	71 (30.3)	27 (38)

* Creatinine quoted in mg/dl
Multiply by 88 to convert to µmol/l

between the various series on these factors. However, there is unequivocal concordance on preoperative renal function as a predictor of renal failure, and the grave adverse significance of postoperative renal failure on both early and long-term survival (Fig. 1) [25].

Renal artery perfusion with cold physiological solutions or by warm perfusion using left heart bypass are techniques employed by several major centers in order to reduce the need for dialysis. In 1989 a retrospective study of 1 125 patients from Crawford's Group in Houston showed no significant reduction in need for dialysis using these methods [26]. However, later analysis by this same group showed significant reduction in acute renal failure with cold renal artery perfusion in patients with thoracoabdominal aneurysm who also had a occlusive visceral artery disease [25]. This group now recommends use of cold perfusion only when there is preoperative renal dysfunction, or renal artery occlusive disease or where clamp times greater than

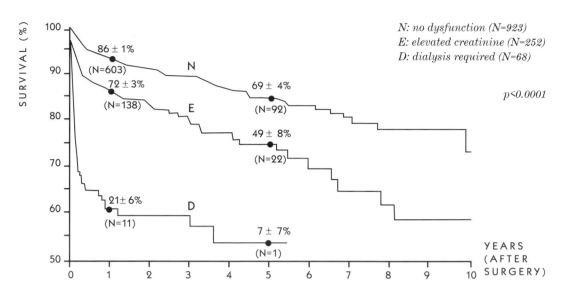

FIG. 1   Effect of postoperative renal dysfunction or dialysis on long-term survival after thoracoabdominal aneurysm repair (No dysfunction, elevated creatinine and dialysis compared) Svensson, 1992 [25].

45 minutes can be anticipated [14]. At the present time the use of renal perfusion either by atriofemoral bypass shunting or cold perfusion seems to be universally in use in the repair of type I, II and most of type III thoracoabdominal aneurysms. The present debate is whether visceral and renal perfusion by atriofemoral shunting is better than cold perfusion in reducing renal failure. Advocates of the single clamp and sew method using cold perfusion emphasize the expeditious nature of this method with clamp times less than 45 minutes. They report renal failure rates which are not significantly different from left heart bypass techniques [20,22].

Multiple logistic regression analysis by Safi et al. of a group of 234 patients showed visceral perfusion to be a predictor of renal failure, being a surprising finding [24]. This was not related to increased clamp times when compared to similar procedures without renal occlusive disease where distal aortic perfusion was used. The possible explanations include athero-embolic showering of the renal parenchyma, and the interesting possibility that non pulsatile renal perfusion (as used by Safi et al. causes increased production of angiotensin II in the kidney causing decreased blood flow) [27].

Jacobs recently reported a series of 52 type I and II thoracic abdominal aneurysm repairs using retrograde aortic perfusion via atriofemoral bypass and selective perfusion of celiac, superior mesenteric and renal arteries [21]. This group used motor-evoked potentials (MEP) to monitor spinal perfusion and in 27% of the patients systemic and distal aortic perfusion pressures were raised to maintain adequate MEP amplitudes. Furthermore, if renal output decreased during the procedure, renal artery catheter pressure was also increased. In common with other centers systemic hypothermia was also used. Despite median cross clamp times of 52 minutes for type I and 130 minutes for type II aortic aneurysms, there was no renal failure found (definition: creatinine increase of 100%, temporary dialysis or complete renal failure). This is the only series, albeit of moderate size, which has completely avoided renal dysfunction in the management of thoracoabdominal aneurysms. Such a logical approach to warm renal perfusion seems to be highly successful and the results of further experience from this group are awaited with interest.

Renal failure following abdominal aortic reconstruction

Many studies have identified age, preoperative pulmonary function and renal function as predictors of death from elective resection of infrarenal abdominal aortic aneurysms. Recently excellent data has been reported from the *UK Small Aneurysm Trial,* a prospective randomized controlled comparison of immediate surgery and surveillance for abdominal aneurysms between 4.0-5.5 centimeters [28]. Risk factor analysis of 13 preoperative variables using univariate associations and multiple logistic regression revealed age, pulmonary function (FEV1) and renal function as significant predictors of 30 day mortality [29]. An adjusted odds ratio for 30 day mortality of 1.41 (1.07-1.85: p< 0.01) per 40 mmol/l increase in creatinine was found giving a virtually linear relationship between death and renal dysfunction (Fig. 2). Observed 30 day death rate varied from 0.9% in younger patients with good lung and renal function to 9.8% in older patients with worse lung and renal function (Table V) [29]. Further clinical testing of the use of a prognostic index based on age, pulmonary and renal function, particularly in larger aneurysms is needed. This well controlled study, however, provides hard data confirming the importance of preoperative renal function on hospital morbidity. Optimization of renal function, including attention to severe renal artery stenosis must be part of the preoperative workup of patients undergoing abdominal aortic aneurysm surgery.

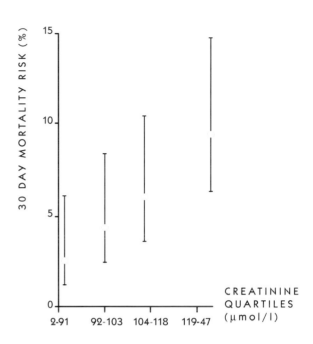

FIG. 2 Relationship between renal dysfunction and mortality in treatment of abdominal aortic aneurysms [29].

Table V	*UK SMALL ANEURYSM STUDY:* OBSERVED RISK OF DEATH WITHIN 30 DAYS BY AGE, RESPIRATORY FUNCTION AND CREATININE LEVEL [29]			
Age	*FEV1*	*Creatinine* μmol/liter	*Observed death*	*Observed risk* %
60 - 69 years	2.2 - 4.4	2 - 103	1/116	0.9
		104 - 473	5/100	5
	0.3 - 2.1	2 - 103	2/89	2
		104 - 473	4/66	6
70 - 80 years	2.2 - 4.4	2 - 103	3/76	4
		104 - 473	10/112	8.9
	0.3 - 2.1	2 - 103	6/114	5.3
		104 - 473	10/102	9.8

Supraceliac or suprarenal clamping?

Patients most at risk of postoperative renal failure are those with disease involving the juxtarenal and suprarenal aorta. In addition to aneurysm, this can be in occlusive disease, inflammatory aneurysms or repeat aortic reconstructions. The problems of athero-embolism and occlusion of the renal artery origins by clamping in this area have been discussed previously. In these situations the clamp can be placed either suprarenally or at the supraceliac level. Suprarenal clamping appears to be safe but only where the juxtarenal aorta is not diseased, where there is no occlusive renal or superior mesenteric artery disease, and where there is 2 centimeters of clear aorta between the superior mesenteric artery and the renal artery origin. In a large series from Brescia, Italy, the use of suprarenal clamping was associated with increased renal dysfunction compared to infrarenal clamping (14% versus 0%) with one patient (2%) requiring permanent dialysis [30]. Ischemic colitis was also found to be significantly increased. Division of the left renal vein is often used in this situation but in most cases this can be avoided. The vein can be easily mobilized and slung, but if divided should be reconstructed to avoid compromise to venous drainage and renal function of the left kidney [31].

Because of the reported complications from suprarenal clamping many authors recommend supraceliac clamping in dealing with juxtarenal surgery. The main complication of supraceliac clamping is renal dysfunction associated mainly with preoperative renal function and prolonged clamp times. The incidence of renal dysfunction is reported to occur between 23-31% being transient in the majority of patients [8,32,33]. An important observation was that suprarenal clamp times less than 30 minutes was not associated with postoperative renal failure of any significance [8].

In the modern vascular era reconstructive surgery for occlusive aortic disease is becoming rare; most surgery in this area is for infrarenal abdominal aortic aneurysm although this also is being encroached upon by the increasing use of endovascular stent repair. Recent analyses of large populations undergoing elective aortic abdominal aneurysm repair confirmed increased mortality rates for patients with preoperative renal failure (11.8% versus 3.4%) [34]. In the State of Maryland, despite advances in peri-operative management and anesthesia comparison of outcome across the last two decades did not show any improvement in mortality rates for either elective or ruptured abdominal aortic aneurysms. Renal failure remained a consistent complication and predictor of death [35]. Valuable data from a prospective study of 470 patients undergoing abdominal aortic aneurysm repair has recently been reported from Paris [36]. Overall mortality in this group was 5.3% but moderate or severe renal dysfunction was shown to be a significant preoperative risk factor increasing death rates to 40% (Table VI). Postoperative renal failure was second only to myocardial ischemia forming 11% of overall postoperative medical complications, with univariate and multivariate analysis confirming renal dysfunction as independent predictors of death.

Mortality in postoperative patients requiring renal replacement therapy is high, with rates of 58-86% reported after ruptured abdominal aortic aneurysm surgery and up to 65% for elective aortic aneurysm surgery. The question of whether renal replacement therapy should be given in such a poor risk group is one that vascular surgeons and intensivists regularly debate. A study from Utrecht shed some light on this difficult problem [37]. Mortality rates in this group were high being 69% overall, 71% for ruptures and 66% for elective, with the ability to wean from ventilator and inotropic support being a positive factor in the management of these patients. Their recommendation is that renal replacement therapy is justified, but subject to daily review and early discontinuation where it becomes clear that multiple organ failure is persisting.

The Leicester Group has prepared a clinical severity score to allow identification of patients requiring renal replacement therapy after ruptured abdominal aortic aneurysm repair. Their score is proposed to identify patients in whom there is a low prospect of survival to facilitate the making of difficult decisions regarding discontinuation of renal replacement therapy and active intensive care [38]. The Leicester scoring system may have the limitations of all similar other systems but certainly warrants further clinical assessment by prospective study.

Renal failure in aortic occlusive disease

Because of the success of iliac angioplasty and stenting, aortic surgery for occlusive disease is much less commonly performed. It is associated with similar incidence of postoperative renal failure as intervention for aneurysmal disease. A particular exception is the management of infrarenal aortic occlusion in at risk patients by the use of extra-anatomical bypasses such as axillofemoral grafting. Thrombus propagation above the renal arteries has been reported by many authors, usually accompanied by superior mesenteric artery occlusion and death from renal failure and mesenteric ischemia. There is controversy about the true frequency of this complication, however, with several other studies reporting no significant increase of thrombus propagation and renal failure [39]. Recent experience of this condition reported from North Carolina reports no incidence of postoperative renal failure using extra-anatomical bypass except in the presence of renal artery stenosis. Their conclusion is that the combination of aortic occlusion and renal artery disease is particularly ominous, and advise that extra-anatomical bypasses are inferior to aortic reconstruction and renal revascularization in this setting.

Renal artery disease and post-reconstruction renal failure

If renovascular disease is high grade causing progressive renal failure, difficult to control hyperten-

| Table VI | PREOPERATIVE RISK FACTORS IN PROSPECTIVE STUDY OF ABDOMINAL AORTIC ANEURYSM REPAIR [36] |

Risk factors	Number of patients (%)		Alive (%)		Deceased (%)	
Population, N = 470						
Severe renal dysfunction	15	(3)	9	(60)	6	(40)
Normal/mild renal dysfunction	455	(97)	436	(96)	19	(4)
Age > 70 years	196	(42)	175	(89)	21	(11)
Age < 70 years	274	(58)	270	(98.5)	4	(1.5)
Previous myocardial infarction	129	(27)	116	(90)	13	(10)
No previous myocardial infarction	341	(63)	329	(96.5)	12	(3.5)
Left ventricular dysfunction	166	(35)	156	(94)	10	(6)
Normal left ventricular function	304	(65)	289	(95)	15	(5)
Coronary artery disease	128	(27)	117	(91.5)	11	(8.5)
No or minor coronary artery disease	342	(63)	327	(95.5)	14	(4.5)
Pulmonary disease	50	(10.6)	43	(90)	5	(10)
No pulmonary disease	420	(89.4)	402	(95)	20	(5)
Obesity	52	(11)	51	(98)	1	(2)
Normal weight	418	(89)	394	(94)	24	(6)
Arrhythmia	31	(6.5)	30	(97)	1	(3)
Normal rhythm	439	(93.35)	414	(94)	25	(6)
Femoral occlusive disease	89	(19)	83	(93)	6	(7)
No femoral occlusive disease	381	(81)	362	(95)	19	(5)

sion or flash pulmonary edema, there is little doubt regarding the need for renal revascularization. Increasingly this is by stent angioplasty and this will not be discussed further. A minority of cases will be unsuitable for endovascular treatment and will come to surgical renal revascularization – this will also not be discussed further. The major difficulty in this area is how to treat asymptomatic but hemodynamically significant renal artery stenosis in patients undergoing aortic reconstruction for aneurysm or occlusive disease. This is because of the recognized natural history of severe renal artery stenosis with its propensity to progression to occlusion. There is evidence from several series that combining aortic and renal reconstruction increases peri-operative mortality up to 31%. Others have argued that in patients with few risk factors, combined revascularization does not increase mortality. Porter's group in Portland, Oregon recently reported a retrospective study of 171 patients undergoing aortic reconstruction in whom 32 patients had significant renal artery stenosis (greater than 70%) found on the preoperative angiogram. A deliberate policy of not revascularizing the renal arteries was employed. They found that the 32 patients with severe renal artery stenosis had no increase in mortality at up to seven years follow-up. They did have higher systolic blood pressure, increased need for antihypertensive medications but no significant increase in serum creatinine [40]. Based on the benign behaviour of the renal artery stenoses in this cohort of patients, their recommendation was that renal revascularization is not indicated. This would seem to be sensible advice but prospective assessment is important before implementation of this policy can be recommended. At the present time each case must be considered on its individual merits and in a patient who has low risk factors with severe renal artery stenosis a policy of combined revascularization should be considered.

Renal failure after peripheral vascular surgery

Preoperative renal function is the most important factor in development of renal failure as a complication. Patients with significant risk factors and preexistent renal dysfunction need careful peri-operative management with hydration, avoidance of nephrotoxicity and of hypovolemia. Lower

limb vascular reconstructions, carotid endarterectomy and other procedures of similar magnitude should have a low risk of postoperative renal complications. However, patients with established severe renal dysfunction and in particular those on dialysis, carry much higher risk of complications of all kinds, in addition to a very reduced lifespan (25% survival at two years after starting dialysis). Selection is of prime importance in this group of patients. Results of femorodistal bypass grafting are poor, and primary amputation is often the safer option. Similarly, carotid endarterectomy should be undertaken only where survival is likely to be longer than one to two years.

Summary

The incidence of renal failure after vascular reconstruction is well documented and strategies to minimize its development are identified. The literature continues to document, however, that this complication is still too common and lethal. Across the board, vascular surgeons could do better by applying the lessons learned by analysis of the clinical evidence in selection and management. Developments focused on strategies to limit the cascade of cellular events resulting from renal ischemia such as the use of endothelin antagonists, exogenous restoration of ATP, and further development of intra-operative renal protection such as improved perfusion protocols, are expected. Meanwhile, large clinical studies of the current methodologies are urgently needed.

REFERENCES

1 Chertow GM, Lazarus JM, Christiansen CL et al. Preoperative renal risk stratification. *Circulation* 1997; 95: 878-884.
2 Chertow GM, Levy EM, Hammermeister KE et al. Independent association between acute renal failure and mortality following cardiac surgery. *Am J Med* 1998; 104: 343-348.
3 Brezis M, Rosen S. Hypoxia of the renal medulla - its implications for disease. *N Engl J Med* 1995; 332: 647-655.
4 Lieberthal W, Koh JS, Levine JS. Necrosis and apoptosis in acute renal failure. *Semin Nephrol* 1998; 18: 505-518.
5 Chonger J. Haemodynamic factors in acute renal failure. *Adv Renal Replace Ther* 1997; 4: 25-37.
6 Solomon R. Radio contrast-induced nephropathy. *Semin Nephrol* 1998; 18: 551-557.
7 Gelman S. The pathophysiology of aortic cross-clamping and unclamping. *Anesthesiology* 1995; 82: 1026-1060.
8 Nypaver TJ, Shepard AD, Reddy DJ et al. Supraceliac aortic cross-clamping: determinants of outcome in elective abdominal aortic reconstruction. *J Vasc Surg* 1993: 17; 868-876.

9 Schmidt CA, Wood MN, Gan KA, Razzouk AJ. Surgery for thoracoabdominal aortic aneurysms. Am Surg 1990; 56: 745-748.

10 Fox AD, Berkowitz HD. Thoracoabdominal aneurysm resection after previous infrarenal abdominal aortic aneurysmectomy. Am J Surg 1991; 162: 142-144.

11 Golden MA, Donaldson MC, Whittemore AD, Mannick JA. Evolving experience with thoracoabdominal aortic aneurysm repair at a single institution. J Vasc Surg 1991; 13: 792-797.

12 Cox GS, O'Hara PJ, Hertzer NR et al. Thoracoabdominal aneurysm repair: a representative experience. J Vasc Surg 1992; 15: 780-788.

13 Hollier LH, Money SR, Naslund TC et al. Risk of spinal cord dysfunction in patients undergoing thoracoabdominal aortic replacement. Am J Surg 1992; 164: 210-214.

14 Svensson LG, Crawford ES, Hess KR et al. Experience with 1509 patients undergoing thoracoabdominal aortic operations. J Vasc Surg 1993; 17: 357-370.

15 Schepens MA, Defauw JJ, Hamerlijnck RP et al. Surgical treatment of thoracoabdominal aortic aneurysms by simple crossclamping. Risk factors and late results. J Thorac Cardiovasc Surg 1994; 107: 134-142.

16 Coselli JS. Thoracoabdominal aortic aneurysms: experience with 372 patients. J Card Surg 1994; 9: 638-647.

17 Acher CW, Wynn MM, Hoch JR et al. Combined use of cerebral spinal fluid drainage and naloxone reduces the risk of paraplegia in thoracoabdominal aneurysm repair. J Vasc Surg 1994; 19: 236-248.

18 Gilling-Smith GL, Worswick L, Knight PF et al. Surgical repair of thoracoabdominal aortic aneurysm: 10 years' experience. Br J Surg 1995; 82: 624-629.

19 Grabitz K, Sandmann W, Stuhmeier K et al. The risk of ischemic spinal cord injury in patients undergoing graft replacement for thoracoabdominal aortic aneurysms. J Vasc Surg 1996; 23: 230-240.

20 Kashyap VS, Cambria RP, Davison JK, L'Italien GJ. Renal failure after thoracoabdominal aortic surgery. J Vasc Surg 1997; 26: 949-957.

21 Jacobs MJHM, Meylaerts SA, de Haan P et al. Strategies to prevent neurologic deficit based on motor-evoked potentials in type I and II thoracoabdominal aortic aneurysm repair. J Vasc Surg 1999; 29: 48-59.

22 Cooley DA, Golino A, Frazier OH. Single-clamp technique for aneurysms of the descending thoracic aorta: report of 132 consecutive cases. Eur J Cardiothorac Surg 2000; 18: 162-167.

23 Martin GH, O'Hara PJ, Hertzer NR et al. Surgical repair of aneurysms involving the suprarenal, visceral, and lower thoracic aortic segments: early results and late outcome. J Vasc Surg 2000; 31: 851-862.

24 Safi HJ, Harlin SA, Miller CC et al. Predictive factors for acute renal failure in thoracic and thoracoabdominal aortic aneurysm surgery. J Vasc Surg 1996; 24: 338-345.

25 Svensson LG, Crawford ES, Hess KR et al. Thoracoabdominal aortic aneurysms associated with celiac, superior mesenteric, and renal artery occlusive disease: methods and analysis of results in 271 patients. J Vasc Surg 1992: 16; 378-390.

26 Svensson LG, Coselli JS, Safi HJ et al. Appraisal of adjuncts to prevent acute renal failure after surgery on the thoracic or thoracoabdominal aorta. J Vasc Surg 1989; 10: 230-239.

27 Watkins L, Lucas SK, Gardner TJ et al. Angiotensin II levels during cardiopulmonary bypass: a comparison of pulsatile and nonpulsatile flow. Surg Forum 1979; 30: 229-230.

28 The UK Small Aneurysm Trial Participants. Mortality results for randomised controlled trial of early elective surgery or ultrasonographic surveillance for small abdominal aortic aneurysms. Lancet 1998; 352: 1649-1655.

29 Brady AR, Fowkes FG, Greenhalgh RM et al. On behalf of the UK Small Aneurysm Trial participants. Risk factors for postoperative death following elective surgical repair of abdominal aortic aneurysm: results from the UK Small Aneurysm Trial. Br J Surg 2000; 87: 742-749.

30 Giulini SM, Bonardelli S, Portolani N et al. Suprarenal aortic cross clamping in elective abdominal aortic aneurysm surgery. Eur J Vasc Endovasc Surg 2000; 20: 286-289.

31 AbuRahma AF, Robinson PA, Boland JP, Lucente FC. The risk of ligation of the left renal vein in resection of the abdominal aortic aneurysm. Surg Gynecol Obstet 1991; 173: 33-36.

32 Qvarfordt PG, Stoney RJ, Reilly LM et al. Management of pararenal aneurysms of the abdominal aorta. J Vasc Surg 1986; 3: 84-93.

33 Breckwoldt WL, Mackey WC, Belkin M, O'Donnell TF. The effect of suprarenal crossclamping on abdominal aortic aneurysm repair. Arch Surg 1992; 127: 520-524.

34 Dardik A, Lin JW, Gordon TA et al. Results of elective abdominal aortic aneurysm repair in the 1990s: a population-based analysis of 2335 cases. J Vasc Surg 1999; 30: 985-995.

35 Heller JA, Weinberg A, Arons R et al. Two decades of abdominal aortic aneurysm repair: have we made any progress? J Vasc Surg 2000; 32: 1091-1101.

36 Becquemin JP, Chemla E, Chatellier G et al. Peroperative factors influencing the outcome of elective abdominal aorta aneurysm repair. Eur J Vasc Endovasc Surg 2000; 20: 84-89.

37 Braams R, Vossen V, Lisman BA, Eikelboom BC. Outcome in patients requiring renal replacement therapy after surgery for ruptured and non-ruptured aneurysm of the abdominal aorta. Eur J Vasc Endovasc Surg 1999; 18: 323-327.

38 Barratt J, Parajasingam R, Sayers RD, Feehally J. Outcome of acute renal failure following surgical repair of ruptured abdominal aortic aneurysms. Eur J Vasc Endovasc Surg 2000; 20: 163-168.

39 Ligush J, Criado E, Burnham SJ et al. Management and outcome of chronic atherosclerotic infrarenal aortic occlusion. J Vasc Surg 1996; 24: 394-405.

40 Williamson WK, Abou-Zamzam AM, Moneta GL et al. Prophylactic repair of renal artery stenosis is not justified in patients who require infrarenal aortic reconstruction. J Vasc Surg 1998; 28: 14-22.

11
105

12

VASCULAR COMPLICATIONS
AFTER KIDNEY TRANSPLANTATION

ALBERT CLARÁ, MANUEL MIRALLES
AUGUST YSA, JOSE ANTONIO BALLESTEROS, MARIA LUISA MIR
FRANCESC VIDAL-BARRAQUER

Since the first successful kidney transplant in 1954, renal transplantation has become one of the cornerstones in the management of patients with end-stage renal disease. For the majority of patients with end-stage renal disease, transplantation results in superior survival, improved quality of life and lower costs compared with chronic dialysis. However, medical problems related to infections and graft dysfunction secondary to rejection or drug toxicity together with vascular or urologic complications following transplantation may affect graft survival and patient well-being. Vascular complications can involve the donor vessels (renal artery thrombosis, renal vein thrombosis, transplant renal artery stenosis), the recipient vessels (iliac artery occlusive disease, pseudoaneurysms and true aneurysms, deep venous thrombosis), or both. Among them, transplant renal artery stenosis (TRAS) is by far the most frequent vascular complication following transplantation. This chapter will present the reader with a general review of this issue. In addition, we will analyze the decision-making and the results of TRAS management at our institution. Finally, a brief discussion at the light of the present knowledge and our experience will allow us to delineate our present opinion on the management of TRAS.

Transplant renal artery stenosis

TRAS is an increasingly recognized complication after kidney transplantation. TRAS occurs in approximately 5%-10% of patients and ranges from 0.6% to 16% depending on the definition of stenosis [1-5]. When angiography has been systematically performed, the incidence increases to 23% [6]. Recognition of this process is important because it represents a potentially reversible cause of hypertension (HT) and allograft loss.

CLINICAL FEATURES

HT is a common complication after renal transplantation which affects 60%-80% of recipients of a kidney graft [7-9], and is associated with low graft survival and accelerated atherosclerosis [8-10]. It is not possible to identify a single etiologic factor for post-transplant HT. The most important contributing factors are impaired renal function, cadaver donor, retained native kidneys and cyclosporine administration. The most common single cause of post-transplant HT is impaired renal function associated with chronic allograft dysfunction. The importance of other factors that promote the development of hypertension varies at different times after transplantation. Recent-onset or refractory HT with or without allograft dysfunction, which becomes apparent between 3 months and 2 years

after transplantation, is the most common presentation of TRAS [2,6,11].

There are four main locations of TRAS (Figs. 1-4). In relation to the arterial anastomotic site the stenosis can be proximal due to recipient atherosclerotic arterial disease, anastomotic, at the main renal artery or distal in the branches [6]. Anastomotic stenosis is generally regarded as secondary to faulty surgical technique and/or postoperative fibrosis [4,12]. The etiology of stenosis at the main renal trunk is less clear but it may be related to mechanical or inmunological damage [4]. Finally, chronic vascular rejection is associated with multiple stenoses in the distal branches.

Several mechanisms have been proposed to explain the development of TRAS: arterial and inmunologic causes. Arterial causes include atheroma in the donor artery and incorrect handling of the graft during preservation and implantation. Examples of such improper handling are: faulty

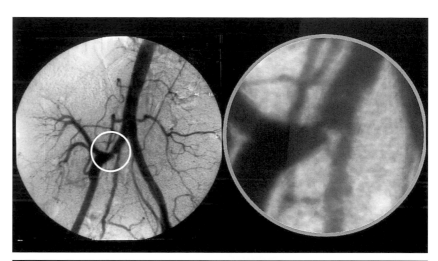

FIG. 1 Pre-anastomotic transplant renal artery stenosis.

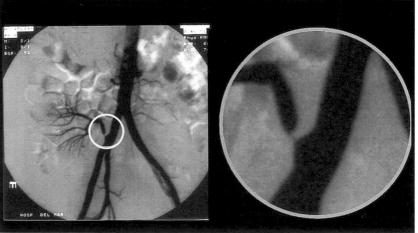

FIG. 2 Para-anastomotic transplant renal artery stenosis.

suture technique, damage to the donor arterial intima by inaccurate cannulation for perfusion, improper apposition of the donor and recipient vessels causing an overacute angle of take-off or a redundant length of renal artery which may cause torsion and angulation. Right kidney allografts have a long renal artery and a short renal vein and make the procedure more complex resulting in an increased incidence of TRAS [13]. End-to-end anastomosis has been associated with TRAS at the suture line by some authors [4,14], but not all [3,15-17]. However, this is particularly true when endarterectomy is required to render a suitable hypogastric artery [18]. Hemodynamic mechanisms may account for some arterial-cause TRAS. The incidence of renal artery stenosis following transplantation of pediatric cadaveric donor kidneys as a single unit is high [17-19]. This finding may be a consequence of increased blood flow and turbulence across the small donor renal artery, faulty suture technique, or mechanical damage to the donor renal artery during procurement and preservation.

Support for an immunological cause of TRAS has come from both experimental and human studies, although some of these data seems equivocal. In humans, histological changes of stenosed arteries may share striking similarities with vascular lesions of renal allograft rejection [6]. In patients with TRAS, a significantly higher incidence of rejection has been found as compared with the control group [20]. TRAS has been found to be equally distributed between living-related and cadaver kidney recipients by many authors [3-21] but not all [13]. Moreover, a similar TRAS incidence in HLA-identical living-related donor grafts has also been referred [15], arguing against immunologic factors as a major etiologic determinant.

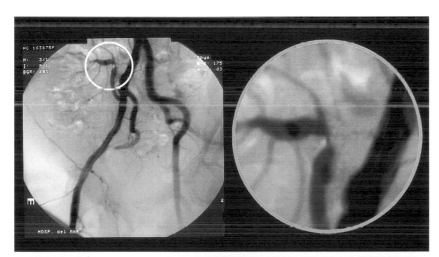

FIG. 3 Stenosis at mid-transplant renal artery.

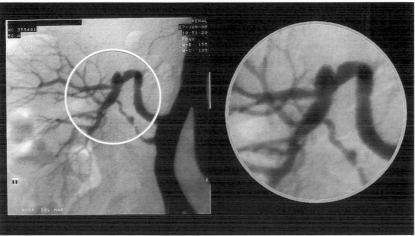

FIG. 4 Stenosis at branches of transplant renal artery.

DIAGNOSIS

A variety of screening tests to detect TRAS have been proposed. These include the measurement of plasma renin activity. Results of measurements of peripheral renin plasma levels in patients with TRAS before and after captopril administration have been variable, and the specificity is low [22]. Isotopic renography performed before and after a dose of captopril has a reported sensitivity of 75% but a specificity of 67% [23], although it may be highly predictive of physiologically significant renal artery stenosis [24]. Duplex is highly sensitive in detecting TRAS but its 75% specificity requires angiographic confirmation [23]. Magnetic resonance angiography may be used to diagnose TRAS, although its reliability is limited to the first 3 cm of the renal artery [24]. Spiral computed tomography may be used to diagnose TRAS with excellent correlation to conventional angiography, avoiding arterial puncture [25,26]. Finally, angiography remains the gold standard for TRAS diagnosis. The catheter may be introduced through the opposite femoral artery to avoid any incidental procedural complication (dissection, hematoma) that could compromise the donor iliac axis. Multiple views have to be performed to properly visualize the renal artery, especially its take-off from the iliac artery. A renal allograft biopsy is sometimes performed before angiography to rule out chronic rejection or other forms of renal parenchymal disease. These findings decrease the likelihood of a successful response to correction of a stenosis and therefore are relative contraindications to intervention [27].

MEDICAL TREATMENT

Although spontaneous regression of TRAS has been described [13,28,29], revascularization seems to be the desirable management option, as hemodynamically significant stenosis is likely to produce poorly controlled hypertension, impairment of renal function and has a tendency to progress towards graft loss. However, some patients may have a TRAS while the HT or renal dysfunction, which was the reason for angiography, may have been caused by the presence of host kidneys or the consequence of damage to the allograft following rejection episodes. Correction of the stenosis in these patients probably would not have improved the hypertension but only have exposed them to the risks of intervention. Merkus et al. reported 24 patients with moderate or significant stenoses, unsuitable for correction, in whom antihypertensive

drug treatment was extended resulting in only one graft loss due to vascular complication at a mean follow-up of 116 months [21].

Similarly, Deglise-Favre et al. reported the outcome of 40 patients with TRAS submitted to medical treatment. At a mean follow-up of 57 months only one graft was lost due to renal artery thrombosis. Actuarial graft survival rate did not significantly differ from that of the angioplasty or surgery group [30]. Therefore patients with a mild to moderate TRAS can be managed with antihypertensive drugs without an increased rate of graft failure or impairment of the long-term renal function. Other indications for medical management include:
1 - poor risk patients,
2 - patients with complications related to immunosuppressive therapy, i.e. malignancy, hepatic dysfunction or sepsis,
3 - patients suffering from diffuse intraparenchymal stenoses which are inaccessible for revascularization procedures.

PERCUTANEOUS TRANSLUMINAL RENAL ANGIOPLASTY

Percutaneous transluminal balloon renal angioplasty (PTRA) is the preferred initial mode of therapy in many institutions [3,5,31,32]. Performance of PTRA for TRAS is based on the techniques described by Gruntzig [33]. The site of the femoral puncture may be chosen according to the type of renal graft artery anastomosis, the angulation of the renal artery and the distance from the femoral artery to the anastomosis. A selective catheter is inserted percutaneously through the appropriate femoral artery and its tip directed toward the lumen of the renal artery. A guidewire (usually 0.035 inch) is then advanced through the catheter and the stenosis. Predilatation systolic pressure gradient may be measured by passing a catheter across the stenosis to measure pressures on both sides of the stenosis. The selective catheter is then exchanged for a short tip balloon catheter. The balloon is inflated with a pressure gauge syringe full of contrast media until the *waist* in the balloon disappears at the lowest pressure possible. The balloon is kept inflated for 15-30 seconds. Repeated inflation may be necessary to achieve satisfactory anatomical results and correction of pressure gradient.

The reported initial technical success rate is above 85%. Recurrent stenosis occurs in 10% to 33% of cases [2,5,13,31,34-38], and 4% to 18% of patients need secondary surgical intervention after failure of

PTA, sometimes for graft salvage. Graft loss as a result of PTA ranges between 0% and 18%. Mortality, usually attributed to other causes, has also been reported [3]. Varying success rates of PTRA may reflect not only technical problems and experience but also differences in the location or type of the stenosis. As usual, the best TRAS candidates for PTRA are short lesions located distal to the anastomosis [13]. Stenosis at the anastomosis line may be better treated surgically, as results of angioplasty are poor and major complications can be frequent [2,18]. PTRA should also be avoided in those patients with arterial kinking, as this has been associated with a 60% failure rate [13,31]. Recurrent TRAS may be amenable to redo-PTRA. In such circumstances, or even in ex-novo treatment of severe anastomotic stenosis, endoluminal stent placement appears to be a promising option [39,40].

SURGICAL REVASCULARIZATION

Surgical revascularization of TRAS may be favored in:
1 - anastomotic stenosis,
2 - stenosis due to twisting or kinking of the transplant artery,
3 - failures of attempted PTRA and
4 - complications of PTRA which might lead to impaired blood flow to the renal graft. Surgical revascularization is not indicated in cases of chronic rejection (histologically confirmed) [42] or when stenoses are diffuse or extended into intrarenal arteries [36].

Surgical approach to the arteries is usually retroperitoneal, although incidental opening of the peritoneum may help to identify the location of the renal vascular pedicle. The lower pole of the kidney and the external iliac artery are dissected. The dissection is followed over the iliac artery until the anastomosis is identified. From this point, the renal artery is identified and isolated at a segment distal to the stenosis. The isolation of the renal artery may be difficult because of the dense scar formation surrounding the allograft and the likelihood of ureteral and renal vein adherence to the renal artery, although through retroperitoneal approach the renal vein is usually avoided. Surgical revascularization techniques should pursue a limited dissection as a goal.

A variety of surgical techniques for correcting TRAS have been proposed. Renal ischemia should be as short as possible. Preservation solution is usually not required. Resection of the stenotic segment and direct arterial reanastomosis may be an appropriate procedure for short-segment stenosis, such as those which may occur in the anastomotic line of end-renal artery to end-hypogastric artery anastomosis. Transection of the transplant artery distal to the anastomosis and end-to-side reimplantation may be recommended for anastomotic stenosis of end-renal artery to side-iliac artery anastomosis type. Saphenous patch angioplasty is a popular repair procedure for stenosis located at any site along the transplant artery or when the stenosis extends to the bifurcation of the main artery (Fig. 5). Finally, a bypass or an interposition graft enable to bridge any type of stenosis when previous procedures have not been considered (Fig. 6). Proximal anastomosis is firstly done end-to-side to the appropriate iliac artery, usually distal to the allograft, to minimize the renal ischemic time. Renal anastomosis can be performed without distal clamping or just with the aid of an occlusion balloon to minimize dissection. The bypass option has the potential advantages of a

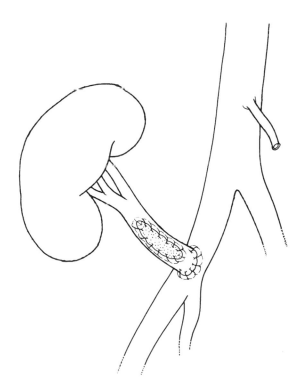

FIG. 5 Patch angioplasty for transplant renal artery stenosis reconstruction.

probably lesser dissection and the maintenance of the original stenosed renal artery that may allow to salvage the kidney in case of bypass thrombosis. Synthetic grafts, for patch or bypass, have been seldom reported.

Immediate technical success rate ranges between 50% and 90% [13,18,42-46]. The reported improvement of renal graft function is between 38.8% and 44.4% and the improvement in hypertension is between 44.4% and 100%. Re-stenoses, graft losses and mortality range from 9.3% to 12%, from 2.4% to 20%, and from 1.6% to 5.5%, respectively.

Other post-transplant vascular complications

Renal artery thrombosis usually occurs early post-transplant, often resulting in graft loss. Most commonly, it occurs as a result of a technical problem such as intimal dissection, kinking or torsion of the vessels. Other causes include hyperacute rejection, unresponsive acute rejection or hypercoagulable states. An acute cessation of urine output is the common presentation. Urgent thrombectomy may be indicated but the majority of grafts are non-salvageable and removal is required.

Renal vein thrombosis is not as common as its arterial counterpart, but again graft loss is the usual end result. Causes include angulation or kinking of the vein, compression by hematoma or lymphocele, anastomotic stenosis or an extension of an underlying deep venous thrombosis. Emergency thrombectomy is rarely successful and nephrectomy is usually required. Lytic therapy for renal allograft vein thrombosis may be efficacious in cases where it results from accompanying deep venous thrombosis [47].

Lymphoceles, from transected lymphatics in the recipient, occur in 0.6% to 18% of patients [48]. These usually do not present until at least 2 weeks post-transplant. Symptoms are generally related to the mass effect and compression of nearby structures. Ultrasound will confirm a fluid collection, though percutaneous aspiration may be necessary to rule out other collections such as urinoma, hematoma or abscess. The standard surgical treatment is creation of a peritoneal window to allow for drainage of the lymphatic fluid into the peritoneal cavity, where it can be absorbed. This can be accomplished by either a laparoscopic or an open

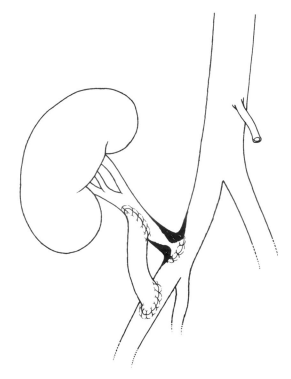

FIG. 6   PTFE bypass graft for transplant renal artery stenosis reconstruction.

approach. Percutaneous insertion of a drainage catheter, with or without sclerotherapy is another option; however, it is associated with a high rate of recurrence and risk of infection [49].

True aneurysm in the transplant renal artery or pseudoaneurysm arising from the arterial anastomosis between the iliac artery and the transplant renal artery are one of the least common vascular complications after kidney transplantation (Fig. 7). Surgical management is mandatory to avoid a catastrophic outcome. Its low incidence, the different patterns of presentation and a redo-surgical field make pseudoaneurysm surgical correction a great challenge to the vascular surgeon in order to preserve allograft function. Technical options may include excision with extracorporeal vascular repair and delayed allograft autotransplantation, or excision with graft interposition.

Personal experience with the management of transplant renal artery stenosis

PATIENTS AND METHODS

Patients undergoing renal transplantation between years 1979 and 2000 in whom postoperative renal artery stenosis developed were identified from a computerized transplant registry. The medical records of these patients were then individually reviewed. Recorded variables included age, sex, cause of native kidney failure, source of the kidney (living related or cadaveric), preservation time, configuration of the arterial anastomosis, rejection episodes, cause of TRAS suspicion, time to diagnosis of TRAS, and blood pressure, number of antihypertensive drugs and creatinine plasma levels at the time of TRAS diagnosis.

Angiography was performed in all cases including lateral and antero-posterior views. Stenosis was categorized according to the reduction of the arterial lumen smaller than 60% and equal or greater than 60%, and to its anatomic location in preanastomotic (recipient iliac artery), para-anastomotic (at anastomotic line or close to it), at mid transplant main renal artery or at its branches. Patients were assigned to follow intensive medical treatment, standard percutaneous transluminal angioplasty (PTA) without stent, or surgical revascularization according to the stenosis location, the degree of stenosis and the impairment of blood pressure and/or renal function once other causes of allograft dysfunction were ruled out. The method of treatment was chosen after discussion among the transplant nephrologist, the urologist and the vascular surgeon. Surgical revascularization procedures were performed by a combined team of an urologist and a vascular surgeon. PTA procedures were performed either by radiologists in another institution or by vascular surgeons at our own institution.

The effect of the selected method of treatment in blood pressure was evaluated at 1 month, 1 year, 2 years and 5 years. For patients with well-controlled diastolic pressure (more than 90 mmHg) at TRAS decision-making, hypertension was considered improved if blood pressure remained controlled and there was a decrease in the number of medications, equal if blood pressure remained controlled with the same number of medications, and deteriorated if diastolic pressure became poorly-controlled (greater than 90 mmHg) and/or there was an increase in number of medications. For patients with poorly-controlled diastolic pressure at TRAS decision-making, hypertension was considered improved if it became well-controlled with the same or less number of medications, equal if there were no change in blood pressure and in the number of medications or when it became well-controlled with an increase of number of medications, and deteriorated if diastolic pressure remained poorly-controlled with an increase in the number of medications. The effect of treatment option on renal function and need of dialysis were evaluated by life-table analyses. Renal function was considered to be worse when plasma creatinine levels increased by more than 20% than the pre-intervention creatinine and remained at these levels for at least six months. Otherwise, renal function was considered stable or improved.

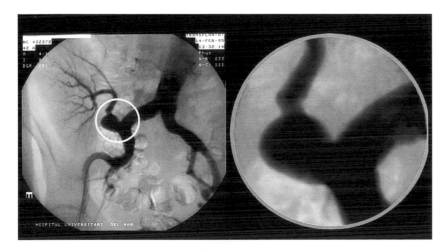

FIG. 7 Transplant renal artery aneurysm.

RESULTS

Between 1979 and 2000, 464 kidney transplants were performed and 30 patients with TRAS were identified. The incidence of TRAS in our recipient population was 6.5% (30 of 464). One case was excluded from the study group because of missing documents in the patient chart that prevented knowledge of complete basal data and response of hypertension and renal function to an iliocorenal bypass performed for TRAS diagnosed 8 months after transplantation. The patient evolution was satisfactory although she entered dialysis 10 years after the surgical procedure due to chronic rejection.

The study group included 23 men and 6 women, aged 24- to 63-years-old (mean age 44.2, standard deviation 11.4). The cause of end-stage renal disease was diabetes mellitus in 6 patients, nephrosclerosis in 6, polycystic kidney disease in 4, glomerulonephritis in 4, interstitial nephropathy in 3, pyelonephritis in 3, and unknown in 3 patients. There were 3 live and 26 cadaver donor kidney transplantations. Mean cold ischemia time for cadaver transplantations was 23.5 hours. The renal artery was anastomosed end-to-end to the recipient hypogastric artery in 5 patients, end-to-side to the recipient external iliac artery in 6 patients and end-to-side to the recipient common iliac artery in 18 patients. Following transplantation 13 patients suffered acute rejection episodes.

TRAS was diagnosed by angiography after clinical suspicion in 25 patients: isolated bruit over the allograft in 2 patients, poor-controlled hypertension in 16 patients, deteriorating kidney function in 3 cases, and the combination of the last two causes in 4 patients. The remaining 4 patients with TRAS were diagnosed by screening methods, angiography or duplex scan. Median time to diagnosis of TRAS since transplantation was 6 months (Fig. 8). The stenotic segment was located proximally to the anastomosis in the recipient iliac artery in 2 patients, para-anastomotic in 17 patients, in the mid transplant main renal artery in 7 patients, in the branches in 1 patient and unknown in 2 patients. Arterial narrowing was more than 60% in 22 patients and less than 60% in the remaining 7 patients. Twenty-three patients underwent primary revascularization procedures (7 PTA and 16 surgical interventions) while six patients were maintained on medical treatment. Complete follow-up, present status, death or dialysis, was recorded in all studied patients (mean 71 months).

MEDICAL TREATMENT GROUP

Six patients received primary medical therapy for TRAS, of whom five had less than 60% stenosis. One patient was not hypertensive and has remained normotensive for a 6-month follow-up period. Two patients had well-controlled diastolic pressure and maintained this status at 1- and 2-year follow-up, respectively. Three patients had poorly-controlled diastolic pressure of whom two remained without any change at 6-month and 5-year follow-up, respectively. One patient had a transient improvement of pressure control for one year but worsened thereafter. Renal function deteriored in four patients at 7, 22, 24 and 46 months, respectively. Three of these patients entered on dialysis at 7 months, 7 years and 14 years, respectively, secondary to chronic rejection

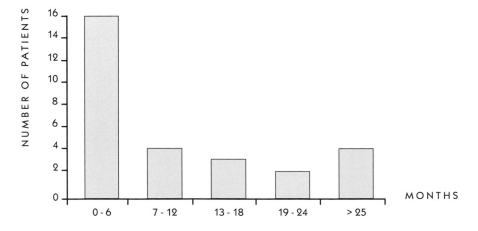

FIG. 8   Time to diagnosis of transplant renal artery stenosis after kidney transplantation.

or recurrent nephropathy. The remaining patient with progressively impairing renal function underwent autotransplantation for hypogastric artery occlusion and remained free of dialysis until his death 5 years later.

REVASCULARIZATION GROUP

Twenty-three patients underwent primary revascularization procedures. Primary PTA was performed in seven patients of whom six had more than 60% stenoses. Lesions were located in the proximal to the anastomosis in 2 patients, para-anastomotic in 2 patients, at mid renal artery in 2 patients and unknown in 1 patient. No procedure-related complications, graft losses or deaths were observed in the post-procedure period.

Primary surgical revascularization was performed in 16 patients of whom 15 had more than 60% stenoses. Lesions were located para-anastomotic in 12 patients, at mid renal artery in 3 patients and unknown in one patient. Seven patients underwent polytetrafluoroethilene (PTFE) patch angioplasty, 9 patients underwent PTFE bypass grafts, 3 from common iliac artery and 6 from external iliac artery. One patient had his bypass anastomosed to the renal artery proximal to the stenosis. Bypass was redone one month later and results of this patient are referred to in this last procedure. One patient had a postoperative branch occlusion with moderate worsening of the renal function. No other complications, graft losses or deaths were recorded in the postoperative period. One patient required a PTA after the development of a new stenosis proximal to a surgical PTFE patch at 14-month follow-up with good result. Finally, one patient required the interposition of a dacron graft after the development of an aorto-iliac and renal artery aneurysm 11.5 years after a TRAS correction with a PTFE patch with good result.

At the time of the revascularization procedure, surgical or PTA, 8 patients had their diastolic pressure well-controlled. After the procedure (Table I), 87.5% of patients did not modify diastolic blood pressure control while some 12.5% improved. This situation remained stable until the second year after the procedure. However, at 5-year follow-up 33.3% patients worsened their diastolic blood pressure control. Fifteen patients had their diastolic pressure poorly-controlled at time of the revascularization procedure. Subsequently (Table II), 80% patients

Table I	CHANGES IN DIASTOLIC BLOOD PRESSURE IN WELL-CONTROLLED HYPERTENSIVE PATIENTS WITH TRANSPLANT RENAL ARTERY STENOSIS AFTER REVASCULARIZATION PROCEDURE			
Change	*1 month*	*1 year*	*2 years*	*5 years*
Better	12.5 % (1/8)	0	14.3 % (1/7)	16.7 % (1/6)
No changes	87.5 % (7/8)	100 % (8/8)	85.7 % (6/7)	50 % (3/6)
Worse	0	0	0	33.3 % (2/6)

Table II	CHANGES IN DIASTOLIC BLOOD PRESSURE IN POOR-CONTROLLED HYPERTENSIVE PATIENTS WITH TRANSPLANT RENAL ARTERY STENOSIS AFTER REVASCULARIZATION PROCEDURE			
Change	*1 month*	*1 year*	*2 years*	*5 years*
Better	80 % (12/15)	66 % (10/15)	82 % (7/9)	88 % (7/8)
No changes	13 % (2/15)	27 % (4/15)	18 % (2/9)	12 % (1/8)
Worse	7 % (1/11)	7 % (1/15)	0	0

improved their blood pressure control, 13.3% remained without change and 6.7% worsened. At 5 years, 87.5% patients had better diastolic pressure control than that observed before procedure.

Renal function after revascularization procedure was improved or stable in 91.3% patients at 1 year, 82.2% at 2 years and 75.6% at five years (Fig. 9). Pre-procedure plasma creatinine levels did not modify the response of renal function after intervention. In patients with serum creatinine before procedure smaller than 2 mg/dL and equal or greater than 2 mg/dL, renal function stability or improvement was achieved in 92.9% and 88.9% patients at 1 year, 85.7% and 77.8% at 2 years, and 73.5% and 77.9% at 5 years, respectively (p>0.05). Six patients entered on dialysis at long-term follow-up due to chronic rejection or recurrent nephropathy. Dialysis-free survival of patients that underwent revascularization procedures was 100% at 1 year, 95.5% at 2 years, 89.8% at 5 years and 59.9% at 10 years (Fig. 10).

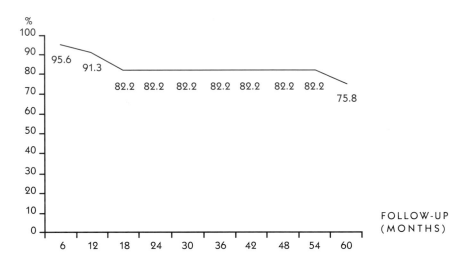

FIG. 9 Percentage of patients with plasma creatinine levels stable or improved after transplant renal artery stenosis revascularization.

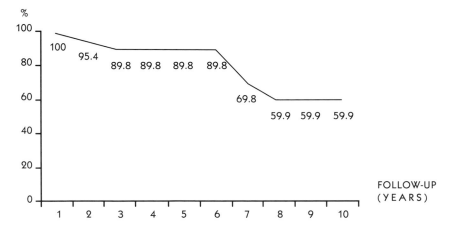

FIG. 10 Dialysis-free survival after transplant renal artery stenosis revascularization.

Discussion

PRELIMINARY ISSUES

At present, the natural history of TRAS has still not been well documented. Therefore it is necessary to schedule periodical screening tests after kidney transplantation, for instance duplex scanning, even in the absence of TRAS suspicion. This may help to evaluate the development of TRAS, to determine its prevalence, to identify if there is a cause-effect relationship between TRAS and allograft dysfunction, and to establish the real risk of spontaneous evolution of TRAS.

At present, all TRAS management options have been associated with excellent results, even the intensive medical treatment. However, the results of these reports are often difficult to interpret and compare, because investigators have used different methods of analyzing and presenting their data. Therefore it is necessary to establish recommended standards for analyzing and reporting on TRAS management options.

DECISION-MAKING IN TRAS

To the present knowledge it may be advisable to choose for a revascularization procedure for TRAS in those patients with a stenosis greater than 60% associated with hypertension resisting to medical therapy or decline in renal function. Other causes of allograft dysfunction should be ruled out in order to maximize the benefit/risk ratio of the procedure.

In case of poor-controlled hypertension or renal dysfunction associated with less than 60% stenosis, a comprehensive study of other potential causes has to be performed. Even in the absence of other explanation, TRAS revascularization should be indicated very cautiously.

REVASCULARIZATION OPTIONS AND RESULTS

We favor PTA as a first line interventional treatment when TRAS is located in the iliac artery, at the mid-portion of the main transplant renal artery or at its branches. Otherwise, TRAS para-anastomotic or associated to renal artery kinking, we favor primary surgical revascularization.

Many surgical options have been proposed for TRAS correction. Our preferred techniques are patch angioplasty and bypass. The reasons for this are:

1 - lesser need for exposure,

2 - greater experience, for a vascular surgeon, in bypass or patch techniques rather than reimplantation options,

3 - maintenance of the stenosed artery, in bypass grafting, which may allow to salvage the kidney in case of graft thrombosis. Surgical revascularization can be performed with minimal risk of morbidity and mortality.

Although synthetic grafts may be at risk of infection in these immunocompromized patients, we decided in earlier years to preserve the saphenous vein just in case of graft loss and need to use the vein for an hemodialysis A-V shunt. Later on we abandoned the saphenous vein for A-V shunts but at that time we had observed good results with PTFE patches or bypasses. Therefore we found no reason to abandon this synthetic graft.

Poorly-controlled diastolic pressure, but not well-controlled, is clearly improved by means of a revascularization procedure in patients with TRAS. This benefit is observed even at 5-year follow-up.

Renal function after TRAS revascularization remains stable or improves in the majority of patients at 5-year follow-up. Increased basal creatinine levels are not associated with a worse evolution of renal function after TRAS revascularization.

Dialysis-free survival of subjects submitted to TRAS correction is similar to that observed in patients without any TRAS diagnosis.

REFERENCES

1 Margules RM, Belzer FO, Kountz SL. Surgical correction of renovascular hypertension folowing renal allotransplantation. *Arch Surg* 1973; 106: 13-16.

2 Roberts JP, Asher NL, Fryd DS et al. Transplant renal artery stenosis. *Transplantation* 1989; 48: 580-583.

3 Greenstein S, Verstandig A, McLean GK et al. Percutaneous transluminal angioplasty. The procedure of choice in the hypertensive renal allograft recipient with renal artery stenosis. *Transplantation* 1987; 43: 29-32.

4 Smith RB, Cosimi AB, Lordon R et al. Diagnosis and management of arterial stenosis causing hypertension after successful renal transplantation. *J Urol* 1976; 115: 639-642.

5 Raynaud A, Bedrossian J, Remy P et al. Percutaneous transluminal angioplasty of renal transplant arterial stenosis. *Am J Roentgenol* 1986; 146: 853-857.

6 Lacombe M. Arterial stenosis complicating renal allotransplantation in man: a study of 38 cases. *Ann Surg* 1975; 181: 283-289.

7 Luke RG, Curtis JJ. Biology and treatment of transplant hypertension. In: Laragh JH and Brenner BM (eds.) *Hypertension*. New York: Raven Press 1994 : pp 2471-2483.

8 Raine AE. Hypertension and ischemic heart disease in renal transplant recipients. *Nephrol Dial Transplant* 1995; 10 (suppl 1): 95-100.

9 Ponticelli C, Montagnino G, Aroldi A et al. Hypertension after renal transplantation. *Amer J Kidney Dis* 1993; 21 (suppl 2): 73-78.

10 Vianello A, Mastrosimone S, Calconi G et al. The role of hypertension as a damaging factor for kidney grafts under cyclosporine therapy. *Amer J Kidney Dis* 1993; 21 (suppl 2): 79-83.

11 Gray DW. Graft renal artery stenosis in the transplanted kidney. *Transplantation Rev* 1994; 8: 15-21.

12 Chandrasoma P, Aberle AM. Anastomotic line renal artery stenosis after transplantation. *J Urol* 1986; 135: 1159-1162.

13 Benoit G, Moukarzel M, Hiesse C et al. Transplant renal artery stenosis: experience and comparative results between surgery and angioplasty. *Transplant Int* 1990; 3: 137.

14 Fung LC, McLorie GA, Khoury AE et al. Donor aortic cuff reduces the rate of anastomotic arterial stenosis in pediatric renal transplantation. *J Urol* 1995; 154: 909-913.

15 Grossman RA, Dafoe DC, Shoenfeld RB et al. Percutaneous transluminal angioplasty treatment of transplant renal artery stenosis. *Transplantation* 1982; 34: 339-343.

16 Munda R, Alexander JW, Miller S et al. Renal allograft artery stenosis. *Am J Surg* 1977; 134: 400-403.

17 Sankari BR, Geisinger M, Zelch M et al. Post-transplant renal artery stenosis: impact of therapy on long-term kidney function and blood pressure control. *J Urol* 1996; 155: 1860-1864.

18 Sutherland RS, Spees EK, Jones JW et al. Renal artery stenosis after renal transplantation: the impact of the hypogastric artery anastomosis. *J Urol* 1993; 149: 980-985.

19 Stanley P, Malekzadeh M, Diament MJ. Post-transplant renal artery stenosis: angiographic study in 32 children. *Am J Roentgenol* 1987; 148: 487-490.

20 Wong W, Fynn SP, Higgins RM et al. Transplant renal artery stenosis in 77 patients – does it have an immunological cause? *Transplant* 1996; 61: 215-219.

21 Merkus JW, Huysmans FT, Hoitsma AJ et al. Renal allograft artery stenosis. Results of medical treatment and intervention: a retrospective analysis. *Transplant Int* 1993; 6: 111-115.

22 Idrissi A, Fournier H, Renaud B et al. The captopril challenge test as a screening test for renovascular hypertension. *Kidney Int* 1988; 34: S 138-141.

23 Erley CM, Duda SH, Wakat JP et al. Noninvasive procedures for diagnosis of renovascular hypertension in renal transplant recipients: a prospective analysis. *Transplantation* 1992; 54: 863-867.

24 Shamlou KK, Drane WE, Hawkins IF et al. Captopril renography and the hypertensive renal transplantation patient: a predictive test of therapeutic outcome. *Radiology* 1994; 190: 153-159.

25 Lewin JS, Laub G, Hausmann R. Three-dimensional time-of-flight MR angiography: applications in the abdomen and thorax. *Radiology* 1991; 179: 261-264.

26 Rubin GD, Dake MD, Napel SA et al. Three-dimensional spiral CT angiography of the abdomen: initial clinical experience. *Radiology* 1993; 186: 147-152.

27 Mell MW, Alfrey EJ, Rubin GD et al. Use of spiral computed tomography in the diagnosis of transplant renal artery stenosis. *Transplantation* 1994; 57: 746-748.

28 Mammen NI, Chacko N, Ganesh G et al. Aspects of hypertension in renal allograft recipients. A study of 1000 live renal transplants. *Br J Urol* 1993; 71: 256-258.

29 Chan YT, Ng WD, Ho CP et al. Reversible stenosis of the renal artery following renal transplantation. *Br J Surg* 1985; 72: 454-455.

30 Fontaine E, Beurton D, Barthelemy Y et al. Renal artery stenosis following pediatric renal transplantation. *Transplant Proc* 1994; 26: 293-294.

31 Deglise-Favre A, Hiesse C, Lantz O et al. Long-term follow-up of 40 untreated cadaveric kidney transplant renal artery stenosis. *Transplant Proc* 1991; 23: 1342-1343.

32 Fauchald P, Vatne K, Paulsen D et al. Long-term clinical results of percutaneous transluminal angioplasty in transplant renal artery stenosis. *Nephrol Dial Transplant* 1992; 7: 256-259.

33 Sniderman KW, Sprayregen S, Sos TA et al. Percutaneous transluminal dilatation in renal transplant artery stenosis. *Transplantation* 1980; 30: 440-444.

34 Gruntzig A. Percutaneous transluminal recanalization with the double-lumen dilatation catheter. In: Zeitler E, Gruntzig A, Shoop W (eds.). *Percutaneous vascular recanalization.* Berlin, Springer-Verlag, 1978, p 17.

35 Clements R, Evans C, Salaman JR. Percutaneous transluminal angioplasty of renal transplant artery stenosis. *Clin Radiol* 1987; 38: 235-237.

36 Bover J, Montana J, Castelao AM et al. Percutaneous transluminal angioplasty for treatment of allograft renal artery stenosis. *Transplant Proc* 1992; 24: 94-95.

37 Thomas CP, Riad H, Johnson BF et al. Percutaneous transluminal angioplasty in transplant renal arterial stenoses: a long-term follow-up. *Transplant Int* 1992; 5: 129-132.

38 Matalon TA, Thompson MJ, Patel SK et al. Percutaneous transluminal angioplasty for transplant renal artery stenosis. *J Vasc Interv Radiol* 1992; 3: 55-58.

39 McMullin ND, Reidy JF, Koffman CG et al. The management of renal transplant artery stenosis in children by percutaneous transluminal angioplasty. *Transplantation* 1992; 53: 559-563.

40 Chan HW, Ho YW, Chan CM et al. Treatment of anastomotic ostial allograft and renal artery stenosis with the Palmaz stent. *Transplantation* 1995; 59: 436-439.

41 Martin LG, Price RB, Casarella WJ et al. Precutaneous angioplasty in clinical management of renovascular hypertension: initial and long-term results. *Radiology* 1985; 155: 629-633.

42 Tilney NL, Rocha A, Strom TB et al. Renal artery stenosis in transplant patients. *Ann Surg* 1984; 199: 454-460.

43 Sagalowsky AI, Peters PC. Renovascular hypertension following renal transplantation. *Urol Clin North Am* 1984; 11: 491-502.

44 Dickerman RM, Peters PC, Hull AR et al. Surgical correction of post-transplant renovascular hypertension. *Ann Surg* 1980; 192: 639-644.

45 Lacombe M. Renal artery stenosis after renal transplantation. *Ann Vasc Surg* 1988; 2: 155-160.

46 Palleschi J, Novick AC, Braun WE et al. Vascular complications of renal transplantation. *Urology* 1980; 16: 61-67.

47 Killewich LA, Pais SO, Sandager G et al. Salvage of renal allograft function and lower extremity venous patency with thrombolytic therapy: case report and review of the literature. *J Vasc Surg* 1995; 21: 691-696.

48 Thomalla JV, Lingeman JE, Leapman SB et al. The manifestation and management of late urological complications in renal transplant recipients: use of the urological armamentarium. *J Urol* 1985; 134: 944-948.

49 Zincke H, Woods JE, Leary FJ et al. Experience with lymphoceles after renal transplantation. *Surgery* 1975; 77: 444-450.

12
118

13

NEUROLOGIC COMPLICATIONS
OF CAROTID SURGERY

RAOUF AYARI, BERTRAND EDE
MICHEL BARTOLI, ALAIN BRANCHEREAU

Early postoperative neurologic complications, reflecting their different aspects of incidence, mechanism, predictive and preventive factors determine the major problem of carotid artery surgery. Since the beginning of carotid surgery and during the second half of the twentieth century we have observed two developments related to this problem. On one hand the complication rate decreased significantly, from 10%-20% in the early years of carotid surgery [1], to less than 5% at present time. On the other hand, both vascular surgeons and neurologists acknowledged the true importance of neurologic complications. These developments have inspired several controversial publications, alerting the scientific community towards the potential dangers of this surgery [2]. Furthermore, scientific societies have launched recommendations to define neurologic complication rates above which surgery is not acceptable as a prophylactic procedure [3].

In this chapter we do not address cranial nerve injuries, long-term neurologic complications, or restenosis because they are discussed elsewhere in this book.

Impact of neurologic complications

Between the early 1980s and the present time the mortality of carotid surgery induced by general causes and cardiac origin in particular has substantially diminished [4]. In our recent personal experience we have not encountered cardiac induced

mortality (see below). These advancements are the result of improved medical care of cardiac diseases in general and coronary artery disease in particular.

In 1415 patients evaluated in the NASCET study, two mortal myocardial infarctions (0.14%) were observed [5]. Two other patients suddenly died, probably due to cardiac causes, and 11 non-mortal myocardial infarctions occurred. Therefore, the main cause of carotid surgical failure is nowadays determined by neurologic complications. In fact it is rather paradoxal and tragic to realize that the same procedure to prevent a stroke can cause the same cerebral vascular accident in an unharmed patient at the moment of surgery. In addition to this psychologic dimension, the neurologic complication rate implies major statistical consequences to determine the actual prophylactic role of surgery in a given category of patients. Figure 1 shows the principle on which all the large, prospective randomized studies are based, and explains the fundamental role of the neurologic complication rates.

Knowing the indisputable harmful character of carotid stenosis it is evident that the existence of a carotid stenosis determines more neurologic events than in the absence of a stenosis. The dotted curves in Figure 1 (operated patients) are less steep (indicating fewer neurologic events) than the curve of the non-operated patients. The removal of a carotid stenosis requires a surgical procedure, which in itself causes neurologic complications during the procedure. As a consequence, from the day of the procedure the operated population is not free from neurologic events and can be considered at the first postoperative day as 100% of the initial population minus the neurologic complication rate related to the procedure. Since neurologic events prevented by surgery are distributed over time, the benefit of

surgical treatment is reached as late as neurologic complication rate is higher. As can be seen in figure 1, it is obvious that preventive surgery, of which the effect will appear after 8 to 10 years, in a population aged over 70 years, is difficult to justify. The NASCET study has demonstrated that in carotid stenoses between 70% and 99% the curves cross at three months if the stroke and death rate is 5.8% [6]. The ACAS study shows this crossing around nine months with a stroke and death rate of 2.3% [7].

Epidemiology

The knowledge and interpretation of the neurologic complication rates of carotid surgery has been a matter of debate. The opponents of surgery have underlined the differences observed according to the method of compiling the results [8]. It appears that the neurologic complication rate increases depending on considering individual series, retrospective surveys or prospective randomized studies (Table I A, B, C); possibly due to the quality of the collected data. Another explanation is that the collective and multicenter studies report on the results of diverse surgical teams who might have different surgical expertise. Furthermore, patient categories also influence the neurologic complication rates.

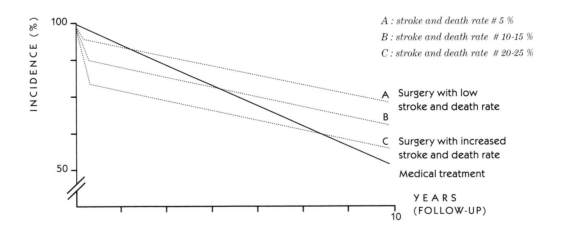

FIG. 1 Theoretical aspects of stroke-free survival curves of therapeutic studies comparing surgery versus medical treatment. The three dotted lines represent three different curves of surgical treatment with early postoperative neurologic deficits.

For example, the surgical risk is increased in symptomatic patients and in patients operated shortly after a minor stroke. Evaluation of the surgical results in the NASCET study has allowed to identify several predictive factors for increased surgical risks:

hemispheric rather than ocular symptoms, left carotid artery repair, ipsilateral ischemia on computer tomography (CT) and irregular or ulcerated plaque [5]. In our personal experience we have observed that the diffusion of the atherosclerotic

Table I A	RESULTS OF CAROTID SURGERY. INDIVIDUAL SERIES					
1st author [ref.]	*Year of publication*	*Study period*	*Number of interventions*	*Stroke %*	*Death %*	*Stroke + death %*
Rockman [9]	1996	1985-1994	1 414	1.2	0.9	NA
Hertzer [10]	1997	1989-1995	1 924	1.8	0.5	2.1
Archie [11]	1999	1990-1997	697	2.2	0.8	2.7
Naylor [12]	2000	1995-1999	500	1.6	1.2	2.2
Personal experience	2001	1997-2000	364	1.4 * 3.8 **	1.2 1.2	2.3 * 5.0 **

NA: not availabe

* Disabling and lethal stroke
** Disabling and minor stroke

In our personal experience the stroke rates are calculated on the number of interventions (N = 364) whereas the death rate and CMMR are calculated on the number of patients (N = 339).

Table I B	RESULTS OF CAROTID SURGERY. COLLECTIVE SERIES					
1st author [ref.]	*Year of publication*	*Study period*	*Number of interventions*	*Stroke %*	*Death %*	*Stroke + death %*
AURC [13]	1988	1987	927	3.6	1.5	4.1
ARCHIV [14]	1988	1987	710	2.3	0.6	2.6
Rubin [15] *	1988	1973-1985	8 535	2.1	1.6	3.2
Yates [16] **	1997	1991-1993	986	NA	1.5	2.3
Cao [17] ***	1998	1994-1997	1 353	2.1	0.6	2.4
Kantonen [18] •	1998	1991-1995	1 600	2.1	1.2	2.3
Troeng [19] ••	1999	1994-1996	1 518	2.9	1.4	4.3

ARCHIV: joint French, non-university vascular surgeons
AURC: joint French, university vascular surgeons
NA: not available

* Cleveland Vascular Society
** Kentucky Vascular Surgery Society Study Group
*** Joint Italian vascular surgeons (EVEREST study)
• Finnvasc Study Group
•• Swedish Vascular Registry

Origin [ref.]	Year of publication	Study period	Number of interventions	Stroke %	Death %	Stroke + death %
Symptomatic stenoses						
ESCT [20] •	1991	1981-1991	455	NA	0.9	
NASCET [5] ••	1999	1988-1996	1415	1.8 *	1.1	6.5
					3.7 **	
Asymptomatic stenoses						
ACAS [7]	1995	1988-1993	825	2.1	0.4	2.3

Table I C RESULTS OF CAROTID SURGERY. PROSPECTIVE RANDOMIZED TRIALS

* Disabling stroke
** Non-disabling stroke
• Irrespective of the degree of stenosis
•• Stenosis between 70 - 99%

cerebrovascular disease demonstrated by symptoms of vertebrobasilar insufficiency represent a significant risk factor for the occurrence of neurologic complications [21].

Different indications for surgery, especially the existence of neurologic symptoms also explain the differences of reported results in the literature. It is important to correctly interpret the results in the literature and subsequently evaluate the different complication rates. It is obvious that the most valuable information is deduced from prospective randomized studies (Table IC), in which a large number of centers participated, authenticated by external observers.

Personal experience

In 1987 we published a study on neurologic complications after carotid surgery performed between 1980 and 1987 [22], the results of which are included in Table II. We have updated our experience and collected the neurologic complications encountered between January 1997 and June 2000. During this period we performed 364 surgical procedures in 339 patients: 166 classic endarterectomies (25 with patch), 145 eversion endarterectomies, and 53 bypasses (35 vein, 18 PTFE). Thirty-day morbidity and mortality included 4 deaths, 4 disabling strokes, 9 non-disabling strokes with minimal or resolved aftereffects, and 5 transient ischemic attacks. The

causes of death were one stroke, one acute respiratory failure, one septic shock, and one mesenteric ischemia following aortic surgery one month after carotid artery repair. The stroke and death rate was 5% for patients and 4.7% for cases. Considering only death and disabling stroke these rates were 2.4% and 2.2% respectively. Neurologic deficits occurred in 19 patients: 1 mortal stroke, 4 disabling strokes, 9 non-disabling strokes, and 5 transient ischemic attacks. The etiology of these neurologic complications included thromboembolism in 10 patients (8 embolizations, 2 thromboses), intolerance during crossclamping in 8, and reperfusion injury in 2 patients.

Mechanisms of neurologic complications

It is important to understand that multiple mechanisms are responsible for the development of neurologic complications during carotid surgery. These mechanisms can be separated in three categories: thromboembolic complications, intolerance to carotid clamping, and reperfusion injury. These mechanisms should be known and understood in order to apply adequate preventive measures. It is surprising to notice the limited number of studies addressing the identification and comprehension of these mechanisms compared to the extensive scientific attention which is

Table II		MECHANISMS OF POSTOPERATIVE NEUROLOGIC ACCIDENTS						
1er author [ref.]	Year of publication	Study period	Number of interventions	Number of neurologic accidents (%)	Mechanisms of neurologic accidents			
					Thrombo-embolic (%)	Clamping (%)	Hemorrhage or reperfusion (%)	Others (%)
Steed [23]	1982	1967-1981	345	21*	20	1	NA	NA
Sundt [24]	1986	1972-1984	1935	58*	40	5	13	NA
Branchereau [22]	1987	1980-1987	700	37 (5.2)*	19 (51.4)	8 (21.6)	5 (13.5)	5 (13.5)
AURC [13]	1988	1987	927	52 (5.6)*	21 (40.4)	9 (17.2)	11 (21.2)	11 (21.2)
Riles [25]	1994	1961-1991	3062	66 (2.2)**	25 (37.9)	10 (15.2)	12 (18.2)	19 (28.7)
Ouriel [26]	1999	1992-1997	1471	31 (2.1) *	NA	NA	11 (35.5)	NA
Radak [27]	1999	1985-1997	2250	59 (2.6)**	40 (67.8)	1 (1.7)	10 (17)	8 (13.5)
Rockman [28]	2000	1985-1997	2024	28 (1.9) *	24 (63.2)	5 (13.2)	5 (13.5)	4 (10.4)
Personal experience	2001	1997-2000	364	19 (5.2) *	10 (52.6)	7 (36.8)	2 (10.6)	-

NA: not available
 * Postoperative TIA and stroke
** Postoperative stroke

13
123

focused on cerebral monitoring related to the problem of intolerance of carotid clamping. The main studies in the literature reporting on the relative incidence of these different mechanisms in the occurrence of neurologic complications are summarized in Table II. All these prospective or retrospective studies are based on the analysis of neurologic symptoms, the moment of occurrence of symptoms, information of the surgical procedure and/or reintervention, and sometimes the data on angiography, duplex scanning and CT scanning. Local regional anesthesia with monitoring of consciousness is an excellent method of assessing the mechanisms of neurologic complications, as clearly demonstrated by Steed et al. [23].

THROMBOEMBOLIC COMPLICATIONS

According to the studies in Table II, thromboembolic processes are the most frequent causes of neurologic complications, varying between 38% and 95%. Overall it can be stated that more or less half of the neurologic complications are caused by this mechanism. Thromboembolic processes can be divided in two categories: embolism characterized by migration of thrombolic material from the carotid bifurcation towards the cerebral circulation, and postoperative thrombosis represented by complete occlusion of the internal carotid artery (ICA) starting at the level of the surgical repair.

Embolization can occur at all stages of the surgical procedures. Before clamping, surgical dissection and mobilization of the carotid bifurcation can potentially initiate cerebral embolization. This risk is particularly increased in ulcerated lesions and soft plaques, which can preoperatively be assessed by means of ultrasonography. The prevention of these accidents is based on meticulous dissection without mobilization of the carotid artery. Furthermore, the ICA should be clamped first, cranial to the pathologic lesion in a plaque-free segment of the artery. During clamping, embolization can occur if an intraluminal shunt is introduced, subsequently dislodging atherosclerotic debris. Finally, inadequate flushing prior to declamping can cause embolization of atheromatous debris, thrombus, or air. Following declamping, embolies are due to non-occlusive thrombus formation at the inner surface of the repaired artery. The appearance of such a thrombus is most frequently caused by technical defaults, more or less stimulated by hypercoagulability or platelet hyperaggregability. The acute postoperative thrombosis obstructs the blood supply at the level of the ICA with appearance of a thrombus cranial to the surgical repair, extending to the level of the intracerebral circulation. In case of an adequate contralateral ICA blood supply, such a postoperative thrombosis can occur without symptoms. Similar to embolic complications, acute postoperative thrombosis is mainly due to technical failures, combined with hypercoagulability or platelet hyperaggregability.

A stenotic suture line is a frequently occurring technical default, explaining the superior results with patch plasty [29]. Other technical failures responsible for thromboembolic events include a remaining intimal flap, dissection of the ICA cranial to the removed plague (Fig. 2), disorder at the proximal limit of the endarterectomy (Fig. 3), and a stenotic kinking generally occurring at the distal border of the endarterectomy. Plasmatic or platelet hyperthrombogenicity might play a role in the occurrence of these complications, however, this is certainly less contributing to complications than the surgical imperfections. The latter are sometimes

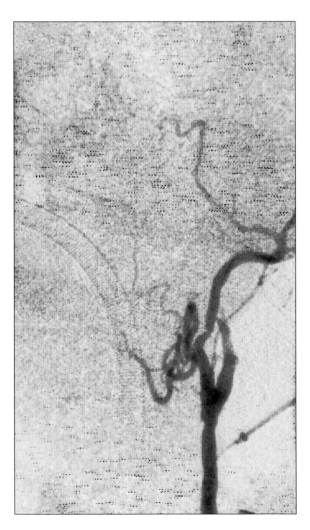

FIG. 2 Stoppage of contrast in the internal carotid artery at a postoperative angiography. Surgical reintervention revealed a dissection at the distal edge of the endarterectomy.

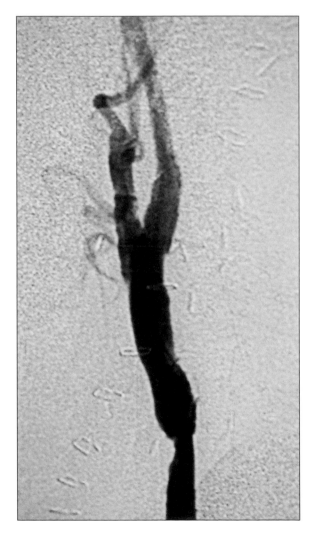

FIG. 3 Technical defect at the proximal border of the endarterectomy of the common carotid artery.

unnoticed or underestimated in the absence of intra-operative assessment of the surgical reconstruction. In exceptional cases, however, hematologic factors probably play a decisive role: all surgeons with extensive experience in carotid surgery have reoperated on patients for acute postoperative thrombosis, observing a fresh thrombus at the level of the repaired arterial segment without any detectable technical default.

The importance of preoperative treatment with aspirin has recently been demonstrated [30]. Since 1999 all our patients receive 250 mg aspirin during or at least one week prior to the procedure. The neutralization of heparin and the amount of protamine can cause a rebound effect with subsequent thrombosis of the ICA. Refraining from neutralization provides a prolonged but progressively decreased anticoagulant effect during the immediate postoperative phase, but augments hemorrhagic complications. Some authors have proposed a sophisticated method to calculate the optimal dose of protamine to avoid acute thrombosis; this method appears appealing but is rather complex and difficult to implement [31]. In practice we inject 200 UI/kg of heparin before carotid clamping. This substantial amount of heparin is administered to prevent all possible phenomena of thrombosis during clamping. After declamping and inspection of the surgical repair we apply a dose of protamine which equals two thirds of the dose of heparin. This empiric approach is based on postoperative coagulation analyses in patients receiving different amounts of protamine (unpublished data).

Intolerance to clamping

In contrast to what the extensive literature on this subject suggests, clamp intolerance is not the most frequent cause of neurologic complications. In fact, it is the second after thromboembolic complications. The concept of clamp intolerance is based on the knowledge of the pathophysiologic response of the brain to ischemia. The normal cerebral blood flow (CBF) is approximately 50 cc/100g/minute. If CBF decreases to 18 cc/100g/minute, the so-called *grey area* of cerebral ischemia, reversible cellular dysfunction develops, without cellular alterations. Below 5 cc/100g/minute, irreversible changes occur with subsequent cellular death [32].

The primary and most obvious mechanism is purely hemodynamic: cellular hypoxic distress sec-

ondary to the decreased CBF. This phenomenon of clamp intolerance encounters two different grades: reversible ischemia without cerebral damage and irreversible ischemia with cerebral lesions. The first stage corresponds to the grey area of cerebral ischemia. Clinical features include neurologic deficit despite normal awakening, which spontaneously disappears within one hour. If this phenomenon is recognized during carotid surgery under local anesthesia, a shunt should be considered. The second stage of ischemia is accompanied by irreversible lesions with stroke and detectable cerebral damage at CT-scanning. The prevention of these neurologic complications is based on the use of an intraluminal shunt providing sufficient CBF during clamping.

The second mechanism, described by Moore et al. [33], is an hemodynamic phenomenon but specifically occurs in patients with cerebral lesions related to a recent stroke. In this situation the area of the cerebral substance around the infarction is composed of a neurologic tissue which is still viable with vascular network where, due to inflammatory alterations, the peripheral vascular resistance is abnormally elevated. During clamping, the decreased arterial pressure associated with augmented peripheral resistance determines a significant decreased perfusion pressure in the affected area, resulting in an enlarged infarction and subsequent aggravated neurologic deficit (Fig. 4). The prevention of this complication is based on the use of a shunt and/or respecting a time delay between the initial neurologic deficit and surgical procedure of at least four to six weeks.

The third mechanism of neurologic complications caused by carotid clamping is the occurrence of acute arterial thrombosis of the intracerebral arterial network (Fig. 5). Thrombosis of a cerebral artery is provoked by diminished blood flow during clamping and is generally associated with preexisting distal arterial lesions. This type of vascular accident induces a local infarction in a cerebral territory distal to the thrombosed area with irreversible neurologic features. Besides the use of a shunt, we believe that high dose heparinization reduces the risk of thrombosis related to circulatory stasis.

13

125

Reperfusion injury

Postoperative reperfusion injury is a less known and uncommon cause of neurologic complications. These injuries are secondary to a hyperperfusion phenomenon which is due to an insufficient autoregulation in certain cerebral territories subjected to a prolonged time of low blood flow. Two clinical aspects exist. Postoperative edema generally appears at the end of the procedure or within one hour after declamping. The clinical signs include blurred consciousness, coma with homolateral neurologic deficit, and epileptic movements with EEG abnormalities. CT-scanning (or MRI) is essential because it can precociously demonstrate signs of edema with closure of the cortical grooves, possibly associated with a deviation of profound, central structures, without hemorrhage. The edema can cause cerebral damage by itself, demonstrable at CT-scanning after a few days: the patient might die if the stroke is extensive, or may survive, generally after a long period of coma, with major neurologic deficits. If the edema does not induce cerebral dam-

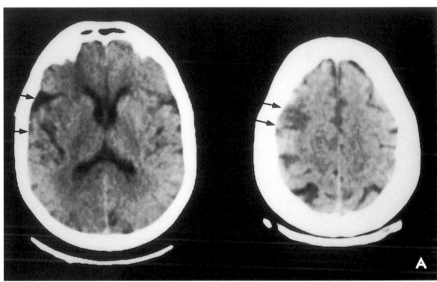

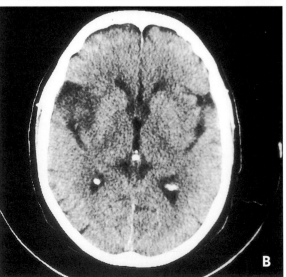

FIG. 4   Intra-operative aggravation of a recently, unnoticed cerebral infarction. A - Preoperative CT-scan. B - Postoperative CT-scan.

age and resolves in several days, complete recovery without neurologic deficit is possible. The treatment of this complication is purely symptomatic: strict control of arterial pressure, heparinization, and anti-edema treatment in the intensive care unit. Cerebral metabolic activity might be achieved with barbiturates.

Hemorrhagic accidents determine the second aspect of revascularization syndromes. They probably represent the most seldom but also the worst neurologic complications following carotid surgery. In a meta-analysis of 9449 carotid artery repairs, Connolly et al. found an incidence of hemorrhagic accidents of 0.5% [34]. The prognosis is much worse than the outcome of edema formation; 50% of the patients die. The early clinical symptoms in the first postoperative hour might be similar, however, they can also develop during the postoperative days. Transcranial doppler might demonstrate specific signs of hyperemia, fastening suspicion on reperfusion syndrome and initiating symptomatic treatment. Besides the

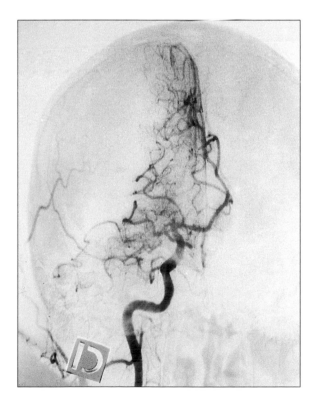

FIG. 5 Acute arterial thrombosis of the middle cerebral artery visualized by means of a postoperative angiography in a patient with a severe neurologic deficit. Intra-operative angiography did not show any defects.

above described reperfusion injuries, other reperfusion-induced headaches without neurologic deficit are noted in approximately 20% of patients following carotid surgery.

RISK FACTORS

The most certain and best known predictive risk factor of reperfusion injury is the presence of severe carotid artery lesions: bilateral tight stenosis or a tight stenosis associated with a contralateral occlusion. Besides assessment of the carotid lesions by means of angiography and/or duplex scanning, associated vertebro-subclavian arterial pathology and low cerebral blood flow shown by transcranial doppler, MRI, SPECT or PET scanning are also predictive elements determining the risk of reperfusion injury. Cerebral blood flow studies demonstrating loss of autoregulation with decreased hemodynamic reserve capacity probably allow to identify patients at highest risk to develop a reperfusion injury. These investigations, however, are not routinely performed.

The presence of a cerebral infarction is also a well known risk factor. The hypothesis is that the vascular walls of the arteries crossing the infarcted area are altered: the increased arterial pressure following endarterectomy subsequently causes a vascular rupture which transforms an ischemic infarction into an hemorrhagic infarction. The contrast uptake in the infarcted areas, visible on CT-scanning, reflects an increased porosity of the blood-brain barrier with consequential augmented hemorrhagic risks (Fig. 6).

Severe and/or uncontrolled hypertension represents a risk factor because of increased arterial pressures during and after the procedure and because these patients might suffer from arteriolar pathology secondary to the hypertension. Intra-operative monitoring of cerebral blood flow might determine the level of increased flow at which reperfusion injury develops. Beside some anecdotal experiments no reliable method is currently available to assess these critical values. In contrast, intra-operative transcranial doppler might be useful to detect the risk of hyperperfusion. In a retrospective study of 233 cases, Jansen et al. [35] have demonstrated that a peak velocity increase greater than 175% and a pulsatility index augmentation greater than 100% at the level of the middle cerebral artery, was associated with a cerebral hemorrhage in 80% of cases. The duration of carotid clamping might be considered as a risk factor because it can determine a relative cerebral

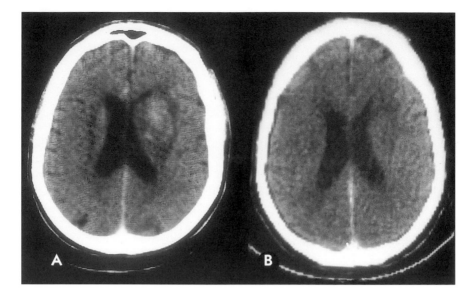

FIG. 6   A - Recent stroke with improving deficit: CT-scanning shows signs of increased porosity at the blood-brain barrier. B - Same patient, 4 weeks later.

ischemia, which is prolonged with extended clamping and even more pronounced in case of a poor collateral network. The latter would be an argument to routinely use an intraluminal shunt, however, the scientific benefit has never been proven.

The occurrence of sudden rise of arterial pressure during the postoperative phase is a risk factor for cerebral hemorrhage. This risk is even increased if the contralateral side is operated simultaneously or a few days later because bilateral dissection at the baroreceptors can provoke arterial hypertension.

PREVENTION

Prevention of neurologic complications is obviously based on the knowledge and identification of all risk factors. A carotid procedure should be postponed in case of unstable hypertension or recent stroke (Fig. 6). An intraluminal shunt should be inserted if hemodynamic monitoring demonstrates significant reduction of cerebral blood flow during clamping. In patients with risk factors it is recommended to invasively monitor the arterial pressure during at least 24 hours, and in case of hypertension to aggressively treat the patient, preferably in the intensive care unit. The occurrence of severe headache should initiate investigations to assess and identify cerebral hyperperfusion (transcranial doppler, MRI) and, if required, activate medical treatment before the occurrence of a hemorrhagic complication.

Comments

The main purpose of this chapter is to show that the mechanisms of neurologic complications following carotid surgery are determined by multiple factors which require different strategies for their prevention. So far, no surgical technique or monitoring method has been developed to solve these problems and significantly diminish the stroke and death rate. The improvement of the outcome has been the sum of the several steps of carotid surgery evolution: indication, timing of the procedure, surgical technique, monitoring, and postoperative management.

The majority of neurologic complications are caused by thromboembolic processes, mainly due to technical errors. In contrast to certain surgical teams who consistently perform a standard arterial reconstruction technique, usually a patch [29] or eversion endarterectomy [17], we prefer to master all available techniques and adapt the method of reconstruction to the type of lesion or specific intra-operative circumstances.

In this respect we consider the carotid bypass, which we have used for 20 years [36] and which comprises 14.5% of our recent experience, a serious option in the presence of an arterial defect at the intra-operative completion angiography or in case of diffuse and complex atherosclerotic lesions (Fig. 7). We have been performing a completion angiography since 1990, and it is one of the contributing components to our improved results. In the last 364 interventions, completion angiography demonstrated 54 defects (15%), the details of which are summarized in Table III. In all cases therapeutic measures were taken. Regarding the 36 defects at the internal carotid artery, 12 arterial spasms could be resolved with local papaverine infiltration, and in 4 cases the excessive spasm required mechanical dilatation after reclamping. The remaining 20 cases needed surgical reintervention: 8 additional endarterectomies of the distal artery, 11 bypasses, and 1 restoration of a patch suture. Sixteen lesions were encountered in the external carotid artery (ECA)

which were subsequently revised: 12 additional endarterectomies of the ECA without clamping the ICA, 2 extended endarterectomies of the ECA with complete reclamping of the carotid bifurcation, and 2 ligations of the ECA. The final two lesions were

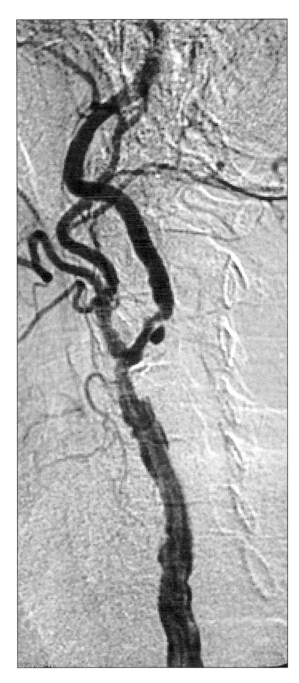

FIG. 7 Extensive atherosclerotic lesions which in our experience are treated with a carotid bypass.

13

Table III	ENCOUNTERED TECHNICAL DEFECTS BY COMPLETION ANGIOGRAPHY IN OUR EXPERIENCE OF 364 CAROTID OPERATIONS (1997-2000)	
Defects in internal carotid artery		N = 36
Spasm		16
Irregular edges of endarterectomy		9
Distal flap		7
Kinking		3
Patch stenosis		1
Defects in external carotid artery		N = 16
Intimal flap		14
Complete thrombosis		2
Defects in common carotid artery		N = 2
Remaining plaque at the proximal border of the endarterectomy		2

observed in the common carotid artery requiring additional endarterectomy. The overall intra-operative reintervention rate was 11%, which is in accordance with the results in the literature, showing a surgical revision rate based on intra-operative angiography between 4% and 23% (Table IV). Angiography is actually rarely performed. Angio-

scopy is advantageous in patients with renal failure or if angiography is not available. The accuracy, however, is less than in angiography [40]. Intra-operative duplex scanning is a noninvasive method with a high accuracy [42,43], however, it requires specific set-up in the operating room and specially trained technicians.

Table IV INCIDENCE OF SURGICAL REVISIONS BASED ON INTRA-OPERATIVE ASSESSMENT

1er author [ref.]	Year of publication	Study period	Number of interventions	Method of assessment	Observed defects %	Corrected defects %
Courbier [37]	1986	NA	100	AG	NA	5
Bandyk [42]	1988	NA	250	AG (n = 250) Duplex (n = 250)	4 8	4
Donaldson [38]	1993	1983-1991	410	AG	16	14
Kinney [43]	1993	1984-1990	461	Duplex (n = 410)	5.6	5.6
Lohr [39]	1995	1984-1991	131	AG	28	23
Branchereau [40]	1995	1992-1993	103	AS	35	5
Zanetti [41]	1999	1994-1997	1305	AG (n = 1004) AS (n = 229) Duplex (n = 2)	9	5
Naylor [12]	2000	1995-1999	500	AS	NA	7
Personal experience	2001	1997-2000	364	AG	15	11

AG: angiography
AS: angioscopy
NA: not available

13
130

REFERENCES

1 Easton JD, Sherman DG. Stroke and mortality rate in carotid endarterectomy: 228 consecutive operations. *Stroke* 1977; 8: 565-568.
2 Warlow C. Carotid endarterectomy: does it work? *Stroke* 1984; 15: 1068-1076.
3 Biller J, Feinberg WM, Castaldo JE et al. Guidelines for carotid endarterectomy: a statement for healthcare professionals from a special writing group of the Stroke Council, American Heart Association. *Stroke* 1998; 29: 554-562.
4 Magnan PE, Caus T, Branchereau A et al. Internal carotid artery surgery: ten-year results. *Ann Vasc Surg* 1993; 7: 521-529.
5 Ferguson GG, Eliasziw M, Barr HW et al. The North American Symptomatic Carotid Endarterectomy Trial: surgical results in 1415 patients. *Stroke* 1999; 30: 1751-1758.
6 Anonymous. North American Symptomatic Carotid Endarterectomy Trial. Beneficial effect of carotid endarterectomy in symptomatic patients with high-grade stenosis. *N Engl J Med* 1991; 325: 445-453.

7 Anonymous. Executive Committee for The Asymptomatic Carotid Atherosclerosis Study. Endarterectomy for asymptomatic carotid artery stenosis. *JAMA* 1995; 273: 1421-1428.

8 Easton JD, Wilterdink JL. Carotid endarterectomy: trials and tribulations. *Ann Neurol* 1994; 35: 5-17.

9 Rockman CB, Riles TS, Gold M et al. A comparison of regional and general anesthesia in patients undergoing carotid endarterectomy. *J Vasc Surg* 1996; 24: 946-956.

10 Hertzer NR, O'Hara PJ, Mascha EJ et al. Early outcome assessment for 2228 consecutive carotid endarterectomy procedures: the Cleveland Clinic experience from 1989 to 1995. *J Vasc Surg* 1997; 26: 1-10.

11 Archie JP. Carotid endarterectomy outcome with vein or dacron graft patch angioplasty and internal carotid artery shortening. *J Vasc Surg* 1999; 29: 654-664.

12 Naylor AR, Hayes PD, Allroggen H et al. Reducing the risk of carotid surgery: a 7-year audit of the role of monitoring and quality control assessment. *J Vasc Surg* 2000; 32: 750-759.

13 L'AURC et Becquemin JP, Souadka F, Meunier J. Risque opératoire actuel de la chirurgie carotidienne: expérience du groupe vasculaire de l'AURC. In: Kieffer E, Bousser MG (eds). *Indications et résultats de la chirurgie carotidienne.* Paris, AERCV, 1988: pp 41-50.

14 Joyeux A et le groupe ARCHIV. Risque opératoire actuel de la chirurgie carotidienne: expérience du groupe ARCHIV. In: Kieffer E, Bousser MG (eds). *Indications et résultats de la chirurgie carotidienne.* Paris, AERCV, 1988: pp 35-39.

15 Rubin JR, Pitluk HC, King TA et al. Carotid endarterectomy in a metropolitan community: the early results after 8535 operations. *J Vasc Surg* 1988; 7: 256-260.

16 Yates GN, Bergamini TM, George SM Jr et al. Carotid endarterectomy results from a state vascular society. Kentucky Vascular Surgery Society Study Group. *Am J Surg* 1997; 173: 342-344.

17 Cao P, Giordano G, De Rango P et al. A randomized study on eversion versus standard carotid endarterectomy: study design and preliminary results: the Everest Trial. *J Vasc Surg* 1998; 27: 595-605.

18 Kantonen I, Lepantalo M, Salenius JP et al. Influence of surgical experience on the results of carotid surgery. The Finnvasc Study Group. *Eur J Vasc Endovasc Surg* 1998; 15: 155-160.

19 Troeng T, Bergqvist D, Norrving B, Ahari A. Complications after carotid endarterectomy are related to surgical errors in less than one-fifth of cases. Swedvasc-The Swedish Vascular Registry and The Quality Committee for Carotid Artery Surgery. *Eur J Vasc Endovasc Surg* 1999; 18: 59-64.

20 Anonymous. European Carotid Surgery Trialist's Collaborative Group. MRC European carotid surgery trial: interim results for symptomatic patients with severe (70-99 %) or mild (0-29 %) carotid stenosis. *Lancet* 1991; 337: 1235-1243.

21 Branchereau A, Ondo N'Dong F, Bordeaux J, Sambuc R. Neurologic complications following carotid artery surgery: pathophysiology and predictive factors. *Ann Vasc Surg* 1986; 1: 79-85.

22 Branchereau A, Ondo N'Dong F, Scotti L. Mécanismes des complications neurologiques postopératoires en chirurgie carotidienne. In: Kieffer E, Natali J (eds). *Aspects techniques de la chirurgie carotidienne.* Paris, AERCV, 1987: pp 317-331.

23 Steed DL, Peitzman AB, Grundy BL, Webster MW. Causes of stroke in carotid endarterectomy. *Surgery* 1982; 92: 634-641.

24 Sundt TM Jr, Ebersold MJ, Sharbrough FW et al. The risk-benefit ratio of intraoperative shunting during carotid endarterectomy. Relevancy to operative and postoperative results and complications. *Ann Surg* 1986; 203: 196-204.

25 Riles TS, Imparato AM, Jacobowitz GR et al. The cause of perioperative stroke after carotid endarterectomy. *J Vasc Surg* 1994; 19: 206-220.

26 Ouriel K, Shortell CK, Illig KA et al. Intracerebral hemorrhage after carotid endarterectomy: incidence, contribution to neurologic morbidity, and predictive factors. *J Vasc Surg* 1999; 29: 82-89.

27 Radak D, Popovic AD, Radicevic S et al. Immediate reoperation for perioperative stroke after 2250 carotid endarterectomies: differences between intraoperative and early postoperative stroke. *J Vasc Surg* 1999; 30: 245-296.

28 Rockman CB, Jacobowitz GR, Lamparello PJ, et al. Immediate reexploration for the perioperative neurologic event after carotid endarterectomy: is it worthwhile? *J Vasc Surg* 2000; 32: 1062-1132.

29 Counsell CE, Salinas R, Naylor R, Warlow CP. A systematic review of the randomised trials of carotid patch angioplasty in carotid endarterectomy. *Eur J Vasc Endovasc Surg* 1997; 13: 345-699.

30 Taylor DW, Barnett HJ, Haynes RB et al. Low-dose and high-dose acetylsalicylic acid for patients undergoing carotid endarterectomy: a randomised controlled trial. ASA and Carotid Endarterectomy (ACE) Trial Collaborators. *Lancet* 1999; 353: 2179-2342.

31 Levison JA, Faust GR, Halpern VJ et al. Relationship of protamine dosing with postoperative complications of carotid endarterectomy. *Ann Vasc Surg* 1999; 13: 67-72.

32 Berguer R. Analyse critique des différentes méthodes de monitorage au cours de l'endartériectomie carotidienne. In: Branchereau A, Magnan PE (eds). *Méthodes de contrôle peroperatoire des restaurations vasculaires.* CVN, Marseille 1994: pp 179-184.

33 Moore WS, Yee JM, Hall AD. Collateral cerebral blood pressure. An index of tolerance to temporary carotid occlusion. *Arch Surg* 1973; 106: 521-524.

34 Connolly Jr ES, Salomon RA. Hyperperfusion syndrome following carotid endarterectomy In: Lofthus CM, Kresowik TF (eds). *Carotid artery surgery,* Thieme, New York, 2000: pp 493-500.

35 Jansen C, Sprengers AM, Moll FL et al. Prediction of intracerebral haemorrhage after carotid endarterectomy by clinical criteria and intraoperative transcranial doppler monitoring. *Eur J Vasc Surg* 1994; 8: 303-311.

36 Branchereau A, Pietri P, Magnan PE, Rosset E. Saphenous vein bypass: an alternative to internal carotid reconstruction. *Eur J Vasc Endovasc Surg* 1996; 12: 26-30.

37 Courbier R, Jausseran JM, Reggi M et al. Routine intraoperative carotid angiography: its impact on operative morbidity and carotid restenosis. *J Vasc Surg* 1986; 3: 343-393.

38 Donaldson MC, Ivarsson BL, Mannick JA, Whittemore AD. Impact of completion angiography on operative conduct and results of carotid endarterectomy. *Ann Surg* 1993; 217: 682-689.

39 Lohr JM, Albers B, Roat TW et al. Effects of completion angiography on the outcome of carotid endarterectomy. *Cardiovasc Surg* 1995; 3: 299-305.

40 Branchereau A, Ede B, Magnan PE, Rosset E. Value of angioscopy for intraoperative assessment of carotid endarterectomy. *Ann Vasc Surg* 1995; 9 Suppl: S67-75.

41 Zannetti S, Cao P, De Rango P et al. Intraoperative assessment of technical perfection in carotid endarterectomy: a prospective analysis of 1305 completion procedures. Collaborators of the EVEREST study group. Eversion versus standard carotid endarterectomy. *Eur J Vasc Endovasc Surg* 1999; 18: 52-60.

42 Bandyk DF, Kaebnick HW, Adams MB, Towne JB. Turbulence occuring after carotid bifurcation endarterectomy: a harbinger of residual and recurent carotid stenosis. *J Vasc Surg* 1988; 7: 261-274.

43 Kinney EV, Seabrook GR, Kinney LY et al. The importance of intraoperative detection of residual flow abnormalities after carotid artery endarterectomy. *J Vasc Surg* 1993; 17: 912-934.

13

131

14

CRITICAL ASPECTS OF CEREBROVASCULAR PROTECTION AND MONITORING DURING CAROTID SURGERY

JEAN-MICHEL JAUSSERAN, BERNARD LALANNE, RAYMOND PADOVANI
ANDRÉ MERY, NICOLAS VALERIO, MICHEL REGGI

Cerebral protection during carotid surgery comprises a multifactorial prevention with the aim of minimizing the risks of the surgical approach, arterial clamping, and restoration of the internal carotid artery (ICA) circulation. Owing to these measures, the surgical results are superior to medical treatment, as shown by the NASCET [1] and ECST [2] studies.

The occurrence of a stroke or transient ischemic attack (TIA) during the carotid procedure is caused by embolization during dissection or following declamping the carotid artery. The second cause of ischemia is determined by intracerebral hemodynamic disturbances due to the carotid clamping. Mechanisms to compensate for the carotid occlusion include anastomotic collateral pathways and cerebral circulatory autoregulation. The extra-intracerebral vascular network is provided by branches of the external carotid artery and plays a decisive role in chronic ICA occlusions. The intracerebral collateral network is essentially based on the circle of Willis, of which the functional value depends on the afferent supra-aortic arteries, the diameter and presence of communicating arteries, as well as potential atherosclerotic lesions in the supra-aortic arteries.

The cerebral circulation is accommodated with an autonomy related to the systemic circulation, stabilizing the cerebral blood flow (CBF) with arterial pressures ranging between 70 mmHg and 170 mmHg. The CBF is approximately 750 mL/min (15% of the total blood flow) or 52 to 56 mL per 100 g brain tissue per minute in a young adult. The cerebral circulation can decrease to 50% of normal values before ischemic dangers occur. A drop of 50%-80% can cause reversible ischemia, however, more than 80% induces irreversible damage with tissue necrosis. Carotid clamping contralateral to a chronic ICA occlusion exposes the brain to increased ischemia because the acute hypoperfusion is associated with occlusion of the collateral network via the external carotid artery. The formation of irreversible ischemia during clamping, potentially occurring at very low CBF (17-18mL/100g/min) is greatly depending on the duration of ischemia [4,5].

Preoperative assessment of ischemic risks

Preoperative assessment of ischemic risks is basically focused on the risk of carotid clamping. Contributing elements in this assessment are the degree of symptomatology (amourosis fugax, TIA, minor stroke) and the time period between the neurologic event and surgery [6].

Carotid compression tests under electroencephalographic (EEG) monitoring are no longer performed. Arteriography allows visualization of the cerebral vessels other than the target ICA, the intracerebral arteries and the polygon configuration of the circle of Willis. In the near future magnetic resonance angiography and three-dimensional scanning will allow similar assessment in a less invasive manner.

Cerebral contrast enhanced computer tomographic (CT) scanning can demonstrate non-healed ischemic lesions, characterized by a blushy contrast filling through the blood-brain barrier. In these circumstances, carotid clamping might aggravate the ischemic infarction and subsequent neurologic deficit. Nuclear medicine techniques like photon-emission-tomography and positron-emission-tomography provide accurate information on CBF and regional perfusion as well as metabolic activity in the different areas of the brain. The application is reserved for patients with stroke, and access to these techniques remains difficult and limited [7,8]. At present, ultrasonic techniques like continuous wave doppler, duplex scanning, and transcranial doppler (TCD) have an essential role in the evaluation of ischemic risks.

Duplex scanning enables one to diagnose a carotid lesion and to accurately assess the degree of stenosis [9]. A tight carotid stenosis observed by duplex scanning combined with patent flow in the ophtalmic artery carries a low cerebral ischemic risk during clamping. Plaque morphology can be analyzed by means of ultrasound, identifying soft and ulcerated lesions as well as floating thrombus, carrying a higher risk of embolization and subsequently guiding the surgeon in meticulous dissection. Biasi et al. [11] have performed a study with B-mode imaging, analyzing the plaque by the computer according to shades of grey, representing the different echogenicity of the different components of the plaque. They concluded that the morphology of the plaque and its echogenicity should be considered as a predictive factor for cerebral embolism and that this technique can be included in the therapeutic decision (surgery or angioplasty).

Transcranial doppler, feasible in up to 85% of patients because of problems with temporal bone penetration, constitutes an important technique to evaluate the intracerebral vascular network, especially for surgeons who do not perform preoperative angiography. Carotid compression during TCD allows one to evaluate the functionality of the polygon of Willis. Cerebrovascular reserve capacity can be assessed with ultrasound and pharmacologic provocation, providing potential information with regard to expected ischemic risks during carotid clamping. In patients operated under EEG monitoring, Pistolese et al. observed that clamping was poorly tolerated in 86% of patients who suffered from an impaired autoregulation as compared to 2.8% in patients with a preserved autoregulation [13].

Intra-operative monitoring

The intra-operative monitoring techniques can be divided in direct methods based on controlling cerebral function (consciousness, EEG, somatosensory evoked potentials [SSEP]) and indirect techniques assessing hemodynamic changes during ICA clamping and its subsequent cerebral metabolism.

MONITORING CONSCIOUSNESS

Local- or locoregional anesthesia permits the surgeon to determine the state of consciousness and motor function of the patient during the intervention, especially during clamping. This is obviously a simple and direct method, not requiring any equipment. It allows the surgeon to indicate the use of an intraluminal shunt if consciousness or motor function deteriorate. The series published in the literature do not show differences in mortality and morbidity between patients operated on with or without a shunt [14,15]. The studies using a shunt selectively under locoregional or general anesthesia have shown that a shunt was applied considerably less in patients under local anesthesia. In a series of 208 endarterectomies under regional anesthesia and EEG monitoring, Stoughton et al. [16] have demonstrated that the EEG carried a significant number of false positive (6.7%) and false negative (4.5%) results.

Locoregional anesthesia is a rather uncomfortable method for the surgeon, especially in noncooperative and anxious patients. We prefer to use general anesthesia in difficult cases, particularly if the surgical access requires cranial extension. For other authors, carotid endarterectomy under locoregional anesthesia is a psychological matter of safety, which should not be underestimated [17]. Locoregional anesthesia has not proven its superiority in patients with coronary artery disease, allowing more appropriate oxygenation and better neurovegetative protection. The same accounts for cerebral complications because general anesthesia permits the use of medication to reduce cerebral metabolism and to avoid reactive edema [18].

INTRA-OPERATIVE EEG MONITORING

EEG monitoring, one of the oldest techniques to assess cerebral function in patients operated under general anesthesia, is performed in a bipolar setting and registered on 16 or 20 channels. It is essential to start registration prior to induction of anesthesia in order to compare the pre- and postoperative EEG and evaluate possible changes induced by anesthetic drugs. In the experience of Pistolese et al. [19], the EEG is one of the most frequently applied techniques during carotid surgery, showing a 90% accuracy in the detection of cerebral ischemia. Carotid clamping can basically induce two types of EEG alterations: an amplitude decrease of the cerebral activity or an augmentation of the amplitude associated with a reduction of the fast-rhythm frequency.

These changes can appear at the ipsilateral or bilateral sides, usually within one minute after carotid clamping. If focal alterations occur not related to carotid clamping, embolization or thrombosis should be suspected. The electric modifications are considered as severe changes if the amplitude decreases more than 75% or delta activity increases. Several studies have shown the correlation between EEG changes and alterations of cerebral blood flow. We have demonstrated that no EEG changes occur if CBF remains higher than 23 mL/100g/min; that minor modifications appear if CBF lowers to 18-23 mL/100g/min and major alterations develop if CBF drops below 18 mL/100g/min [20]. All authors agree to stress the EEG modifications induced by barbiturates, which can distort the results [21].

EVOKED POTENTIALS

Monitoring SSEP is an accurate method to evaluate cerebral function [22], also enabling assessment of the responses of both hemispheres. SSEP are usually measured at the median nerve but the tibial nerve can also be used. Similar to EEG, it is important to start SSEP monitoring prior to anesthesia because responses can be influenced by anesthetic agents, like depression of evoked potentials by increased latency times or reduced amplitudes. During carotid clamping, the occurrence of cerebral ischemia is characterized by extension of the latency of the response to stimulation. These changes appear within the first five minutes after clamping, indicating a CBF decrease below 15 mL/100g/min. Three consecutive stimulations are necessary to confirm the delayed latency. Following a marked interest for SSEP during the last years it appears that many surgeons regain the preference for EEG monitoring [13]. In contrast to SSEP, the advantage of EEG is the rapid reaction to clamping or cerebral hemodynamic problems. The set-up and installation of EEG equipment is much easier than the SSEP technique.

STUMP PRESSURE

Measuring the stump pressure after clamping the external and common carotid artery reflects cerebral collateral hemodynamics. In 1969 Moore [23] demonstrated that a stump pressure below 25 mmHg was associated with an increased risk of cerebral ischemia. The threshold pressure level above which the intervention can be safely performed without a shunt is still a matter of debate.

Furthermore, this technique only provides an instantaneous measurement, not allowing continuous monitoring, thereby failing to notice hemodynamic changes. This method has been criticized because of the lack of correlation with other monitoring techniques. Whitley [24] has demonstrated that a stump pressure lower than 35 mmHg induced EEG changes in only 34% of patients. In contrast, if the stump pressure decreased below 25 mmHg, in only 25% of patients EEG readings remained normal. In a study of 443 patients operated under locoregional anesthesia, Fiorani et al. [25] have shown false positive and negative results in 2.7% and 8.8%, respectively. For the majority of surgeons this technique has only an indicative value and should be combined with modern monitoring techniques. We, however, still use stump pressure measurements and apply the following criteria for insertion of an intraluminal shunt: difference between the systemic pressure and stump pressure less than 100 mmHg as well as disappearance of the pulsatile pattern of the stump pressure curve. In practice we recommend to use a shunt in patients with a stump pressure below 40 mmHg or if the pulsatile pattern vanishes.

TRANSCRANIAL DOPPLER

The TCD monitors CBF at the middle cerebral artery during the procedure and detects flow alterations at the ipsilateral side. Due to limited penetration through the temporal bone, TCD can not be performed in 10%-20% of patients [12]. Comparative studies between TCD and EEG have shown an increased correlation if cerebral blood flow decreased below 70% with a sensitivity and specificity for TCD of 84% and 96%, respectively. The advantage of TCD is the rapid response to hemodynamic changes which precede EEG alterations [19].

In the experience of Visser et al. [26], TCD allows the surgeon to identify those patients in whom an intravascular shunt is not necessary. Another advantage of TCD is the ability to monitor the efficacy of the shunt and potential problems like kinking of the shunt or arterial thrombosis with subsequent collapse of CBF. Furthermore, TCD can detect micro-embolization during carotid endarterectomy. In a series of 76 patients undergoing carotid endarterectomy, Cantelmo et al. [27] have found signals corresponding to micro-embolization in 95% of cases. These signals appear during different phases of the procedure and correlate with the existence of parenchymatous lesions identified by magnetic resonance imaging. A recent study of Jordan et al. [28] described TCD monitoring during carotid surgery and angioplasty, showing an eight-fold increased embolization rate during angioplasty as compared to surgical treatment. The contribution of TCD in the early diagnosis of postoperative reperfusion injury enables immediate therapeutic action in the prevention of hemorrhagic complications [29].

MISCELLANEOUS MONITORING TECHNIQUES

Regional CBF can be studied after injection of Xenon 133 and allows identification of critical drops in flow during carotid clamping, however, the technique is difficult to apply. Surgeons who have used this technique have encountered an increase of 30%-40% in the insertion of a shunt. In the experience of Rehncrona et al [30], the Xenon 133-TCD technique did not provide intra-operative advantages as compared to continuous EEG registration. All noting together determines that these isotope techniques are no longer in clinical use. More recent methods are based on the study of cerebral oxymetry, which indirectly gathers information on oxygen concentration and cerebral metabolism. Oxygen saturation measurement of jugular blood is obtained by means of an optic fiber catheter positioned in the jugular vein that emits infrared light. This catheter assesses venous oxymetry during the intervention and the indication to insert a shunt is based on a decrease of venous saturation of more than 50%. The degree of saturation and clinical outcome do not always correlate and the oxygen saturation can not be modified if ischemia occurs: neurologic deficits have been observed with a oxygen saturation greater than 60% [31]. Cerebral oxymetry is performed with a probe which contains a transmitter and receiver of infrared beams, applied to the frontal region at the skull. It emits infrared beams which are transmitted to the cerebral cortex. The degree of absorption allows to calculate the concentration of oxygenated hemoglobine, desoxygenated hemoglobin, and cytochrome oxydasis. The concentration of oxydated cytochrome oxydasis is of particular interest because this metabolite represents the last level of electron transport. The latter is a very accurate evaluation of tissue oxygenation, comprising the potential value as an indicator of early anoxia. These promising techniques directly evaluating cerebral metabolism are currently under clinical investigation [32,33].

Methods of cerebral protection

CAROTID SHUNT

The use of an intraluminal shunt during carotid clamping represents an essential element of cerebral protection, solving the hemodynamic problems of the circulatory interruption [34].

The application of an internal shunt can be performed according to three different attitudes: systematic use, systematic refrain, and selective use. Thompson et al. [14] recommended systematic use, providing optimal cerebral protection. If the time to insert the shunt does not exceed two minutes, ischemic lesions are unlikely to develop. The shunt provides a flow of 100 to 300 mL/min, depending on the type of shunt. Javid et al. [35] propose four arguments to justify systematic use:

1 - reduction of ischemia-induced neurologic complications and improved cerebral hemodynamic protection,
2 - no time restraint, allowing an adequate surgical reconstruction,
3 - the complication rate caused by insertion of a shunt is very limited,
4 - the cost of a shunt is comparable to the costs of monitoring techniques or cerebral protection.

In a study comprising 1800 patients, Javid et al. were not able to insert a shunt in less than 1% of the patients.

The surgeons opposing the use of a shunt appeal to the technical difficulties related to the anatomy of the carotid bifurcation and the type of lesions as well as the potential complications: emboli or dissection and thrombosis of the shunt [36].

Our personal experience contains two comparable groups of 50 patients with a carotid stenosis having a stump pressure of less than 50 mmHg [37]. In the first series all patients where shunted and no neurologic deficit occurred. In the second series, intraluminal shunts were not applied and four patients (8%) developed a temporary neurologic deficit. In contrast, Whitney et al. [38] encountered a postoperative stroke rate of 1.6% and transient neurologic complications in 3.9% in 128 patients with a carotid stenosis and contralateral occlusion; they concluded that intolerance to clamping is a rare cause of stroke, even in patients with a contralateral occlusion, and that the use of a shunt is unnecessary.

Selective use of a shunt, proposed more than twenty years ago, seems to be the most appropriate strategy [23,39,40]. Imparato et al. [39] have recommended the following indications for the use of a shunt:

1 - intolerance to clamping as assessed by intra-operative monitoring techniques,
2 - contralateral ICA occlusion,
3 - impaired neurologic status with recent cerebral ischemia.

These criteria remain perfectly valid and are presently still applied.

INTRA-OPERATIVE HEPARINIZATION

Intra-operative heparinization during carotid surgery is performed at a dose of 50 to 100 UI/kg. Certain surgical teams administer 300 UI/kg as a single measure of cerebral protection, which is subsequently neutralized with protamine at the end of the procedure. Administration of low molecular weight heparine at a dose of 30 UI/kg is recommended by some authors [3], reporting a comparable complication rate as in heparinized patients: this strategy does not require the use of protamine.

ROLE OF GENERAL ANESTHESIA

General anesthesia favors cerebral protection, offering numerous advantages because it facilitates ventilatory control and oxygenation and reduces metabolic demands of the brain [3]. It is more comfortable for the patient and ameliorates the technical precision of the surgeon. Cerebral and myocardial protective agents can be administered and blood pressure control is significantly better as compared to locoregional anesthesia. Pistolese et al. [19] stated that general anesthesia assures superior cerebral pharmacologic protection, especially in patients with a compromised cerebral vasomotor activity.

MISCELLANEOUS MEASURES OF CEREBRAL PROTECTION

All elements of surgical techniques to improve the procedure and limit the neurologic complications should be included in the strategy for cerebral protection. Branchereau et al. [41] emphasize on the risk of embolization during dissection of the carotid bifurcation and recommend clamping of the ICA at the start of the carotid dissection. These suggestions have been confirmed in patients operated on with TCD monitoring [21], showing micro-embolization immediately after the start of the procedure. The

14

137

technical perfection of the surgical procedure remains an essential prerequisite for obtaining good results. The technique of eversion endarterectomy [42], which we have used since 1992 [43], appears to offer excellent anatomic results. The speed of the intervention and limited clamp time, which were positive factors in carotid surgery, are no longer considered as important determinants [44]. Intra-operative anatomic control to detect technical errors allows to correct defaults and reduces the early reintervention rate for thrombosis or residual stenosis. Intra-operative control can be performed by means of arteriography, duplex scanning or angioscopy. Courbier et al. [45] revised 5% of their reconstructions based on completion angiography and experienced a significant reduction of postoperative neurologic complications. Intra-operative duplex scanning, requiring large equipment in the surgical suite, is an excellent technique to assess the surgical intervention; however, duplex experience is mandatory.

Steinmetz et al. [46] describe four possible errors in increasing severity and recommend surgical revision in stages III and IV (tight stenoses and thromboses), comprising 2% of their experience.

Angioscopy is a reliable method of intra-operative control. Branchereau et al. [47] performed a comparative study between angioscopy and angiography and found a correlation rate of 94.1% and a false negative angioscopy in 5.9%.

Carotid angioplasty and cerebral protection

Carotid angioplasty carries a high risk of cerebral embolization during all phases of the procedures [48]. Jordan et al. [28] recently showed by means of TCD that the embolization rate of angioplasty was eight times higher than during carotid surgery. Several technical procedures have been developed to diminish the embolic risks during angioplasty, of which stent placement to anchor the embolic particles to the arterial wall is the most commonly used [49]. Théron et al. [50] were the pioneers of cerebral protection during angioplasty by means of an intra-carotid balloon. Several devices are currently used to improve the clinical outcome of angioplasties [51]. In a recent study, Henry et al. [52] only encountered one neurologic complication in 48 patients.

Conclusion

The extensive literature and multiplicity of the applied monitoring techniques emphasize the intensive psychological burden for the surgeon, especially now the international studies NASCET and ECST have proven the indisputable justification of the surgical procedure. Among protective measures we underline the intra-operative administration of heparin and performance of meticulous surgery, respecting selective indications. Furthermore, we advocate the use of selective shunting based on intra-operative monitoring and general anesthesia.

REFERENCES

1 Barnett HJ, Taylor DW, Eliasziw M et al. Benefit of carotid endarterectomy in patients with symptomatic moderate or severe stenosis. North American Symptomatic Carotid Endarterectomy Trial Collaborators (NASCET). N Engl J Med 1998; 339: 1415-1425.

2 Anonymous. European Carotid Surgery Trialists Collaborative Group. Randomised trial of endarterectomy for recently symptomatic carotid stenosis: final results of the MRC European Carotid Surgery Trial. Lancet 1998; 351: 1379-1387.

3 Thevenet A. Chirurgie des carotides. Editions techniques Encycl Med Chir (Paris, France). Techniques chirurgicales, Chirurgie Vasculaire 43140, 9-1990: p 5.

4 Boysen G, Engell HC, Pistolese GR et al. On the critical lower level of cerebral blood flow in man with particular reference to carotid surgery. Circulation 1974; 49: 1023-1025.

5 Norris JW, Krajewski A, Bornstein NM. The clinical role of cerebral collateral circulation in carotid occlusion. J Vasc Surg 1990; 12: 113-118.

6 Courbier R. Classification des maladies artérielles cérébro-vasculaires In: Kieffer E (ed). Indications et résultats de la chirurgie carotidienne. AERCV, Paris 1988, pp 17-24.

7 Lewis DH, Cohen WA, Kuntz CD, Winn HR. White matter is ischemia on brain SPECT. J Nucl Med 1994; 35: 1476-1481.

8 Soricelli A, Postiglione A, Cuocolo A et al. Effect of adenosine on cerebral blood flow as evaluated by single-photon emission computed tomography in normal subjects and in patients with occlusive carotid disease. A comparison with acetazolamide. Stroke 1995; 26: 1572-1578.

9 Griewing B, Morgenstern C, Driesner F et al. Cerebrovascular disease assessed by color-flow and power doppler ultrasonography. Comparison with digital substraction angiography in internal carotid stenosis. Stroke 1996; 27: 95-100.

10 Park AE, McCarthy WJ, Pearce WH et al. Carotid plaque morphology correlates with presenting symptomatology. J Vasc Surg 1998; 27: 872-879.

11 Biasi GM, Mingazzini P, Baronio L et al. Carotid plaque characterization using digital image processing and its potential in future studies of carotid endarterectomy and angioplasty. J Endovasc Surg 1998; 5: 240-246.

12 Benichou H, Bergeron P, Ferdani M et al. Doppler transcranien pré et peropératoire: prévision et surveillance de la tolérance au clampage carotidien. *Ann Chir Vasc* 1991; 5: 21-25.

13 Pistolese GR, Appolloni AL, Ronchey S. Techniche di monitorragio cérébrale in chirurgia carotida. In: Chiesa R, Melissano G (eds). *La chirurgia dei tronchi sopra aortici*. Europa Scienze Umane Editrice, Milano 1997; pp 238-246.

14 Thompson JE. Carotid endarterectomy, 1982. The state of the art. *Br J Surg* 1983; 70: 371-376.

15 Sundt TM Jr, Ebersold MJ, Sharbrough FW et al. The risk-benefit ratio of intra-operative shunting during carotid endarterectomy. Revelancy to operative and postoperative results and complications. *Ann Surg* 1986; 203: 196-204.

16 Stoughton J, Nath RL, Abbott WM. Comparison of simultaneous electroencephalographic and mental status monitoring during carotid endarterectomy with regional anesthesia. *J Vasc Surg* 1998; 28: 1014-1023.

17 Love A, Hollyoak MA. Carotid endarterectomy and local anesthesia: reducing the disasters. *Cardiovasc Surg* 2000; 8: 429-435.

18 Berguer R. Analyse critique des différentes méthodes de monitorage au cours de l'endartériectomie carotidienne. In: Branchereau A, Magnan PE (eds). *Méthodes de contrôle peropératoire des restaurations vasculaires*. CVN, Marseille 1994; pp 179-184.

19 Pistolese GR, Appolloni A, Ronchey S et al. Update on cerebral monitoring and protective methods. *Ann Ital Chir* 1997; 68: 441-451.

20 McGrail KM. Intra-operative use of electroencephalography as an assessment of cerebral blood flow. *Neurosurg Clin N Am* 1996; 7: 685-692.

21 Arnold M, Sturzenegger M, Schaffler L, Sciler RW. Continuous intra-operative monitoring of middle cerebral artery blood flow velocities and electroencephalography during carotid endarterectomy. A comparison of the two methods to detect cerebral ischemia. *Stroke* 1997 Jul; 28: 1345-1350.

22 Horsch S, Ktenidis K. Intra-operative use of somatosensory evoked potentials for brain monitoring during carotid surgery. *Neurosurg Clin N Am* 1996; 7: 693-702.

23 Moore WS, Hall AD. Carotid artery back pressure: a test of cerebral tolerance to temporary carotid occlusion. *Arch Surg* 1969; 99: 702-710.

24 Whitley D, Cherry KJ Jr. Predictive value of carotid artery stump pressure during carotid endarterectomy. *Neurosurg Clin N Am* 1996; 7: 723-732.

25 Fiorani P, Sbarigia E, Speziale F et al. General anaesthesia versus cervical block and perioperative complications in carotid artery surgery. *Eur J Vasc Endovasc Surg* 1997; 13 : 37-42.

26 Visser GH, Wieneke GH, Van Huffelen AC, Eikelboom BC. The use of preoperative transcranial doppler variables to predict wich patients do not need a shunt during carotid endarterectomy. *Eur J Vasc Endovasc Surg* 2000; 19: 226-232.

27 Cantelmo NL, Babikian VL, Samaraweera RN et al. Cerebral microembolism and ischemic changes associated with carotid endarterectomy. *J Vasc Surg* 1998; 27: 1024-1031.

28 Jordan WD Jr, Voellinger DC, Doblar DD et al. Microemboli detected by transcranial doppler monitoring in patients during carotid angioplasty versus carotid endarterectomy. *Cardiovasc Surg* 1999; 7: 33-38.

29 Dalman JE, Beenakkers JC, Moll FL et al. Transcranial doppler monitoring during carotid endarterectomy helps to identify patients at risk of postoperative hyperperfusion. *Eur J Vasc Endovasc Surg* 1999; 18: 222-227.

30 Rehncrona S, Algotsson L. Mesure du débit sanguin cérébral au cours de la chirurgie carotidienne. In: Branchereau A, Magnan PE (eds). *Méthodes de contrôle peropératoire des restaurations vasculaires*. CVN, Marseille 1994; pp 121-128.

31 Chan KH, Miller JD, Dearden NM et al. The effect of changes in cerebral perfusion pressure upon middle cerebral artery blood flow velocity and jugular bulb venous oxygen saturation after severe brain injury. *J Neurosurg* 1992; 77: 55-61.

32 Samra SK, Dy EA, Welch K et al. Evaluation of a cerebral oximeter as a monitor of cerebral ischemia during carotid endarterectomy. *Anesthesiology* 2000; 93: 964-970.

33 De Letter JA, Sie TH, Moll FL et al. Transcranial cerebral oximetry during carotid endarterectomy: agreement between frontal and lateral probe measurements as compared with an electroencephalogram. *Cardiovasc Surg* 1988; 6: 373-377.

34 Halsey JH Jr. Risks and benefits of shunting in carotid endarterectomy. The International Transcranial Doppler Collaborators. *Stroke* 1992; 23: 1583-1587.

35 Javid H. Intraluminal shunting during carotid endoarterectomy. In: Bergan JJ, Yao JST (eds). *Cerebrovascular insufficiency*. Grune et Stratton, New York 1982: pp 309-325.

36 Moore WS. Selective shunting of the carotid artery: an overview. In: Moore WS (ed) *Surgery for cerebrovascular disease*. Churchill Livingstone, New-York 1987; pp 475-476.

37 Jausseran JM, Lalanne B, Bergeron P et al. Les indications du shunt intra-luminal en chirurgie carotidienne. *J Chir* 1987; 124: 459-463.

38 Whitney EG, Brophy CM, Kahn EM, Whitney DG. L'intolérance au clampage carotidien: une cause rare d'accident vasculaire cérébral péri-opératoire. *Ann Chir Vasc* 1997; 11: 109-114.

39 Imparato AM, Ramirez A, Riles T, Mintzer R. Cerebral protection in carotid surgery. *Arch Surg* 1982; 117: 1073-1078.

40 Sundt TM, Sharbrough FW. The use of electroencephalographic monitoring to determine shunt requirement. In: Moore WS (ed). *Surgery for cerebrovascular disease*. Churchill Livingstone, New York 1987: pp 481-489.

41 Branchereau A, Ondo N'Dong F, Bordeaux J, Sambuc R. Complications neurologiques de la chirurgie carotidienne; mécanismes et facteurs prédictifs. *Ann Chir Vasc* 1986; 1: 79-85.

42 Vanmaele RC, Van Schil PE, DeMaeseneer MG et al. Endarteriectomy and remplantation for carotid stenosis In: Chang JB (ed). *Modern vascular surgery*, Vol 6. Springer Verlag, New York 1994: pp 85-95.

43 Jausseran JM, Ferdani M, Houel F et al. Endartériectomie carotidienne par éversion. *J Mal Vasc* Paris 1998; 23: 7-12.

44 Jausseran JM, Lalanne B, Bergeron P et al. Protection cérébrale en chirurgie carotidienne. Le rôle du shunt intraluminal. Résultats d'une enquête nationale. *Presse Med* 1998; 17: 428-431.

45 Courbier R, Jausseran JM, Reggi M et al. Routine intra-operative carotid angiography: its impact on operative morbidity and carotid restenosis. *J Vasc Surg* 1986; 3: 343-350.

46 Steinmetz OK, MacKenzie K, Nault P et al. Intra-operative duplex scanning for carotid endarterectomy. *Eur J Vasc Endovasc Surg* 1998; 16: 153-158.

47 Branchereau A, Ede B, Magnan PE, Rosset E. Contrôle angioscopique de l'endartériectomie carotidienne. In Branchereau A, Magnan PE (eds). *Méthodes de contrôle peropératoire des restaurations vasculaires*. CVN, Marseille 1994: pp 169-177.

48 Coggia M, Goëau-Brissonnière O, Duval JL et al. Embolic risk of the different stages of carotid bifurcation balloon angioplasty: an experimental study. *J Vasc Surg* 2000; 31: 550-557.

49 Bergeron P, Chambran P, Benichou H, Alessandri C. Recurrent carotid disease: will stents be an alternative to surgery? *J Endovasc Surg* 1996; 3: 76-79.

50 Théron J, Courtheoux P, Alachkar F et al. New triple coaxial catheter system for carotid angioplasty with cerebral protection. *Am J Neuroradiol* 1990; 11: 869-877.

51 Ohki T, Roubin GS, Veith FJ et al. Efficacy of a filter device in the prevention of embolic events during carotid angioplasty and stenting: an ex vivo analysis. *J Vasc Surg* 1999; 30: 1034-1044.

52 Henry M, Amor M, Henry I et al. Carotid stenting with cerebral protection: first clinical experience using the PercuSurge Guard Wire system. *J Endovasc Surg* 1999; 6: 321-331.

14

139

15

CRANIAL NERVE INJURY
AFTER CAROTID ARTERY SURGERY

MASSIMO D'ADDATO, MICHELE MIRELLI

Peripheral cranial nerve injuries after carotid artery surgery are frequently neglected in clinical experience and are rarely subject to clinical studies. The prevalence of these complications is quite variable: literature reports vary between 3% and 80% [1,2]. The variability of these data depends on the retrospective or prospective character of the study, and the sensitivity of the diagnostic techniques applied in the pre- and postoperative evaluation of the cranial nerves. The anatomical complexity of the neck and the close anatomic relations between the carotid bifurcation and the cranial nerves explain the high incidence of neural lesions after carotid artery surgery. A profound knowledge of the surgical anatomy together with a meticulous surgical skill are paramount in the prevention of complications due to cranial nerve damage.

Facial nerve, VII (Fig. 1)

The facial nerve, which emerges trough the stylomastoid foramen, splits into the posterior auricular nerve (the motor nerve of the auricular muscles and the occipital part of the occipitofrontal muscle, and the sensory nerve of the skin of the auricle), the digastric nerve (the motor nerve of the stylohyoid muscle and posterior belly of the digastric muscle), and finally into the temporofacial and cervicofacial branches.

The cervicofacial branch, which suffers most frequently from iatrogenic lesions, emerges from the anterior side of the parotid gland, proceeds forward between the masseter muscle and the ascending branch of the mandible, crosses the facial artery and vein, and innervates through its facial part the lower lip and the muscles of the corner of the mouth. The cervical part innervates the platysma muscle.

Clinical manifestations of cervicofacial branch lesions are weakness of the corner of the mouth, possibly with loss of saliva and accidental biting of the lower lip. The neurologic deficit may be confused with a central facial paralysis, which mainly affects the upper lip. The position of the head during surgery (hyperextension and rotation) pulls down the cervicofacial branch, which may cause a direct lesion of this nerve while approaching the carotid artery. Such a lesion may be due to transection of the nerve in case of a high incision of the skin, traction or compression from the retractor, or electrocoagulation. In their experience with carotid endarterectomy under local anesthesia, Imparato et al. found that anesthetizing the cervical skin could also cause damage to this nerve [3]. The incidence of this complication varies in the literature between 0% and 12.5% [1-15] (Tables I and II). The prognosis is good, as it is nearly always a temporary lesion. Hertzer et al. found restoration within 12 months in all cases [4].

The lesions of the posterior auricular nerve and the nerves to the digastric and stylohyoid muscles, which may occur when approaching a high carotid bifurcation, are rare and clinically unsuspicious.

Prevention of damage to the mandibular branch of the facial nerve requires some precautionary techniques, for example:
- do not use a transverse incision to approach the carotid bifurcation;

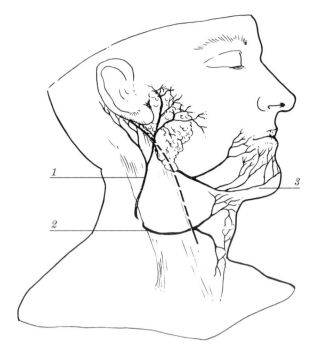

1. Great auricular nerve
2. Transverse cervical nerve
3. Mandibular branch of the facial nerve

FIG. 1 Cutaneous nerves of the cervical plexus and mandibular branch of the facial nerve.

Table I	INCIDENCE OF PERIPHERAL NERVE LESIONS AFTER CAROTID ENDARTERECTOMY IN THE LITERATURE (PROSPECTIVE STUDIES)									
1st author [ref.]	*Publication year*	*Number of patients*	*VII*	*IX*	*X Inf*	*XSup*	*XII*	*Aur*	*Σ*	*Total*
Hertzer [4]	1980	240	2.5		5.8	2.1	5.4			16
Liapis [5]	1981	40	5		27		20	7.5		59
Evans [6]	1982	128		1.5	35		11			47
Astor [7]	1983	133			5.9	1.3	5.8			13
Forsell [8]	1985	162	0.6	1.2	3.1		10.5	6.8	1.2	23
Aldoori [2]	1988	52	5.8		5.8		15.8	42		69
Forsell [9]	1995	689		0.3	1.2	0.3	10.7			12
Ballotta [10]	1995	200	1		4	1	5.5	1		12
Schauber [11]	1997	183	1.1		7.7		4.4	1.1		14

X inf: inferior or recurrent laryngeal nerve
X sup: superior laryngeal nerve
Aur: great auricular nerve
Σ: cervical sympathetic chain

| Table II | INCIDENCE OF PERIPHERAL NERVE DAMAGE AFTER CAROTID ENDARTERECTOMY IN THE LITERATURE (RETROSPECTIVE STUDIES) | | | | | | | | | |

| 1st author [ref.] | Publication year | Number of patients | Incidence of peripheral nerve damage in % | | | | | | | Total |
			VII	IX	X Inf	XSup	XII	Aur	Σ	
Ranson [12]	1969	267	11.2		1.1		4.1		2.2	19
Krupski [13]	1985	300	2.3		7.7		4.3	2.7	0.3	17
D'Addato [14]	1987	300	3	0.6	4		9.3	1.6		18
Maniglia [15]	1991	336	2.4		6		4.8			13

X inf: inferior or recurrent laryngeal nerve
X sup: superior laryngeal nerve
Aur: great auricular nerve
Σ: cervical sympathetic chain

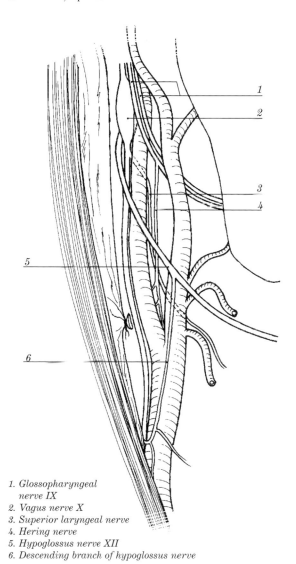

1. Glossopharyngeal
   nerve IX
2. Vagus nerve X
3. Superior laryngeal nerve
4. Hering nerve
5. Hypoglossus nerve XII
6. Descending branch of hypoglossus nerve

FIG. 2 Deep cervical nerves exposed during carotid endarterectomy.

- push the upper part of the longitudinal skin incision backward towards the ear;
- perform hemostasis by compression and ligation instead of electrocoagulation.

Glossopharyngeal nerve, IX
(Fig. 2)

This nerve emerges from the skull through the jugular foramen and advances upwards and forwards while making a concave curve. It progresses between the internal jugular vein and the carotid artery around the vagal nerve, then between the internal and external carotid arteries, and finally between the styloglossal and stylopharyngeal muscles to arrive at the base of the tongue. It contains:
- sensory fibers for the pharynx, auditory canals, the middle ear, the tonsils, and the posterior parts of the tongue;
- motor fibers for the striated muscle of the pharynx;
- parasympathetic fibers for the parotid gland.

The incidence of complications in the literature (prospective studies) varies between 0% and 1.5% [4,6] (Table I). As with the facial nerve, the highest incidence occurs in high dissections of the internal carotid artery and when a subluxation of the mandible is conducted. After this procedure Sandmann et al. [16] as well as Sekhar et al. [17] found an incidence of the IXth cranial nerve lesions in 52% and 45% of the cases, respectively. In one prospective study performed in 12 patients, the pharyngeal function was analyzed by means of cineradiography before and after surgery and showed the presence of a pharyngeal dysfunction in five cases (40%) of which two were permanent [18]. These neural lesions occurred more frequently in patients operated on using a shunt, which requires a more extensive dissection and traction.

Clinically a unilateral lesion of the IXth cranial nerve may be silent, while a bilateral lesion causes dysphagia and false routing. When symptomatic, it causes nasal regurgitations, hypersalivation, and rhinolalia. Objectively it is characterized by a hemiparalysis of the soft palate. In general, patients present this lesion after an extended upward access of the internal carotid artery beyond the digastric muscle. In this situation, however, it is difficult to know whether the cause of these troubles is due to a lesion of the IXth cranial nerve, sympathetic fibers of the Xth, or even of the XIIth cranial nerve.

The Hering nerve, the important collateral branch of the glossopharyngeal nerve innervating the carotid sinus, is located in the carotid bifurcation. Lesions of this nerve may provoke fluctuations in the arterial blood pressure and heart rate. To prevent episodes of hypertension or bradycardia during surgery, it is wise to infiltrate the carotid bifurcation with a local anesthetic. The baroreceptor function after surgery has been studied by various authors. Dehn and Angell-James [19] showed an increased baroreceptor function in 32% of the cases, a decreased function in 8%, and no change in 60% of the cases. Hirschl et al. [20] found an increased baroreceptor function after carotid endarterectomy in 50% of the hypertensive patients, while the normotensive patients did not show any significant change in blood pressure.

Vagus nerve, X (Fig. 2)

The vagus nerve leaves the skull through the jugular foramen, forms the inferior vagal ganglion and proceeds in the neck behind and around the internal and common carotid arteries in the plane formed by these arteries and the internal jugular vein. The vagal nerve may show an abnormal anatomical path: in about 2% of the cases it runs anteriorly to the carotid artery [1,21]. From the terminal part of the inferior ganglion emerge pharyngeal branches, which form a plexus together with the branches from the glossopharyngeal nerve, close to the pharyngeal wall.

From the cervical part of the Xth cranial nerve originates the superior laryngeal nerve, which sub-

divides into two branches at the level of the hyoid cartilage: one external and one internal branch. The external branch, which has a diameter of about 1 to 2 mm, shows a variable course. In 70% of the cases it runs through the visceral sheath, while in 30% it is located on the pretracheal sheath, in close relation with the superior thyroid artery. This external, motor branch innervates the lower pharyngeal sphincter muscle and the cricothyroid muscle of the larynx, while the internal, sensory branch innervates the laryngeal mucosa. The role of the cricothyroid muscle of the larynx is to fine-tune the vocal cords to emit high sounds.

From the thoracic part of the vagal nerve originates the inferior laryngeal nerve (or recurrent laryngeal nerve), which crosses below the right subclavian artery and the aortic arch and runs along the oesophagotracheal fossa up to the larynx to innervate all its other intrinsic muscles. Upon contraction of these muscles the vocal cords are thickened to produce low sounds. In rare cases the inferior laryngeal nerve may originate from the cervical part of the vagal nerve, near the carotid bifurcation, which increases the risk of a direct trauma. From this nerve, as well as from the cervical part of the vagal nerve, emerge cardiac nerves. A lesion of these can cause postoperative tachycardia. According to the literature, the incidence of superior laryngeal nerve lesions varies between 0% and 2% [4,8]. They occur during carotid access or clamping. Ligation and transection of the superior thyroid artery, as proposed by Verta et al. [22] to improve mobilization of the external carotid artery, increases the risk of traumatizing the nerve. Lesions of the vagal nerve may occur in any operation area during preparation of vessels or due to poor usage of wound retractors. The branches of the pharyngeal plexus contain motor fibers for the sphincter muscles of the pharynx and lesions of these collateral branches may cause serious dysphagia.

Lesions of the superior laryngeal nerve are insidious and symptoms are often difficult to diagnose. Disturbances subjectively present with a change in quality and weakness of the voice and difficulty producing high tones, which can be particularly clear while singing. Objectively it presents with a reduced sensibility of the laryngeal orifice and a paralysis and median position of the ipsilateral vocal cord. These symptoms are essentially transitory, and usually recover completely within 12 months after surgery [4]; however, they may also be permanent [23,24].

Lesions of the recurrent laryngeal nerve cause a paralysis and paramedian position of the ipsilateral vocal cord due to an insufficiency of the complete intrinsic musculature of the larynx, except for the cricothyroid muscle. Clinically the disturbance of the recurrent laryngeal nerve is responsible for a severe dysphonia with a bitonal or hoarse, weak voice accompanied by a rapid tiredness of speech. The dysphonia may be accompanied by hoarseness with loss of the coughing mechanism. Finally, the lesion may be asymptomatic or may pass unnoticed. The latter possibility is particularly dangerous in case of bilateral surgery, as the bilateral character of such a lesion may provoke a complete obstruction of the airway. Hence, it is important to conduct an ENT investigation of the vocal cords before performing surgery on the second side. Damage to the vagal nerve and its branches occurs most often after reinterventions or in cases of periarterial infection or fibrosis. In these circumstances exposition of the vessels should be performed meticulously in order to avoid neural damage. Preparation of the carotid bulb in particular should be done as close to the arterial wall as possible [21]. Isolation and clamping of the superior thyroid artery should be conducted very attentively.

Damage to the superior laryngeal nerve may pass unnoticed if one does not actively search for it. Prospective studies showed these lesions have a low incidence, in the order of 0% to 2% [4,8]. Other prospective studies showed that the incidence of lesions of the recurrent laryngeal nerve vary between 1.5% and 35% [6]. This large variability can be explained by the different pre- and postoperative diagnostic techniques used in the different studies. The studies by Evans et al. [6] and Liapis et al. [5] presented the highest incidences (27% and 35%, respectively) of these lesions, which were diagnosed by means of clinical examination and spectral voice analysis before and after surgery. Forssel et al. used voice recording and stroboscopic vocal cord examination and found recurrent laryngeal nerve lesions in 1.2% of the patients [8]. While this lesion could present minimal symptoms or none at all, postoperative dysphonia as single diagnostic criterion identifies only the clearly symptomatic cases, irrespective of the kind of retrospective studies. One should be aware that voice changes after carotid surgery may be provoked by other causes than nerve lesions. Actually, postoperative speech problems may also be due to a tracheal intubation trauma or a direct trauma with hematoma formation of the

larynx following the use of autostatic retractors [25]. Damage to the vagal nerve may be due to crushing of the nerve by inadvertent clamping or by compression through a retractor or a hematoma. In case of a nerve lesion above the origin of the superior laryngeal nerve, laryngoscopy shows a weak adduction of the ipsilateral vocal cord. A more distal lesion initially yields the same laryngoscopic findings, but eventually abduction of the vocal cord will occur due to compensation by the superior laryngeal nerve.

Like the lesions of the VIIth and IXth cranial nerve, preparation of the vessels close to the base of the skull increases the risk of vagus nerve lesions, especially in case of subluxation of the mandible. Sandmann et al. [16] and Sekhar et al. [17] found vagus lesions in 23% and 43%, respectively.

The majority of patients who present damage of the vagus nerve or its branches show a spontaneous recovery of symptoms [2,4]. As opposed to the majority of authors, Imparato et al. [3] and AbuRahma et al. [26] confirmed that persistence of a paralysis of one vocal cord of more than 4 months indicates an irreversible lesion, for which an injection of a plastic substance into the vocal cord would be useful.

Accessory nerve, XI

The eleventh pair of cranial nerves emerge from the jugular foramen and divides into an internal branch (efferent preganglionary visceral fibers) and an external branch. The latter passes beneath the posterior belly of the digastric muscle, runs laterally towards the internal side of the sternocleidomastoid muscle and through the occipital triangle, and reaches the internal side of the trapezius muscle. This external, motor branch innervates the trapezius muscle, which is also innervated by the cervical plexus.

A lesion of this nerve, which is rare in carotid endarterectomies (Table I), is due to transection, compression of the nerve by means of retractors, or an electrical trauma when the anterior side of the sternocleidomastoid muscle is mobilized close to its mastoid insertion. Tucker et al. [27] have described some cases of late postoperative lesions, which appeared 20 to 60 days after surgery, supposedly due to postoperative fibrosis. The lesion becomes manifest clinically through a paralysis of the sternocleidomastoid muscle and paresis of the trapezius muscle. The latter is accompanied by an ipsilateral dropping shoulder with a painful acromioclavicular joint, which is often the first symptom reported by the patients.

Hypoglossus nerve, XII (Fig. 2)

It emerges from the hypoglossal canal, runs between the internal jugular vein and the internal carotid artery with a forward and upward curve, and passes before the external carotid artery close to the digastric muscle towards the base of the tongue. Here, it innervates the muscles of the ipsilateral half of the tongue. Generally, it passes 2 to 5 cm above the carotid bifurcation and is rarely located near the bifurcation itself. Below and slightly in front of the carotid bifurcation it yields the descending branch, which anastomosis through a loop with a branch of the superficial cervical plexus and innervates the infrahyoidal muscles. In case of a high carotid bifurcation, a short neck or distal carotid lesions, it may be necessary to transect the digastric muscle at the level of its tendon and to mobilize the hypoglossal nerve. This mobilization requires division of the descending branch, which should take place close to the origin in order to avoid damage to the motor innervation of the infrahyoidal muscles. During this maneuver it is useful to ligate and transect the descending branch of the XIIth nerve, the sternocleidomastoid artery and vein, and the venous plexus around the nerve. A lesion of this nerve may actually be caused by direct traction or indirectly by ligation or electrocoagulation of its venous plexus.

Clinically unilateral damage to this nerve causes a contralateral deviation of the tongue, disartria, and chewing difficulties. In case of bilateral damage in patients who underwent bilateral carotid endarterectomy within a short interval, an airway obstruction due to weakness of the lingual muscles may occur in the patient in the supine position [28]. This deficit, when attributable to reversible lesions, always restores within 12 months after surgery [9]. The incidence of this complication varies in the literature between 1.2% and 15% [1,2] (Table I), but in some studies it is as high as 20% [5]. Permanent lesions of the XIIth cranial nerve are rare and in the majority of cases the symptoms recede in the four to six months following the intervention.

Cervical plexus (Fig. 1)

The cutaneous branches of the cervical plexus that may be involved are the great auricular and transverse cervical nerve. The great auricular nerve originates from the second and third cervical nerves. After having crossed the deep cervical aponeurosis it appears on the outer side of the sternocleidomastoid muscle while running upwards from its posterior to its anterior side beneath the platysma colli muscle. At the level of the mandibular angle it subdivides into an anterior branch (for the skin in the parotid region) and a posterior branch (for the skin of the auricle and mastoid region).

Damage to this nerve may occur directly by transection through a longitudinal or high transversal cervical incision, or indirectly by electrocoagulation of the veins around the nerve. Clinically it becomes manifest by a hypestesia or anesthesia of the auricle and the posteroinferior part of the cheek.

The transverse cervical nerve emerges from the cervical plexus, runs forward and crosses horizontally the lateral side of the sternocleidomastoid muscle beneath the platysma colli muscle. This is the sensory nerve to the skin of the supra and infrahyoidal region. Damage to this nerve, inevitable with longitudinal incisions laterally in the neck along the anterior side of the sternocleidomastoid muscle, results in an area of anesthesia located within the area of the cutaneous incision. The incidence of lesions of branches of the cervical plexus varies in the literature between 0% and 7.5% [4,5]. Some prospective studies describe a much higher incidence of 42% [19] to 60% [30] for great auricular nerve lesions, and from 69% [19] to 89% [29] for transverse cervical nerve lesions. The deficit recedes completely in the majority of the cases in the 6 to 12 months following the intervention. The disturbance persists in 20% of the patients [19].

Cervical sympathetic chain

Anterior to the long neck muscle and posterior to the large vessels, the cervical sympathetic nerve runs from the base of the skull (external orifice of the carotid canal) to the anterior side of the posterior third of the first rib. Its damage is very rare in carotid endarterectomy and is manifested clinically by a Horner's syndrome. Its incidence in the literature varies between 0.3% and 2.2% [12,13]

Discussion

Lesions of the cranial nerves after carotid surgery occur frequently, but can be avoided easily. The neurological deficits that result are reversible in the majority of cases in the weeks or months following surgery. The etiopathology of the peripheral nerve lesions determines the clinical evolution of the postoperative neurological deficit. Different degrees of nerve lesions correspond with different traumatic mechanisms, which are reflected by the classification as proposed by Sunderland [30]. Traction, compression, electrocoagulation, destruction by a clamp during surgery, or postoperative hematoma formation cause ischemia or mechanical deformation of the axons and are responsible for a temporary neurologic deficit (first, second or third degree lesions according to Sunderland's classification). In such cases clinical restoration may occur after a period of several weeks or months. In contrast, ligation or transection of a nerve causes a permanent deficit which is, from an pathoanatomical point of view, characterized by a degeneration of axons at the site of the lesion (neuroma proximally and glioma distally) as well as a wallerian degeneration of the distal end (fourth and fifth degree lesion according to Sunderland's classification).

The neural formations most frequently affected are the great auricular nerve, the hypoglossus nerve (XII), the mandibular branch of the facial nerve (VII), the vagus nerve (X), and the recurrent laryngeal nerve. Less frequently, a deficit is observed of the superior laryngeal nerve, the glossopharyngeus nerve (IX), and accessory nerve (XI). Lesions of peripheral nerves during carotid endarterectomy depends on different factors, like anomalies of the course of the nerve, the kind of access, and the technique used (Fig. 3).

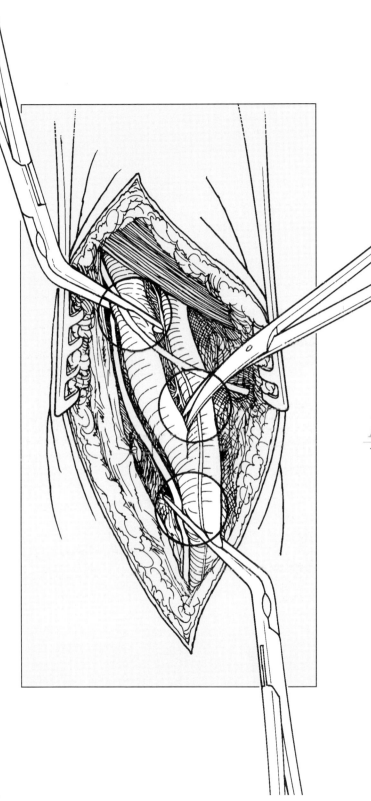

FIG. 3 Causes of peripheral nerve damage during carotid endarterectomy.

ABNORMAL COURSE

Anomalies of the course result in preoperative lesions of the recurrent laryngeal and hypoglossus nerves. In some cases, indeed, these nerves are closely related to the carotid bifurcation. This is the reason why the phase of the dissection of the carotid arteries comprises a particular risk of nerve damage.

The recurrent laryngeal nerve, which usually originates from the thoracic portion of the vagus nerve, sometimes emerges from the cervical portion in the neighborhood of the carotid bifurcation. In this anatomically unusual situation along the posterior side of the common carotid artery, it may easily be damaged due to maneuvers to expose the vessels.

The hypoglossus nerve is normally located between 2 and 5 cm above the carotid bifurcation. In some cases this nerve descends down close to the carotid bifurcation where it can easily be damaged. Moreover, the hypoglossus nerve is bridled and fixed by small venous plexus, by its descending branch, by the sternocleidomastoid artery and vein, and by the occipital artery. Because mobilization of the hypoglossus nerve can occur by simple traction, a temporary paresis of the hemitongue may occur postoperatively. Traction without mobilization causes a lesion due to nerve compression which may lead to a first, second or third degree lesion, according to Sunderland's classification. Hence, mobilization of the nerve by ligation and transection of the venous plexus and perineural vessels has an important prophylactic value.

In some cases an aberrant course may also provoke a lesion of the vagus nerve. This nerve is usually located behind the common carotid artery, but may sometimes be in front of and around it, as well as around the internal jugular vein. This location facilitates direct preoperative damage.

SURGICAL ACCESS

The route of access plays an important role in the occurrence of lesions of the mandibular branch of the facial nerve and the cutaneous nerves of the cervical plexus. The anatomical localization and the superficiality of these nerves makes them vulnerable to transection or compression by a retractor. The laterocervical surgical access route may be transverse or, more often, longitudinal. The different risks of a postoperative neurologic deficit depend on the route of access. The transverse approach facilitates transection of the great auricular nerve as well as compression by a retractor of the mandibular branch of the facial nerve. In contrast, the lon-

gitudinal approach always facilitates transection of the transverse cervical nerve and may also ease transection of the great auricular nerve, and sometimes even the mandibular branch of the facial nerve. The surgical position (hyperextension of the neck with rotation of the head) is very important because, while moving the facial nerve downward, it facilitates its transection in case of a high cutaneous incision. The incidence of this lesion may be reduced by modifying the longitudinal access route in that the upper part of the cutaneous incision is directed backward towards the mastoid process and the auricle.

Access routes extended upwards to the level of the subparotideal space increase the risk of complications at the level of the cranial nerves, in particular the IXth and Xth.

SURGICAL TECHNIQUE

The application of retractors, hemostasis, preparation of vessels, carotid clamping and the need for reintervention play a fundamental role in the occurrence of various cranial nerve lesions. The legs of a retractor may cause a compression lesion of the great auricular nerve, the mandibular branch of the facial nerve, the hypoglossus nerve, and more seldom of the accessory nerve. When the retractor is positioned too deeply into the incision, it may cause damage to the vagus nerve and the recurrent laryngeal nerve, even in the absence of an aberrant route. In some cases the neurologic deficit may be the consequence of an indirect mechanism. This is the case when venous hemostasis is performed by means of electrocoagulation. This provokes a temporary neurologic lesion by increasing the local temperature. Therefore, compression or ligation of the perineural vessels is the method of choice for hemostasis in these procedures. The use of low-voltage bipolar coagulation and, if possible, conducting the coagulation in cold serum reduces this risk as compared with unipolar coagulation and with the use of too high electrical voltages.

Carotid clamping is an important moment in the occurrence of a possible lesion of the vagus nerve. The close relationships between this nerve and the carotid arteries require meticulous preparation before clamping and a unambiguous localization of the nerve.

In the preparation of the superior thyroid artery the same care should be taken to avoid ligation or transection of the superior laryngeal nerve. Some investigators propose it is more worthwhile to avoid ligation or transection of collaterals of the external carotid artery [21].

Redo surgery, which greatly upsets the operation area, enhances the risk of damage to peripheral nerves to such an extent that the incidence of peripheral nerve lesions during carotid endarterectomy increases from 19.8% to 28.5% in this situation. For this reason some authors [31] advocate the choice of a venous carotid graft in this situation, which allows access to the common and internal carotid arteries below and above, respectively, the area previously operated in, so as to avoid all repeated dissection.

This strategy is not always without complications for the cranial nerves, particularly at the level of the IXth and superior laryngeal nerves, which are regularly exposed and retracted with this technique. This problem of cranial nerve lesions during redo surgery of the carotid artery is one of the reasons for the interest in balloon angioplasty in this situation [32].

REFERENCES

1 Rogers W, Root HD. Cranial nerve injuries after carotid artery endarterectomy. *South Med J* 1988; 81: 1006-1009.

2 Aldoori MI, Baird RN. Local neurological complication during carotid endarterectomy. *J Cardiovasc Surg* 1988; 29: 432-436.

3 Imparato AM, Riles TS, Ramirez AA, Lamparello PJ. Early complications of carotid surgery. *Int Surg* 1984; 69: 223-229.

4 Hertzer NR, Feldman BJ, Beven EG, Tucker HM. A prospective study of the incidence of injury to the cranial nerves during carotid endarterectomy. *Surg Gynecol Obstet* 1980; 151: 781-784.

5 Liapis CD, Satiani B, Florance CL, Evans WE. Motor speech malfunction following carotid endarterectomy. *Surgery* 1981; 89: 56-59.

6 Evans WE, Mendelowitz DS, Liapis C et al. Motor speech deficit following carotid endarterectomy. *Ann Surg* 1982; 196: 461-464.

7 Astor FC, Santilli P, Tucker HM. Incidence of cranial nerve dysfunction following carotid endarterectomy. *Head Neck Surg* 1983; 6: 660-663.

8 Forssell C, Takolander R, Bergqvist D et al. Cranial nerve injuries associated with carotid endarterectomy: a prospective study. *Acta Chir Scand* 1985; 151: 595-598.

9 Forssell C, Kitzing P, Bergqvist D. Cranial nerve injuries after carotid artery surgery. A prospective study of 663 operations. *Eur J Vasc Endovasc Surg* 1995; 10: 445-449.

10 Ballotta E, Da Giau G, Renon L et al. Cranial and cervical nerve injuries after carotid endarterectomy: a prospective study. *Surgery* 1999; 125: 85-91.

11 Schauber MD, Fontenelle LJ, Solomon JW, Hanson TL. Cranial/cervical nerve dysfunction after carotid endarterectomy. *J Vasc Surg* 1997; 25: 481-487.

12 Ranson JH, Imparato AM, Clauss RH et al. Factors in the mortality and morbidity associated with surgical treatment of cerebrovascular insufficiency. *Circulation* 1969; 39: I 269-274.

13 Krupski WC, Effeney DJ, Goldstone J et al. Carotid endarterectomy in a metropolitan community: comparison of results from three institutions. *Surgery* 198; 98: 492-499.

14 D'Addato M. Complications neurologiques périphériques de la chirurgie carotidienne. In: Kieffer E, Natali J (Eds) *Aspects techniques de la chirurgie carotidienne*. Paris, AERCV, 1987, pp 351-358.

15 Maniglia A, Han DP. Cranial nerve injuries following carotid endarterectomy: an analysis of 336 procedures. *Head Neck Surg* 1991, 13: 121-124.

16 Sandmann W, Hennerici M, Aulich A et al. Progress in carotid artery surgery at the base of the skull. *J Vasc Surg* 1984; 1: 734-743.

17 Sekhar LN, Schramm VL Jr, Jones NF et al. Operative exposure and management of the petrous and upper cervical internal carotid artery. *Neurosurgery* 1986; 10: 967-982.

18 Ekberg O, Bergqvist D, Takolander R et al. Pharyngeal function after carotid endarterectomy. *Dysphagia* 1989; 4: 151-154.

19 Dehn TC, Angell-James JE. Long-term effect of carotid endarterectomy on carotid sinus baroreceptor function and blood pressure control. *Br J Surg* 1987; 74: 997-1000.

20 Hirschl M, Hirschl MM, Magometschnigg D et al. Arterial baroreflex sensitivity and blood pressure variabilities before and after carotid surgery. *Klin Wochenschr* 1991; 69: 763-768.

21 Towne JB. Nonneurological complications of carotid artery surgery. In: Bernard VM, Towne JB (Eds). *Complications in vascular surgery*. Orlando, Grune & Stratton, 1980 pp 235-244.

22 Verta MJ Jr, Applebaum EL, McClusky DA et al. Cranial nerve injury during carotid endarterectomy. *Ann Surg* 1977; 185: 192-195.

23 Faaborg-Andersen K, Jensen M. Unilateral paralysis of the superior laryngeal nerve. *Acta Otoryngol* 1964; 57: 155-159.

24 Droulias C, Tzinas S, Harlaftis N et al. The superior laryngeal nerve. *Am Surg* 1976; 42: 635-638.

25 Holley HS, Gildea JE. Vocal cord paralysis after tracheal intubation. *JAMA* 1971; 215: 281-284.

26 AbuRahma AF, Lim RY. Management of vagus nerve injury after carotid endarterectomy. *Surgery* 1996; 119: 245-247.

27 Tucker JA, Gee W, Nicholas GG et al. Accessory nerve injury during carotid endarterectomy. *J Vasc Surg* 1987; 5: 440-444.

28 Bageant TE, Tondini D, Lysons D. Bilateral hypoglossal nerve palsy following a second carotid endarterectomy. *Anesthesiology* 1975; 43: 595-596.

29 Weiss K, Kramar R, Firt P. Cranial and cervical nerve injuries: local complications of carotid artery surgery. *J Cardiovasc Surg* 1987; 28: 171-175.

30 Sunderland S. The anatomy and physiology of nerve injury. *Muscle Nerve* 1990; 13: 771-784.

31 Branchereau A, Pietri P, Magnan PE, Rosset E. Saphenous vein bypass: an alternative to internal carotid reconstruction. *Eur J Vasc Endovasc Surg* 1996; 12: 26-30.

32 Hobson RW, Goldstein JE, Jamil Z et al. Carotid restenosis: operative and endovascular management. *J Vasc Surg* 1999; 29: 228-235.

15

149

16

RECURRENT CAROTID STENOSIS

PIERGIORGIO CAO, PAOLA DE RANGO
GIANFRANCO CARLINI, SIMONA ZANNETTI

Carotid endarterectomy (CEA) is recognized as one of the most durable vascular reconstructive procedures. Following the initial report by Eastcott, recurrent stenosis was not detected or documented for many years [1]. In 1968, Edwards et al. carried out a long term evaluation in a cohort of 75 patients who had undergone CEA [2]. Three restenoses were identified in 43 operated arteries, indicating an incidence of 7%. Subsequently, numerous reports have described symptomatic and asymptomatic recurrent carotid artery stenoses. This chapter will explore the etiology, incidence, risk factors, prevention, indications and techniques for repair, and outcome of patients undergoing reintervention for carotid restenosis.

Etiology

The occurrence of restenosis may be related to incomplete CEA, myointimal hyperplasia, or recurrent atherosclerosis. A technical error at the time of primary CEA can cause a lesion that compromises the arterial lumen, more accurately defined as residual carotid artery stenosis rather than recurrent carotid artery stenosis. Causes of residual lesions include incomplete CEA with residual atheromatous plaque, intimal flap, or damage of the lumen with primary closure. For optimal identification of residual pathology following CEA, an imaging procedure on the operating table has been used by many surgeons. Otherwise, a residual lesion can be distinguished from a recurrent lesion by an early duplex scan after CEA. In general, duplex scan assessment of a lesion within one month following CEA reveals technical errors rather than recurrent stenosis.

Myointimal hyperplasia is a cause of recurrent stenosis that develops typically between 6 and 18 months following CEA. It is characterized by a thickening of the arterial wall with a firm consistency and a smooth neointimal lining. Microscopically, the lesion consists of myocytes and fibroblasts supported by a gelatinous matrix. Myointimal hyperplasia represents an abnormal myofibroblastic proliferation that occurs in association with a vessel injury. For reasons not yet understood, some arteries are more prone to this exuberant proliferative response.

Recurrent lesions that develop several years after primary CEA are related to new atheromatous proliferation. These lesions can occur at the proximal or distal margins of the prior endarterectomy or be new atheromatous disease that developed in a previously endarterectomized segment.

Incidence

The incidence of restenosis after CEA is variable and depends on the definition employed, the method of detection, the length of follow-up, and the type of analysis (Table I). Regarding the latter, incidence rates are frequently reported as absolute restenosis rates instead of using life-table methods. Calculation of absolute rates generally underestimates the true incidence of restenosis because it is independent from duration and frequency of follow-up [3].

Two recent reviews examined the incidence of recurrent carotid stenosis. Lattimer and Burnand found that the incidence of restenosis ranges from 1% to 37% [8]. Frericks et al. performed a systematic review of the Medline database using the standard meta-analytical technique and identified 20 publications on carotid restenosis [5]. They found that restenosis rates progressively decrease during the years after CEA. The meta-analysis

revealed a restenosis risk of 10% in the first year, 3% in the second year, and 2% in the third year; the long-term risk was about 1%. The Asymptomatic Carotid Atherosclerosis Study (ACAS) confirmed that the high incidence of restenosis occurs in the first 18 months following CEA. Among 645 patients operated for asymptomatic CEA and evaluated for restenosis, the authors found an overall restenosis rate of 12.7%. Stratifying for time intervals, the incidence of restenosis was 4.1% in the first 3 months after operation, 7.6% in the period from 3-18 months, and 1.9% thereafter [6].

A large randomized clinical trial on surgical technique for CEA (EVEREST) showed that in 1353 CEAs the restenosis risk was 4.2% at a mean follow-up of 33 months [7].

Risk factors, prevention, and technical issues related to restenosis

Studies have demonstrated that female gender, continued smoking, and failure to obtain a completion procedure documenting technical success of primary CEA are important factors associated with recurrent carotid stenosis [8]. Several approaches have been recommended for prevention. Since continued smoking is associated with restenosis, a beneficial approach would be to counsel the patient on the importance of stopping smoking.

16

152

Table I	INCIDENCE OF RESTENOSIS AFTER CAROTID ENDARTERECTOMY			
1st author [ref.]	*Year*	*Number of patients*	*Follow-up*	*Restenosis %*
De Grootte [3]	1987	265	2 years	13.3
Gelabert [4]	1994	1232	2 years	6.5
Frericks [5]	1998	7560	1 year	10
Moore (ACAS) [6]	1998	1645	5 years	12.7
			< 3 months	4.1
			13 - 18 months	7.6
			18 - 60 months	1.9
Cao (EVEREST) [7]	2000	1353	33 months	4.2

Various pharmacological approaches have been suggested as a means of preventing restenosis. The most common is the use of aspirin antiplatelet therapy. Yet, there is no evidence that use of aspirin prevents or reduces the incidence of myointimal hyperplasia.

Technical factors have a significant role in the risk of recurrent stenosis. Randomized prospective studies and recent meta-analyses demonstrated that patch angioplasty and eversion technique for CEA are protective against recurrent carotid stenosis [9-17]. A systematic review of the Cochrane database showed that carotid patch angioplasty was associated with significantly fewer perioperative arterial occlusions (odds ratio 0.14; 95% confidence interval [CI] 0.05-0.42) and with significantly fewer arteries developing restenosis greater than 50% during follow-up (odds ratio 0.33; 95% CI 0.18-0.59). However, it is not clear whether these reduced risks are associated with clinical benefit in terms of reduced risk of death or stroke [10].

Archie performed a meta-analysis of six randomized studies on the use of patch plasty in carotid disease: 448 CEA by primary closure and 591 CEA with patch. The restenosis rate in the first year after CEA was significantly higher in the primary closure group than in the patch group (7.4% vs. 2.1% respectively, p < 0.001) [11].

Analysis of the ACAS database showed that use of a patch reduced the overall risk of restenosis from 21% to 7%, the patch being the only negative independent predictor of restenosis on multivariate analysis. Indeed, none of the traditional risk factors (age, hypertension, smoking, diabetes, gender, etc.) had a statistically significant effect on recurrent stenosis [6]. Similarly, AbuRahma et al. recently performed a randomized study on 74 patients undergoing bilateral CEA with primary closure on one side and patch on the contralateral side. They found that patching had a cumulative patency rate significantly greater than primary closure at 24 months (98% vs. 75%; p < 0.001), showing that local factors (i.e., surgical technique) play a significant role in development of carotid restenosis [12].

With respect to patch material and restenosis, there is not sufficient evidence to differentiate between the effect of venous and synthetic patches [13].

Eversion technique for CEA has been shown to prevent carotid restenosis [7,14-20]. Recent randomized studies have shown the protective role of eversion technique for CEA on restenosis. The largest randomized experience was the EVEREST study that analyzed outcomes of 678 eversion CEA vs. 675 non-eversion CEA (patch + primary closure). The cumulative restenosis risk at 4 years was significantly lower in the eversion group with respect to the non-eversion group (3.6% vs. 9.2%; p = 0.01), with an absolute risk reduction of 5.6% and a relative risk reduction of 62% [7].

Clinical manifestations

Clinical significance of restenosis remains controversial. Some authors believe that the clinical course of recurrent stenosis is benign, especially when caused by myointimal hyperplasia. However, there is also evidence that supports the hypothesis that recurrent carotid disease is causally related to late ipsilateral stroke after CEA.

Evidence from international trials suggests that after successful CEA, the risk of ipsilateral late stroke is about 1%-2% per annum [21,22]. Approximately one-third of late post CEA strokes appear to be related to recurrent stenosis [23]. According to published series, the risk of restenosis-related symptoms varies widely. Indeed, data are extremely heterogeneous, reflecting the retrospective fashion of most studies and lack of consistent follow-up of patients. In addition, length of follow-up and definition of events varied among series.

In an extensive review of the literature by Lattimer and Burnand the incidence of symptoms related to recurrent stenosis was only 0%-8% [8]. A recent systematic overview by Frericks et al. of 20 publications examining the incidence and clinical significance of recurrent carotid stenosis showed that the risk of stroke with restenosis was moderately increased (5.5% vs. 3.3% at 3 years; RR 2.0). However, the presence of significant heterogeneity in relative risk of stroke among studies (ranging from 0.10% to 10%) implies the difficulty in calculating an overall estimate of the true relative risk [5]. The results of ACAS showed that of 136 patients with recurrent carotid stenosis, only one underwent reoperation for symptoms [6]. Similarly, data from the EVEREST trial show that of 56 restenoses detected at a mean follow-up of 33 months, only one patient had an ipsilateral stroke subsequent to restenosis [7]. Among nine patients with a previous asymptomatic carotid restenosis followed conservatively because of advanced age or significant comorbidities, O'Donnell et al. found that three of nine patients had neurological events (two stroke and one TIA). In addition, 30% of patients whose recurrent stenosis progressed to occlusion suffered a stroke. In the same experience, patients with moderate (50%-75%) carotid restenoses did not experience neurological events [23].

It is difficult to determine the risk of ipsilateral stroke in patients with recurrent carotid stenosis because many undergo prophylactic redo-operations during the course of follow-up. Neurological events in patients with a restenosis are rare in the first 2 to 3 years after the primary CEA and appear more often several years after CEA [5,24-26]. This may be related to the underlying pathology of recurrent atherosclerotic lesions, characterized by friable plaques more prone to embolization. Yet, Rockman et al. found that 28.1% of the patients with myointimal hyperplasia at reoperative surgery manifested preoperative symptoms [27].

To date, there are no evidence-based data on how to manage patients with recurrent carotid stenosis. Crucial issues are whether recurrent carotid stenosis significantly increases the risk of ipsilateral stroke and whether the risks of reintervention outweigh the risk of late stroke.

In the absence of randomized controlled trials on the management of patients with recurrent carotid disease, indications for revascularization for restenosis should be given considering the natural history of recurrent stenosis and outcome of surgical or endovascular reintervention.

Indications for treatment

Debate in favor of conservative management of recurrent carotid stenosis is not only based on the presumed increased risk of perioperative neurological complications but also on cranial and cervical nerve injuries in redo cases [28]. Indications for repairing recurrent carotid stenosis are relatively similar to those for primary repair: patients who develop symptoms related to the recurrent lesion are candidates for repair. On the other hand, asymptomatic recurrent stenosis involves a more complex assessment. Generally, if recurrence is early and therefore secondary to myointimal hyperplasia, it is safe to follow-up patients with periodic duplex scan evaluation. The lesion may stabilize and not progress further. In case the lesion continues to

progress, surgical intervention should be considered. Late recurrence due to atherosclerosis should be treated in the same way as primary atherosclerotic stenoses in the asymptomatic patient.

In summary, reoperation should be considered in the presence of a high-grade recurrent carotid stenosis and carotid territory symptoms and in asymptomatic patients with progressing lesions or contralateral carotid occlusion.

Management and postoperative outcome

Two therapeutic attitudes are possible in the presence of recurrent carotid stenosis: open surgical reoperation or endoluminal treatment with carotid angioplasty and stenting (Figure). Presently, consistent data comparing endovascular management with carotid endarterectomy are lacking, thus creating controversies on the choice of treatment in patients with carotid restenosis.

Surgical treatment

Few surgeons have vast experience in redo-carotid surgery. Surgical repair of recurrent carotid stenosis is more difficult than primary operation and has higher morbidity and mortality. The operation is similar to the primary surgical procedure. The incision can be made on the line of the old scar.

A more proximal and distal carotid artery exposure should be performed with respect to the original procedure. Dissection may be easier by exposing the common carotid artery to an area not previously dissected. Routine use of shunting and general anesthesia is suggested by some authors [29].

Endarterectomy cleavage may be very difficult due to adhesion of early recurrent lesions to the vascular wall (myointimal hyperplasia). Late atherosclerotic recurrences might be easier to re-endarterectomize on the subadventitial plane. Yet, subadventitial planes may be obscured distally and proximally and end-point feathering can be difficult. It would be better to leave some diseased intima and media and protect the reconstruction with a patch closure rather than risking a deep dissection plane with the possibility of damaging the integrity of the arterial wall. Patch angioplasty (with or without endarterectomy) is necessary in most reoperations for recurrent carotid artery disease. In patients with extensive, long segment recurrent disease, carotid bypass with an interposition graft should be the treatment of choice.

With respect to complications, different authors report conflicting results (Table II). Reintervention carries an increased risk of stroke and/or cranial nerve injuries when compared to the original procedure. Several studies showed that operation for recurrent carotid stenosis can be performed without a significantly increased risk of perioperative stroke and death, except for the incidence of cranial nerve injury [25,30-34]. O'Donnell et al. reported 48 reinterventions for carotid recurrences with only one perioperative death (2.1%) and one perioperative stroke (2.1%): the overall perioperative mortality/morbidity rate was not low (4%) when compared to results for primary CEA [23]. An incidence of failure (cumulative rate of stroke, carotid occlusion, and TIA) after redo carotid surgery up to 19.9% has also been reported [27,30]. A recent study by AbuRahma showed that repeat CEA is associated with a high incidence of

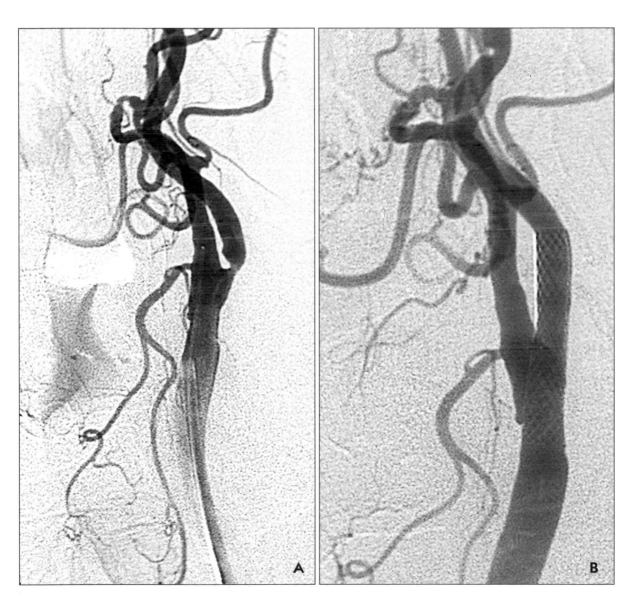

FIGURE. Recurrent stenosis of the internal carotid artery prior to (A) and after (B) endoluminal treatment.

1st author [ref.]	Year	Number of patients	Stroke (%)	Death (%)	Cranial nerve injury (%)
Treiman [33]	1992	102	2 (1.9)	1 (1)	0
Gagne [30]	1993	41	0	0	2 (5)
AbuRahma [31]	1994	46	3 (7)	0	3 (7)
Mensour [32]	1997	69	4 (5.8)	0	6 (8.7)
Rockman [27]	1999	82	3 (3.7)	0	1 (1.2)
Hill [34]	1999	40	0	0	0

Table II RECURRENT CAROTID STENOSIS: OUTCOME OF REOPERATION

cranial/cervical nerve lesions, some of which have a long healing time and can be permanent with significant disability [35].

Endovascular treatment

Carotid stenting is considered an appealing alternative to operative management of carotid restenosis. It obviates the necessity for dissection of the carotid artery, thus reducing the risk of cranial nerve injury. Symptomatic and asymptomatic carotid restenosis have been considered for endoluminal treatment. Low periprocedural risks (range 0%-3.5%) have been reported, particularly in patients with carotid restenosis caused by myointimal hyperplasia [36-39]. Yet, 12% or more secondary recurrences have been reported in some series [40]. For this reason, long-term follow-up after endovascular treatment for carotid restenosis should be meticulous.

Conclusion

Recurrent carotid stenosis is a relatively uncommon event. Our knowledge of the natural history of recurrent stenosis is still not refined, yet the risk of stroke with recurrent lesions is increased. Surgical or endovascular management should be recommended in the case of symptomatic lesions with ipsilateral hemodynamically significant stenosis, and in asymptomatic lesions with progressing stenosis or contralateral carotid occlusion.

REFERENCES

1 Eastcott HH, Pickering JW, Rob CG. Reconstruction of internal carotid artery in a patient with intermittent attacks of hemiplegia. *Lancet* 1954; 2: 994.
2 Edwards WS, Wilson TA, Bennet A. The long-term effectiveness of carotid endarterectomy in the prevention of strokes. *Ann Surg* 1968; 168: 765-770.
3 DeGroote RD, Lynch TG, Jamil Z, Hobson RW II. Carotid restenosis: long-term noninvasive follow-up after carotid endarterectomy. *Stroke* 1987; 18: 1031-1036.
4 Gelabert HA, El-Massry S, Moore WS. Carotid endarterectomy with primary closure does not adversely affect the rate of recurrent stenosis. *Arch Surg* 1994; 129: 648-654.
5 Frericks H, Kievit J, van Baalen JM, van Bockel JH. Carotid recurrent stenosis and risk of ipsilateral stroke. A systematic review of the literature. *Stroke* 1998; 29: 244-250.
6 Moore WS, Kempczinski RF, Nelson JJ, Toole JF. Recurrent carotid stenosis. Results of the Asymptomatic Carotid Atherosclerosis Study. *Stroke* 1998; 29: 2018-2025.
7 Cao P, Giordano G, De Rango P et al. Eversion versus conventional carotid endarterectomy: late results of a prospective multicenter randomized trial. *J Vasc Surg* 2000; 31: 19-30.
8 Lattimer CR, Burnand KG. Recurrent carotid stenosis after carotid endarterectomy. *Br J Surg* 1997; 84: 1206-1219.
9 AbuRahma AF, Robinson PA, Saiedy S et al. Prospective randomized trial of carotid endarterectomy with primary closure and patch angioplasty with saphenous vein, jugular vein, and polytetrafluoroethylene: long-term follow-up. *J Vasc Surg* 1998; 27: 222-234.
10 Counsell CE, Salinas R, Naylor R, Warlow CP. A systematic review of the randomised trials of carotid patch angioplasty in carotid endarterectomy. *Eur J Vasc Endovasc Surg* 1997; 13: 345-354.
11 Archie JP. Carotid endarterectomy outcome with vein or dacron graft patch angioplasty and internal carotid artery shortening. *J Vasc Surg* 1999; 29: 654-664.
12 AbuRahma AF, Robinson PA, Saiedy S et al. Prospective randomized trial of bilateral carotid endarterectomies. Primary closure versus patching. *Stroke* 1999; 30: 1185-1189.
13 Counsell C, Warlow C, Naylor R. Patches of different types for carotid patch angioplasty. *Cochrane Database of Systematic Reviews* 2000; 2: CD000071.
14 Cao P, Giordano G, De Rango P et al. Eversion versus conventional carotid endarterectomy: a prospective study. *Eur J Vasc Endovasc Surg* 1997; 14: 96-104.

15 Raithel D, Kasprzak PM. The eversion endarterectomy- a new technique. In Greenhalgh R, Hollier L (eds.) *Surgery for stroke.* London, WB Saunders Co. Ltd, 1993; pp 183-191.

16 Cao PG, De Rango P. Zannetti S et al. Eversion versus conventional carotid endarterectomy for preventing stroke (Cochrane Review). In: *The Cochrane Library,* (Issue 1, 2001; Oxford: Update Software).

17 Ballotta E, Da Giau G, Saladini M et al. Carotid endarterectomy with patch closure versus carotid eversion endarterectomy and reimplantation: a prospective randomized study. *Surgery* 1999; 125: 271-279.

18 Darling RC III, Paty PSK, Shah DM et al. Eversion endarterectomy of the internal carotid artery: technique and results in 449 procedures. *Surgery* 1996; 120: 635-640.

19 Koskas F, Kieffer E, Bahnini A et al. Carotid eversion endarterectomy: short and long-term results. *Ann Vasc Surg* 1995; 9: 9-15.

20 Reigner B, Reveilleau P, Gayral M et al. Eversion endarterectomy of the internal carotid artery: midterm results of a new technique. *Ann Vasc Surg* 1995; 9: 241-246.

21 Anonymous. Beneficial effect of carotid endarterectomy in symptomatic patients with high-grade carotid stenosis. North American Symptomatic Carotid Endarterectomy Trial collaborators. *N Engl J Med* 1991; 325: 445-453.

22 Anonymous. MRC European Carotid Surgery Trial: interim results for symptomatic patients with severe (70-99%) or with mild (0-29%) carotid stenosis. European Carotid Surgery Trialists Collaborative Group. *Lancet* 1991; 337: 1235-1243.

23 O'Donnell TF Jr, Rodriguez AA, Fortunato JE. The management of recurrent carotid stenosis: should asymptomatic lesions be treated surgically? *J Vasc Surg* 1996; 24: 207-212.

24 Ricotta JJ, O'Brien-Irr MS. Conservative management of residual and recurrent lesions after carotid endarterectomy: long-term results. *J Vasc Surg* 1997; 26: 963-972.

25 O'Donnell TF Jr, Callow AD, Scott G et al. Ultrasound characteristics of recurrent carotid disease: hypothesis explaining the low incidence of symptomatic recurrence. *J Vasc Surg* 1985; 2: 26-41.

26 Washburn WK, Mackey WC, Belkin M, O'Donnell TF Jr. Late stroke after carotid endarterectomy: the role of recurrent stenosis. *J Vasc Surg* 1992; 15: 1032-1037.

27 Rockman CB, Riles TS, Landis R et al. Redo carotid surgery: an analysis of materials and configurations used in carotid reoperations and their influence on perioperative stroke and subsequent recurrent stenosis. *J Vasc Surg* 1999; 29: 72-81.

28 Avramovic JR, Fletcher JP. The incidence of recurrent carotid stenosis after carotid endarterectomy and its relationship to neurological events. *J Cardiovasc Surg* 1992; 33: 54-58.

29 Fisher DF Jr, Clagett GP, Parker JI et al. Mandibular subluxation for high carotid exposure. *J Vasc Surg* 1984; 1: 727-733.

30 Gagne PJ, Riles TS, Jacobowitz GR. Long-term follow-up of patients undergoing reoperation for recurrent carotid artery disease. *J Vasc Surg* 1993; 991-1001.

31 AbuRahma AF, Snodgrass KR, Robinson PA et al. Safety and durability of redo carotid endarterectomy for recurrent carotid artery stenosis. *Am J Surg* 1994; 168: 175-178.

32 Mansour MA, Kang SS, Baker WH et al. Carotid endarterectomy for recurrent stenosis. *J Vasc Surg* 1997; 25: 877-883.

33 Treiman GS, Jenkins JM, Edwards WH Sr et al. The evolving surgical management of recurrent carotid stenosis. *J Vasc Surg* 1992; 16: 354-362.

34 Hill BB, Olcott C IV, Dalman RL et al. Reoperation for carotid stenosis is as safe as primary carotid endarterectomy. *J Vasc Surg* 1999; 30: 26-35.

35 AbuRahma, Choueiri MA. Cranial and cervical nerve injuries after repeat carotid endarterectomy. *J Vasc Surg* 2000; 32: 649-654.

36 Hobson RW II, Goldstein JE, Jamil Z et al. Carotid restenosis: operative and endovascular management. *J Vasc Surg* 1999; 29: 228-238.

37 Yadav JS, Roubin GS, King P et al. Angioplasty and stenting for restenosis after carotid endarterectomy. Initial experience. *Stroke* 1996; 2075-2079.

38 Bergeron P, Chambran P, Benichou H, Alessandri C. Recurrent carotid disease: will stents be an alternative to surgery? *J Endovasc Surg* 1996; 3: 76-79.

39 Diethrich EB, Ndiaye M, Reid DB. Stenting in the carotid artery: initial experience in 110 patients. *J Endovasc Surg* 1996; 3: 42-62.

40 Lanzino G, Mericle RA, Lopes DK et al. Percutaneous transluminal angioplasty and stent placement for recurrent carotid artery stenosis. *J Neurosurg* 1999; 90: 688-694.

17

COMPLICATIONS OF RECONSTRUCTIVE SURGERY OF THE VERTEBRAL AND SUBCLAVIAN ARTERIES

EUGENIO ROSSET, MATHIEU POIRIER, JEAN-PIERRE RIBAL
BRUNO MACHEDA, AHMED BESBISS, GÉRARD GLANDDIER

Despite the functional and vital importance of the territories supplied by the vertebrobasilar system, the surgery of vertebral arteries and, to a lesser extent, of the subclavian arteries has remained underdeveloped as compared to carotid surgery. Generally, several reasons for this are put forward: the complex pathophysiology induces a discrepancy between the anatomy and clinical findings; presence of a variety of symptoms consisting of functional and, thus, subjective signs; difficult angiographic visualization of the vertebrobasilar system, and finally a difficult surgical access and reconstruction of the vertebral arteries at different levels of their complex anatomic tract [1].

Yet, several groups have recently stressed that a rigorous selection of the surgical indications and techniques could yield interesting results with a minimal risk of complications [2-4]. The indications for vertebral and subclavian surgery are based on retrospective, uncontrolled historical series. Data on the natural history of arterial lesions involved are inaccurate, even when it is clear that serious neurologic complications may occur.

Surgery of these arterial lesions most often aims at curing or reducing chronic symptoms. From this point of view it involves functional surgery, of which the possible occurrence of complications may annul its indication. It is therefore extremely important to know the possible complications, their consequences, and their incidence during this kind of surgery in the series published, and how to prevent them.

Complications concerning access to the vertebral artery

ACCESS TO THE PROXIMAL VERTEBRAL ARTERY (SEGMENT V1)

Peripheral nerve complications

The Claude Bernard Horner syndrome is by far the most frequent complication after surgery of the proximal vertebral artery. Moore observed a frequency of 13% in a literature review on 1,158 vertebral restorations [5]. Branchereau and Magnan [6] reported an incidence of 25% in a series of 148 proximal vertebral reconstructions with one persisting deficit (Table I). It occurs when sympathetic perivertebral fibers are mobilized or transected (Fig. 1). The clinical signs may be very discrete or, in contrast, cause an important functional deficit in case of a marked ptosis or permanent watering of the eyes. Usually these symptoms pass away in a few weeks or months. Permanent syndromes are rarely seen, due to an extended exposition of the vertebral artery at its origin, in particular transection of the nervous plexus close to the subclavian artery and the stellate ganglion. It is therefore recommended to avoid transection of the perivertebral nervous fibers by retracting them, and to avoid as far as possible transection of the nervous fibers at the origin of the vertebral artery.

The paralysis of the recurrent laryngeal nerve can be due to two mechanisms: a direct trauma of this

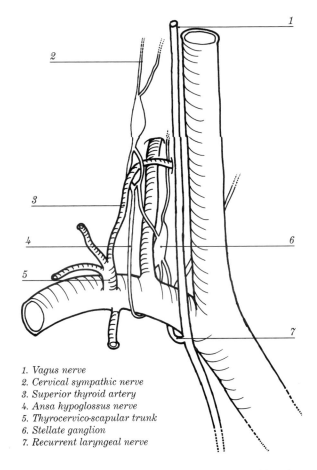

1. Vagus nerve
2. Cervical sympathic nerve
3. Superior thyroid artery
4. Ansa hypoglossus nerve
5. Thyrocervico-scapular trunk
6. Stellate ganglion
7. Recurrent laryngeal nerve

FIG. 1   Relations between the subclavian-vertebral junction and the cervical sympathetic plexus.

Table I	COMPLICATIONS OF THE SURGICAL APPROACH OF THE PROXIMAL VERTEBRAL ARTERY							
1st author [ref.]	Year	Study period	Number of reconstructions	Horner's syndrome	Recurrent laryngeal nerve paralysis	Phrenic nerve paralysis	Lymphatic damage	Dysphagia
Roon [7]	1979	1961-1978	43	0	0	0	1	0
Imparato [8]	1984	1964-1983	109	NS	0	1	0	0
Berguer [9]	1986	1975-1985	35	5	0	1	4	0
Branchereau [6]	1990	1979-1985	148	37 *	3 ●	0	4	0
Thevenet [10]	1992	1964-1991	686	228 ●	0	7 ●	20 ●●	12 ●

NS: not specified
* Permanent syndrome
● Regressive
●● Of which 3 with chylothorax

nerve occurs especially in case of restoration of the right vertebral artery because of the closeness of this nerve and the subclavian artery. Secondly, it may also occur after a trauma to the vagus nerve while exposing the common carotid artery in order to use it as implantation site. In both cases the nerve deficit may show the classical clinical symptoms as seen in vocal cord paralysis: dysphonia and bitonal voice. The recurrent nerve paralysis may occur inconspicuously. That is why one should check systematically the mobility of the vocal cords when a bilateral reconstruction is planned before performing the second reconstruction, in order to avoid the risk of bilateral paralysis, of which the clinical consequences might be dramatic. If a recurrent nerve paralysis is proven by an examination, the planned intervention should be postponed for several months until complete recovery is obtained.

A lesion of the phrenic nerve is observed especially when in the reconstruction performed the subclavian artery has been used as donor site. In this type of reconstruction the phrenic nerve, located adjacent to the anterior scalenus muscle, may be traumatized during exposition of the subclavian artery by means of a retractor positioned laterally, or by excessive traction on a loop around the nerve. Here too, bilateral damage has annoying consequences on respiratory function, and systematic monitoring of the mobility of the diaphragmatic domes on pulmonary X-rays is required before a contralateral cervical reconstruction is planned.

Lymphatic complications

Lymphatic damage may occur during exposition of the vertebral artery in the supraclavicular area due to the abundance of lymphatic vessels in that region. On the right side the most important lymphatic conduit is the great lymphatic vein, formed by the conjunction of three trunks: the subclavian, right anterior mediastinal, and right jugular trunk. It drains into the terminal part of the right subclavian vein and forms, together with its affluents, a lymphatic tree in front of the arterial tree. On the left, the thoracic duct is the most voluminous lymphatic structure that drains the whole subdiaphragmatic region. It makes a curve originating from above the subclavian artery medial to the vertebral artery and drains into the superior part of the venous junction of the jugular and subclavian veins (Fig. 2).

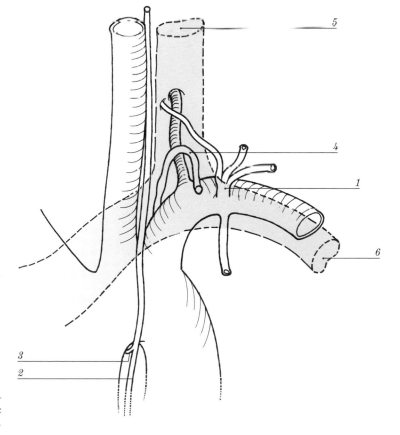

1. *Thyrocervico-scapular trunk*
2. *Vagus nerve*
3. *Recurrent laryngeal nerve*
4. *Thoracic duct*
5. *Internal jugular vein*
6. *Subclavian vein*

FIG. 2 Anterior view of the left supraclavicular cavity showing the relations between the arteries, pleural dome, and thoracic canal.

The clinical signs of lymphatic damage are variable. Most often it concerns a simple lymphorrhea with a direct or delayed occurrence, manifested by a clear or milky fluid in the drainage bottle. The application of a compressing bandage suffices in most cases to stop the lymphorrhea. In more severe cases, prolonged drainage without suction and interruption of oral food may suffice to close the lymphatic leakage.

A lymphocele may occur when the drain is removed too early. As in the other localizations, a simple puncture with a compressive bandage can resolve the problem. Surgical closure of the leakage is seldom necessary. In that case a delay of several days is necessary to allow for organization of the lesions and easy identification of the leak. A chylothorax is exceptional and occurs in case of a pleural lesion together with lymphatic damage or in case of a secondary rupture into the pleura of an expanding lymphocele. Repeated punctures or even drainage are often necessary, with or without parenteral nutrition. When a chylothorax persists and before signs of malnutrition occur, a thoracotomy to ligate the thoracic duct might be indicated. Prevention of this kind of complication is based on careful lymphostasis by using ligatures during the dissection of the lymphatic plexus in front of the vertebral artery.

Pleural lesion

The proximity of the pleural dome explains the possibility of the occurrence of a pleural lesion during the exploration of the vertebral artery. This kind of lesion may occur unnoticed during the procedure and the diagnosis is made when a limited pneumothorax is present, either with or without a discrete pleural effusion, detected by means of a postoperative X-thorax. A considerable pleural effusion indicates another associated complication: lymphatic lesion in the case of a chylothorax; and vascular lesion in the case of a hemothorax.

Hemorrhagic complications

Being very exceptional, the hemorrhagic complications are seldom due to venous bleeding. The proximal vertebral approach requires ligation of not only the superficial cervical veins, but also the vertebral vein, which may be doubled. Veins are rarely the cause of major hematomas. Arterial bleeding mostly comes from the site of reconstruction, particularly when an endarterectomy is performed. Therefore it is preferable, when the deobstructed zone appears too fragile due to a too external cleavage level, to abandon this technique and choose for a technique that is less prone to hemorrhages [3].

ACCESS TO THE DISTAL VERTEBRAL ARTERY (V3)

This technique allows access to the vertebral artery in its suboccipital segment, which describes a typical route, actually between the first and second cervical vertebrae, or more rarely, between the first cervical vertebra and the entrance into the occipital membrane. The access to the distal segment of the vertebral artery is especially liable to the risk of peripheral nerve damage (Table II). The first parts of the approach are the same as those of the carotid access, while the incision is extended up to the mastoid process. Transection of the cutaneous branches of the superficial cervical plexus as well as the auriculotemporal nerve are common, causing a more or less transient postoperative anesthesia of

Table II	COMPLICATIONS OF THE SURGICAL APPROACH OF THE DISTAL VERTEBRAL ARTERY								
1st author [ref.]	*Year*	*Study period*	*Number of cases*	*Horner's syndrome*	*Recurrent laryngeal nerve paralysis*	*Spinal nerve (XI) paralysis*	*Hematoma*	*Infection*	*Humero-scapular peri-arthritis*
Kieffer [10]	1992	1978-1989	241	10	-	21	2	1	-
Koskas [11]	1995	1979-1991	92	4	1	8	3*	1	20
Berguer [12]	1998	1984-1998	100	2	1	-	-	-	-

*2 réinterventions

the ear lobe. The external branch of the spinal nerve is usually marked after incision of the superficial cervical aponeurosis. The variations in the course of this nerve are the reason for a peroperative trauma, leading to paralysis of the trapezius muscle: hampered elevation of the shoulder and pain due to abnormal tension of the accessory elevator muscles of the shoulder [13]. This deficit is usually completely regressive within a few weeks when treated with physical therapy. Damage to the spinal nerve may in exceptional cases lead to the appearance of a scapulo-humeral peri-arthritis. Transection of the anterior branch of the spinal root C2 is common while exposing the distal vertebral artery. It never has clinical sequelae and therefore causes no complications, due to the abundance of anastomoses between the first three cervical nerves [13].

Hemorrhagic complications

Hemorrhagic complications are as exceptional at the level of segment V3 as at the level of segment V1. However, venous bleeding may occur from the perivertebral venous plexus. The consequences are rarely serious. It can be prevented by meticulous hemostasis during exploration of the vertebral artery by using fine bipolar coagulation. Arterial bleeding may occur either from the anastomosis or a transected collateral artery during the access of the vertebral artery. Therefore we take great care during hemostasis of the collateral arteries by means of ligation using monofilament 8/0 sutures. The hemorrhage may also be the result of an infection. Then the occurrence is delayed due to infectious necrosis of the reconstruction. Arterial

hemorrhage from the reconstruction can cause a rapidly growing compressing hematoma like those seen after conventional carotid surgery. An urgent surgical intervention is then imperative.

Infectious complications

Infectious complications are rare at the cervical level. They present with an important hemorrhage in the most serious cases. An in-situ redo procedure is difficult to perform and ligation of the vertebral artery is most often the only solution. If the infection occurs of a proximal reconstruction from the subclavian artery, one might consider a distal reconstruction by means of a distal carotid-vertebral bypass.

Neurologic complications due to vertebral artery reconstructions

Central neurologic complications after surgery of the vertebral artery are more uncommon than those in carotid surgery (Tables III and IV): 1% in a study by Branchereau et al. in a series of 110 isolated proximal reconstructions [4] and 1.9% in a study by Berguer et al. in a series of 154 proximal or distal reconstructions performed since 1991 [2].

These are predominantly due to thromboembolization. Two other common causes of neurologic complications during carotid surgery, ischemia due to clamping and reperfusion syndrome, are very rare for isolated vertebral artery surgery, even virtually theoretical [3].

Table III	CENTRAL NEUROLOGIC COMPLICATIONS AND SURGERY OF THE PROXIMAL VERTEBRAL ARTERY						
1st author [ref.]	*Year*	*Study period*	*Number of cases*	*Mortality*	*CVE*	*TIA*	*Occlusions*
Roon [7]	1979	1961-1978	43	1	2*	-	2
Imparato [8]	1984	1964-1983	109	3	-	-	2
Branchereau [4]	1992	1979-1987	110	1	-	1	5
Thévenet [10]	1992	1964-1991	686	3	1●	-	-

CVE: cerebrovascular event
TIA: transient ischemic attack
*1 hemispheric, 1 vertebrobasilar
● Hemispheric

Table IV CENTRAL NEUROLOGIC COMPLICATIONS AND SURGERY OF THE DISTAL VERTEBRAL ARTERY

1er author [ref.]	Year	Study period	Number of cases	Mortality	CVE	TIA	Thrombosis
Kieffer [10]	1992	1978-89	241	4*	6	-	18
Koskas [11]	1995	1979-91	92	-	-	2	-
Berguer [12]	1998	1984-98	100	4*	5	-	8

CVE: cerebrovascular event
TIA: transient ischemic attack
* All secondary to CVE

Untimely mobilization of an emboligenic lesion or an error while clearing it may cause an embolic event, but in the majority of cases the thromboembolic events are due to technical flaws and, given the small caliber of the vertebral artery, this generally leads to an occlusion of the reconstruction. The surgical procedure chosen may be the reason for a postoperative occlusion: a reconstruction of an artery with too small a caliber or proximal to stenotic lesions in the transverse canal for a proximal reconstruction (segment V1); reconstruction distal to a stenosis at the donor site. Technical failures causing a postoperative occlusion are manifold and vary with the technique: semi-closed endarterectomies may generate a thrombosis in case of a remaining distal intimal flap; open endarterectomies may show a stenosis in case of a direct suture of the deobstructed area. Reimplantations into the common carotid or subclavian artery may show kinking in case of a too long vertebral artery. Hence, a sufficient exposure of the pretransverse segment of the vertebral artery is required. Such an exposure allows for the exact measurement of the required length for an optimal reconstruction. In case of a reimplantation into the common carotid artery the anastomosis should be made at the posterior side of the carotid tree in order to avoid kinking of the vertebral artery (Fig. 3) [14].

Postoperative thrombosis of the reconstruction may have various neurologic sequelae, ranging from a massive infarction in the vertebrobasilar outflow area in case of a poor supply via the circle of Willis to, in the opposite case, the simple, neurologically asymptomatic thrombosis. Then, the persistence or even aggravation of the symptoms of vertebrobasilar insufficiency is seen. The high number of technical failures possible have led some surgeons, albeit experienced in reconstructive surgery of the vertebral artery, to advocate the systematic performance of a peroperative completion angiogram. Since the systematic use of this method, Berguer et al. have observed in a series of 369 vertebral artery reconstructions a reduction of the number of postoperative occlusions from 11% to 2.5% (p =0.002). Simultaneously they found a significant reduction of postoperative neurologic complications, as well as an increased long-term patency [2].

Another possible mechanism for neurologic complications during surgery of the supra-aortic trunks is the ischemia due to cross-clamping. The application of a shunt during vertebral artery surgery has been reported rarely in literature. Berguer et al., in the beginning of their experience, have used it twice in patients presenting with multilevel lesions, with poor results: the hindrance caused by the presence of the shunt resulted in one postoperative occlusion. In the two cases a reintervention was undertaken without a shunt with a good neurologic result [2]. These authors have abandoned the use of shunts and have preferred moderate hypothermia (34°C ± 0.5°C) to protect the brain, which theoretically leads to an 18% reduction of the cerebral metabolism. This choice is based on the fact that clamping the vertebral artery, as opposed to clamping of the internal carotid artery, does not cause a total interruption of the outflow as the vertebral artery has numerous anastomoses along its extracranial course from the ascending cervical artery and costocervical trunk (Fig. 4).

When a reimplantation into the common carotid artery is planned, it is necessary to simultaneously clamp the common carotid and vertebral arteries.

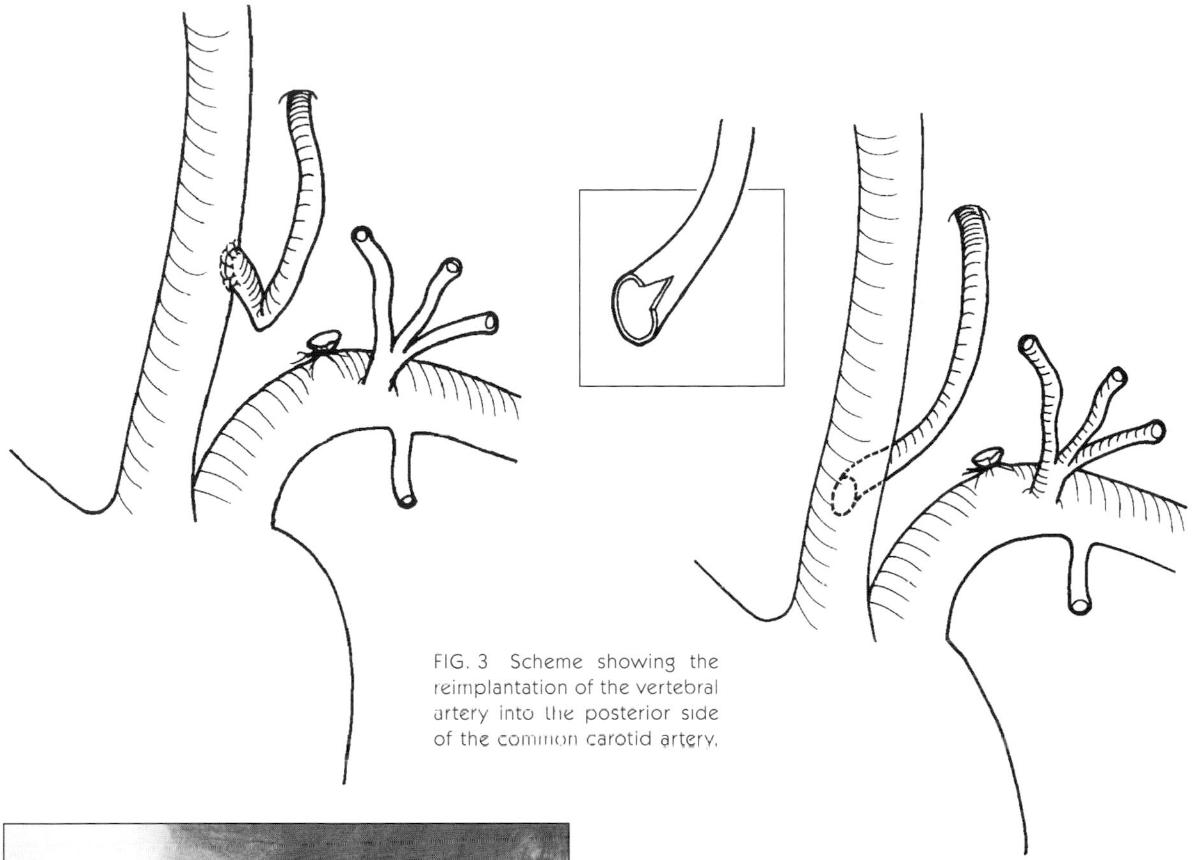

FIG. 3 Scheme showing the reimplantation of the vertebral artery into the posterior side of the common carotid artery.

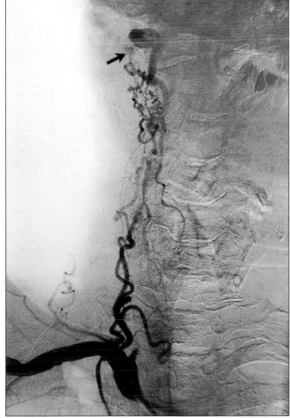

FIG. 4 Arteriogram showing refilling by cervical collaterals of the suboccipital part of the vertebral artery.

In this case, the supply from the internal carotid artery is assured by the external carotid artery. However, if an occlusion of the contralateral internal carotid artery exists, the simultaneous clamping of the carotid and vertebral artery may cause cerebral ischemia. Two solutions are then possible: a venous carotid-vertebral bypass allows sequential carotid-vertebral clamping, but the two anastomoses are difficult to perform and the positioning of such a venous bypass is quite delicate. The other solution consists of a direct reimplantation under the protection of a carotid shunt. In our experience we have used a shunt twice, placed in the common carotid through a short arteriotomy. The direct vertebral reimplantation was performed by means of a second arteriotomy proximal to the area of the shunt. The reimplantation could thus be performed under isolated vertebral clamping, while the vertebral artery was reopened during the removal of the shunt and closure of the carotid arteriotomy (Fig. 5). In the two cases the neurologic result was satisfactory, while we could not confirm the usefulness of this precaution.

The appearance of a reperfusion syndrome has not been described after an isolated vertebral reconstruction. This complication is more commonly seen after multiple reconstructions in patients with multilevel disease suffering from cerebral hypoperfusion [15].

The increase in morbidity and mortality after combined carotid and vertebral surgery as compared with isolated vertebral surgery was noted by Branchereau and Magnan in a series of 191 vertebral reconstructions performed between 1979 and 1985: in this series the cumulative morbidity and mortality risk was 9.7% after combined surgery of the carotid and vertebral arteries and 0.9% after isolated vertebral surgery [6]. The more generalized atherosclerotic disease in these patients as well as the greater complexity of the techniques applied are the two major factors leading to the increased morbidity and mortality [16]. That is why the indications for combined carotid and vertebral surgery should be limited: Berguer et al. did not perform any longer any combined carotid and vertebral procedures in asymptomatic patients concerning their vertebrobasilar perfusion [2], in too old, high-risk patients, and in those at risk of carotid clamping [16].

Clearly exceptionally, one central neurologic complication in the form of a medullary ischemia was seen [1]. It concerned a patient who had undergone a vertebral reconstruction into the left thyro-bicervico-scapular trunk, combined with a carotid reconstruction. The underlying mechanism was that of a thromboembolic event in the area of the anterior spinal artery, of which the anastomoses with the vertebral artery and cervical arteries from the subclavian artery are numerous [13].

Complications concerning access of the subclavian artery

Whether one regards the isolated reconstructions of the subclavian artery via a cervical approach or the combined reconstructions via a thoracic approach, the surgical reconstructions of the subclavian artery have become less frequent since the advent of the endovascular techniques. We will only address the specific complications while discerning the complications related to the mode of access and those related to the arterial reconstruction (Table V).

CERVICOTOMIES

The standard approach is a transversal cervicotomy, which is very similar to the approach of the proximal vertebral artery [17]. Peripheral nerve complications are approximately the same as those seen after accessing the proximal vertebral artery. A Horner's syndrome occurs often, especially when the subclavian-vertebral crossing is exposed and mobilized.

The recurrent laryngeal nerve may also be traumatized either directly, notably in case of a right subclavian approach, or via a trauma to the vagus nerve. The latter is in particular exposed when a reconstruction is performed from the common carotid artery. A lesion of the phrenic nerve occurs especially during surgery of the distal subclavian artery. Its access requires the exposition and transection of the anterior scalenus muscle in the aponeurosis through which the phrenic nerve runs. As in vertebral artery surgery, a paralysis of the phrenic or recurrent laryngeal nerve should cause extreme prudence when a contralateral cervical procedure is planned. Lymphatic complications may also be observed, particularly on the left side because of the proximity of the thoracic canal. The clinical presentation, both the risks and the therapeutic consequences of these different complications have already been described.

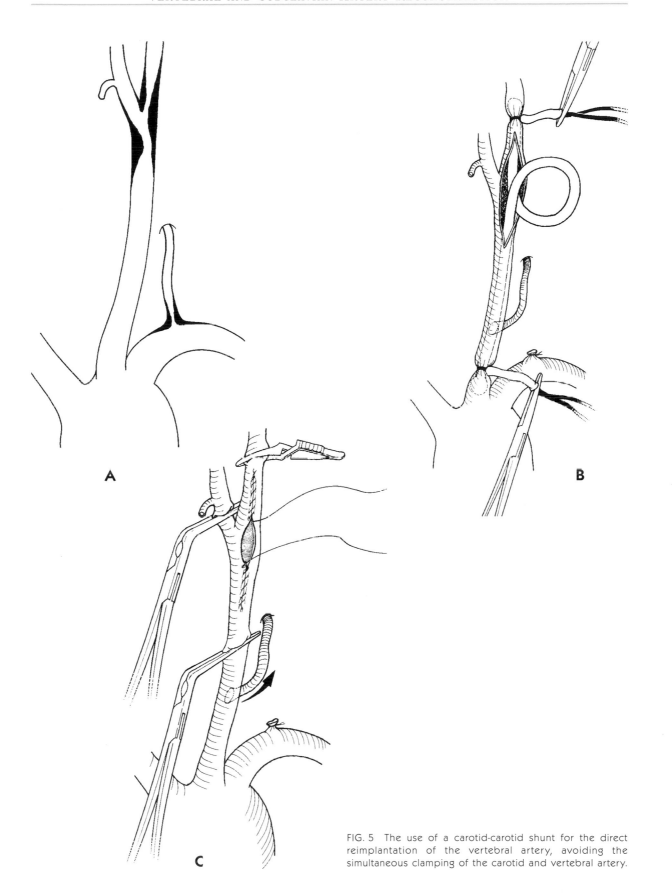

A

B

C

FIG. 5 The use of a carotid-carotid shunt for the direct reimplantation of the vertebral artery, avoiding the simultaneous clamping of the carotid and vertebral artery.

Table V		COMPLICATIONS OF RECONSTRUCTIVE SURGERY OF THE SUBCLAVIAN ARTERY										
1st author [ref.]	*Year*	*Study period*	*Number of cases*	*Death*	*CVE*	*TIA*	*Thrombosis*	*Horner's syndrome*	*Recurrent laryngeal nerve paralysis*	*Phrenic nerve paralysis*	*Thoracic canal lesion*	*Pneumo-thorax*
Sterpetti [18]	1989	1972-1987	46	-	1	1	1	2*	2*	1*	-	-
Perler [19]	1990	1979-1989	31	-	1	-	1	-	1*	1*	-	1
Branchereau [20]	1991	1979-1985	105	1●	4●	-	4	-	-	-	-	-
Vitti [21]	1994	1968-1990	124	1	-	-	-	-	2*	2*	1	-

CVE: cerebrovascular event
TIA: transient ischemic attack
* Regressive lesions
● Simultaneous carotid surgery in both cases

Lesions of the brachial plexus occur more specifically during extended expositions of the subclavian artery, in case of distal subclavian reconstruction or vertebral reconstructions using the subclavian artery as reimplantation site.

In a literature review by Moore, four paralyses of the brachial plexus were found among 1158 vertebral-subclavian reconstructions [5]. The vast majority of the lesions described were partial and recovered within several weeks or months. The postoperative hemorrhagic complications usually have a technical origin: leakage from the anastomosis site, bleeding from a collateral artery of which the hemostasis has been insufficient, unnoticed damage to a collateral artery. Infectious bleedings have a delayed appearance and pose very specific problems. Here too, the occurrence of a compressing hematoma is possible, requiring an acute intervention.

Especially worth mentioning are the preoperative hemorrhages that can occur during the exploration and are of venous or arterial origin. A small incision, notably on the left side where the subclavian artery lies deep, may cause a particularly tricky hemorrhage, especially when one wishes to avoid trauma to the nearby nervous elements. These hemorrhages are mostly due to lesions of the subclavian vein or of collateral venous or arterial branches. The importance of a hemorrhage may, rather than performing an approximate or blind hemostasis, require enlargement of the incision. Partial sterno-cleidomastoidectomy with subluxation of the clavicle may suffice to yield a good exposure of the venous plexus. A proximal approach towards the intrathoracic subclavian artery may necessitate an urgent sternotomy or left thoracotomy to master the brachiocephalic trunk or the intrathoracic part of the left subclavian artery. One should not hesitate to quickly convert the planned procedure in case of these massive hemorrhagic complications, which put at stake the vital prognosis of the patient. Prevention of this event is based on a profound anatomical knowledge of the region, a meticulous surgical technique, a sufficient illumination, and an adequate instrumentation.

Infectious complications may be fostered by a postoperative hematoma. Its consequences are extremely variable, ranging from a simple superficial cellulites to a mediastinitis in case of intrathoracic extension of the infection.

THORACOTOMIES

Except for the painful sequelae related to a parietal trauma, respiratory complications may become manifest after thoracotomies. The treatment is mainly symptomatic, based on correct drainage of the pleural cavity, early postoperative physical therapy, and a specific antibiotic treatment if required. Major respiratory complications that require prolonged ventilatory support should not be treated with a tracheotomy because prosthetic material is usually nearby.

STERNOTOMIES

Sternotomies induce specific complications. Most frequently a venous thrombosis is seen proximal to a ligature of the left innominate venous trunk. This ligation is often necessary when a correct exposure is desired of the left subclavian artery via a sternotomy, e.g. in a complex reconstruction of the supraaortic trunks. Collateral circulation is initiated usually without major clinical consequences. Yet, edema formation of the left upper limb may occur together with a considerable superficial collateral circulation. Restoration of the continuity of the innominate venous trunk is technically difficult, but may in its turn also induce postoperative thrombotic complications. In general, heparin treatment for several days suffices to make the symptoms of acute venous stasis disappear. The sequelae of this kind of event are manifested by edema of the upper limb and a visible collateral circulation. These usually are minimal or even insignificant after a few weeks.

Complications due to reconstruction of the subclavian artery

POSTOPERATIVE OCCLUSION

Postoperative occlusion is usually due to an erroneous indication of technique. It is most often a problem of compression or kinking, leading to an occlusion of the bypass revascularizing the subclavian artery. In that case the occlusion may be delayed and cause late clinical manifestations. Acute upper limb ischemia is rare because of its arterial collateralization. Its treatment requires a reintervention with revision of the reconstruction.

NEUROLOGIC COMPLICATIONS

Central neurologic complications may be seen after subclavian reconstruction, but they are rare (Table V). The mechanism is mostly thromboembolic. A technical failure is usually the cause of a distal embolization or a thrombosis of the reconstruction performed. The occurrence of an embolus causing vertebrobasilar symptoms is rare and may have quite variable consequences. If the embolus occludes the vertebral artery at its origin, the symptoms are generally minimal while the collateral circulation mostly supplies the distal vertebral artery. The only consequence is the loss of the expected benefit of the subclavian reconstruction.

If an embolus migrates distally up to the intracerebral level, the consequences may be an aspecific transient ischemic attack, a Wallenberg syndrome which leaves usually only minimal sequelae in case of obliteration of the terminal part of the vertebral artery and the PICA, a massive, potentially lethal infarction in case of embolization of the basilar trunk. The reconstruction technique most commonly used for the subclavian artery is actually the transposition of the subclavian artery into the common carotid artery. Postoperative thrombosis of such a reconstruction may indicate a thrombosis and/or embolization of the carotid trunk, with as a possible consequence a hemispheric cerebrovascular event.

As in vertebral artery surgery, the combined surgery increases significantly the incidence of central neurologic complications [20]. A reperfusion syndrome may also be observed after a multilevel reconstruction.

Endoluminal reconstructions

Apart from complications specific for the transcutaneous access, the endoluminal angioplasties of the vertebral and subclavian arteries carry a specific risk of neurologic complications. The irregular and heterogeneous character of the lesion to be treated should cause reluctance to decide for a reconstruction and dilatation. The literature does not allow evaluation of this risk, as the majority of the series are limited, heterogeneous, and the results reported with limited precision. In our experience we have observed a cerebellar syndrome in one woman after a transluminal angioplasty of a prevertebral stenotic lesion of the subclavian artery. The symptoms have receded slowly without sequelae.

REFERENCES

1 Rosset E, Ayari R, Magnan PE et al. Résultats à long terme de la chirurgie des artères vertébrales. In: Branchereau A, Jacobs M (eds). *Résultats à long terme des reconstructions artérielles.* Armonk, Futura Publishing Compagny 1997, pp 67-79.
2 Berguer R, Flynn LM, Kline RA, Caplan L. Surgical reconstruction of the extracranial vertebral artery: management and outcome. *J Vasc Surg* 2000; 31: 9-18.

3   Kieffer E. Chirurgie de l'artère vertébrale. *Encycl. Méd. Chir.* (Editions Scientifiques et Médicales Elsevier SAS, Paris), Techniques chirurgicales, Chirurgie vasculaire, 43-130, 34p.

4   Branchereau A, Rosset E, Magnan PE et al. Long term results of proximal vertebral reconstructions. In: Berguer R, Caplan L (eds). *Vertebrobasilar arterial disease.* St Louis, Quality Medical Publishing, 1992; pp 265-279.

5   Moore WS. Complications with repair of the supra-aortic trunks and vertebral arteries In: Bernhard VM, Towne JB (eds). *Complications in vascular surgery.* Saint Louis, Quality Medical Publishing, 1991, pp 456-465.

6   Branchereau A, Magnan PE. Results of vertebral artery reconstruction. *J Cardiovasc Surg* 1990; 31: 320-326.

7   Roon AJ, Ehrenfeld WK, Cooke PB, Wylie EJ. Vertebral artery reconstruction. *Am J Surg* 1979; 138: 29-36.

8   Imparato AM. Vertebral artery reconstruction: a nineteen-year experience. *J Vasc Surg* 1985; 2: 626-634.

9   Berguer R, Feldman AJ. Surgical reconstruction of the vertebral artery. *Surgery* 1983; 93: 670-675.

10 Kieffer E, Koskas F, Rancurel G et al. Long term results of distal vertebral cervical artery reconstruction In: Berguer R, Caplan L (eds). *Vertebrobasilar arterial disease.* St Louis, Quality Medical Publishing, 1992; pp 279-289.

11 Koskas F, Kieffer E, Rancurel G et al. Direct transposition of the distal cervical vertebral artery into the internal carotid artery. *Ann Vasc Surg* 1995; 9: 515-524.

12 Berguer R, Morasch M, Kline RA. A review of 100 consecutive reconstructions of the distal vertebral artery for embolic and hemodynamic disease. *J Vasc Surg* 1998; 27: 852-859.

13 Rosset E, Branchereau A. Artère vertébrale distale: bases anatomiques et technique de l'abord chirurgical. In: Branchereau A (ed). *Voies d'abord des vaisseaux.* Paris, Arnette Blackwell, 1995, pp 34-44.

14 Berguer R, Kieffer E. Reconstruction of the distal vertebral artery. In Berguer R, Kieffer E (eds). *Surgery of the arteries to the head.* New York, Springer-Verlag 1992, pp 141-153.

15 Rosset E, Magnan PE, Branchereau A et al. Hemodynamic vertebrobasilar insufficiency caused by multiple arterial lesions: results of surgical treatment. *Ann Vasc Surg* 1993; 7: 243-248.

16 Magnan PE, Branchereau A. Simultaneous one or two stage restoration of the vertebral and carotid arteries. *J Mal Vasc* 1994; 19 Suppl A: 1-4.

17 Mary H, Marty-Ane C, Fabre D. Artère sous-clavière et axillaire. In: Branchereau A (ed). *Voies d'abord des vaisseaux.* Paris; Arnette Blackwell, 1995, pp 47-60.

18 Sterpetti AV, Schultz RD, Farina C, Feldhaus RJ. Subclavian artery revascularization: a comparison between carotid-subclavian artery bypass and subclavian-carotid transposition. *Surgery* 1989; 106: 624-632.

19 Perler BA, Williams GM. Carotid-subclavian bypass - a decade of experience. *J Vasc Surg* 1990; 12: 716-723.

20 Branchereau A, Magnan PE, Espinoza H, Bartoli JM. Subclavian artery stenosis: hemodynamic aspects and surgical outcome. *J Cardiovasc Surg* 1991; 32: 604-612.

21 Vitti MJ, Thompson BW, Read RC et al. Carotid-subclavian bypass: a twenty-two-year experience. *J Vasc Surg* 1994; 20: 411-418.

17

18

COMPLICATIONS OF PERCUTANEOUS CAROTID ARTERY ANGIOPLASTY

ANDRÉ NEVELSTEEN, HENDRIK LACROIX, GAART MALEUX

Carotid endarterectomy is one of the most commonly performed vascular operations. It is currently advised not only to patients suffering from symptoms of cerebral ischemia, but also to some subsets of patients who are entirely asymptomatic. Although the first operations for carotid artery stenosis were already being performed in the early 1950s [1], recognition of carotid endarterectomy as the gold standard *has required decades and numerous randomized clinical trials. On the other hand, endovascular surgery has undeniably and dramatically changed the possibilities for treatment of both occlusive and aneurysmal arterial disease. It should therefore be no surprise that the first reports on balloon dilatation of internal carotid artery stenoses appeared already some 15 years ago [2-4]. Already since 1992, reports of over 100 patients have been published with an overall stroke-transient ischemic attack (TIA) rate of around 4% [5]. In these early series, treatment was limited to simple balloon angioplasty. In more recent studies, however, primary stent placement became the method of choice, which means that carotid artery angioplasty and carotid artery stenting will be used synonymously in this chapter.*

Recent developments

It is generally agreed that carotid angioplasty has some theoretical advantages over carotid endarterectomy. The procedure can be done under local anesthesia, and even on an outpatient base. There is no need for surgical dissection and the cranial nerves at not at risk. This, however, has to be balanced against the specific and partially unknown risks of angioplasty: plaque manipulation might induce an elevated cerebral embolization rate, while temporary balloon occlusion of the carotid artery might be associated with cerebral ischemia, reflex bradycardia and even episodes of hypotension. In addition, there remains the possible long-term complication of restenosis.

The first carotid angioplasty in our department was performed in 1983 [6]. It concerned a 47-year-old woman with a symptomatic carotid artery stenosis due to fibromuscular dysplasia, which was successfully dilated. After five years she was still asymptomatic without evidence of restenosis. Taking into account our results of carotid endarterectomy [7], we have always favored conventional endarterectomy for atherosclerotic lesions; angioplasty is reserved in our department for patients who are at risk for conventional surgery, as well for cardiopulmonary, as for technical reasons. This means that over the last two years (1999-2000) we performed only 32 carotid angioplasties compared to 301 carotid endarterectomies. We feel that this conservative attitude is still shared by most vascular surgeons, but, in the mean time, carotid angioplasty has gained much more enthusiasm, certainly in the cardiological and radiological world. Recently, Wholey et al. presented a global experience of 4 757 patients who underwent carotid artery angioplasty in 36 major centers worldwide [8]. Strikingly, 57% of these cases were provided by cardiologists, 30% by radiologists, and only 13% by vascular surgeons. Apart from this, they also documented a carotid artery angioplasty annual growth rate of 27% in 1997, 18% in 1998, climbing to 47% in 1999. In this chapter we will focus on the complications and the continuing problems of these procedures.

Early complications of carotid angioplasty

Technical success of carotid angioplasty is defined in most studies as less than 30% to 50% postprocedural residual stenosis over the region of the original lesion. Technical failure includes, however, not only residual stenoses, but also patients with approach problems due to tortuous arteries or in whom it might be not possible to cross the stenosis with a guide wire. This has certainly been a major problem in the early years of carotid angioplasty, with failure rates going up to 10% [9-11]. More recently, with the introduction of newer materials, technical failures have become more exceptional but still occur in 1% to 2% of the cases [8]. Although most of these patients are subjected to subsequent carotid endarterectomy, it is virtually never mentioned whether, as it has been demonstrated in abdominal aortic aneurysms, this failed

angioplasty contributes to a higher operative morbidity rate in these cases.

Despite the fact that most procedures are performed under local anesthesia, carotid angioplasty continues to carry a mortality rate ranging between 0% and 2% (Table I). Most deaths are due to stroke or myocardial infarction. Most authors also state that the most important factor might be a negative patient selection when compared to conventional carotid endarterectomy. Gupta et al., at the other hand, reported a series of 100 elderly patients, more than 65 years old, considered to be inoperable, mostly because of concomitant coronary artery disease [23]. There were no deaths and over 90% of the patients were discharged home within 24 hours.

As for carotid endarterectomy, neurological events are also the most frequent complications of carotid angioplasty. A search in the literature revealed only one study without any complications [14]. All other authors observed neurological events with an incidence of 2% going up to more than 70% [19]. In a collected series of 7 851 cases of carotid angioplasty we defined a mean stroke rate of 4.4% (Table II).

Stroke rates tend to vary clearly in relation to the indication [28]. In the review study presented by Wholey et al. (4 749 patients with 5 210 carotid artery stenoses), the overall stroke rate of 4.8% in symptomatic cases decreased to 3% in case of asymptomatic stenosis [8]. This review study identified also a learning curve of 50 cases in relation to stroke and procedure related deaths. The respective stroke rate decreased from 4.9% in centers under 50 cases to 3.6% in centers performing 200 to 300 cases. Surprisingly, it increased again to 4.4% in centers performing more than 300 procedures. Teitelbaum et al. reported a stroke rate of more than 20% in 22 high risk patients [20]. Gupta et al. only encountered one stroke in a series of 100 patients with inoperable coronary artery disease [23]. Advanced age as an independent risk factor for neurological complications was identified in the series of Mathur et al. [29]. These data were confirmed by Chastain et al., who experienced a 25% neurological complication rate in patients over 80 years of age, decreasing to 8.6% in patients younger than 75 years [30]. Finally, the degree of stenosis has also been recognized as an important prognostic factor. Mathur et al. indeed reported a significantly higher neurological complication rate in the presence of long or multiple stenoses [29].

These data were confirmed by ex vivo experiments of Ohki et al. [31].

MECHANISMS OF COMPLICATIONS

According to Riles et al. [32], there are three major causes of peri-operative stroke after carotid endarterectomy: cerebral embolization during operative dissection or from the endarterectomy surface, hypoperfusion during carotid artery clamping, and cerebral hemorrhage due to postoperative hyperperfusion. Although significant cerebral ischemia can occur during carotid angioplasty, certainly in patients with contralateral occlusion [33], it seems clear that the risk of embolization during plaque mobilization is much greater. This has indeed been demonstrated both in experimental and clinical studies [34-35]. Jordan et al. studied the incidence of micro-embolization as detected by transcranial doppler monitoring during the treatment of 115 carotid bifurcation stenoses [36]. Included were 40 percutaneous carotid angioplasties and 75 conventional carotid endarterectomies. Micro-emboli were noted in 37 (92.5%) of the percutaneous and 46 (61%) of the operative procedures. Percutaneous angioplasty resulted in 4 (10%) neurologic events. Only one (1.4%) of the carotid artery endarterectomy patients was noted to have a stroke. Here also, the nature of the atherosclerotic plaque and the lesion itself might be very important. Ohki et al. noted that certain lesions (echolucent plaques and tight more than 90% stenoses) produce indeed higher numbers of embolic particulates [31]. Several other authors have tried in this regard to correlate plaque morphology, as identified by

Table I	EARLY OUTCOME AFTER CAROTID ANGIOPLASTY				
1st author [ref.]	Year of publication	Carotid arteries	Death (%)	Any stroke or death (%)
Dietrich[12]	1996	116	2	9
Eckert[11]	1996	61	0	3
Gil-Peralta [10]	1996	85	0	4
Kachel [9]	1996	71	0	1
Roubin [13]	1996	147	1	10
Criado [14]	1997	33	0	0
Smedema [15]	1997	33	0	1
Yadav [16]	1997	74	1	8
Gaines[18]	1998	187	3	20
Naylor [19]	1998	7	0	5
Tcitelbaum [20]	1998	25	1	6
Waigand [21]	1998	56	0	2
Bergeron[17] *	1999	96	0	1
Gross [22]	1999	88	0	5
Gupta [23]	2000	100	0	1
Henry [24]	2000	314	0	9
Qureshi [25]	2000	111	0	14
Shawl [26]	2000	190	0	5
Wholey [8] **	2000	5 210	99	299
Yoon [27]	2000	48	0	2
Total		**7 052**	**107 (1.5)**	**405 (5.8)**

* Multicenter study including 36 centers
** European CAST I study including 7 European surgical centers

duplex ultrasound with the potential risk of embolization [37-38]. Until now there is, however, no real evidence on the accuracy of plaque morphology to predict the risk of stroke [39-40].

CEREBRAL PROTECTION

Awareness of these problems led to the introduction of cerebral protection methods. Théron et al. described already in 1990 a special triple coaxial catheter in this regard [41] and reported their results in 1996 [42]. Among 136 patents in whom cerebral protection was used, no embolic complications occurred during angioplasty and two (1%) occurred during or after stent placement. Among 38 patients who underwent angioplasty without cerebral protection, dissection occurred in two

cases (5%) and embolic complications were observed in three cases (8%) during the procedure. Kachel [9] introduced a balloon occlusion technique of the common carotid artery in order to flush the debris by the external carotid. He reported a 4.6% complication rate, which is certainly not convincing when compared to other series without cerebral protection. Albuquerque et al. [43] described a simple method of distal occlusion of the internal carotid artery with a compliant silicone balloon during the angioplasty phase, when the largest number of emboli are generated. After angioplasty, debris is then flushed into the external carotid circulation. Subsequent stent placement is performed with the occlusion balloon deflated. They used this technique in 16 patients. In one patient it proved im-

Table II		EARLY NEUROLOGICAL COMPLICATIONS AFTER CAROTID ANGIOPLASTY				
1st author [ref.]	*Year of publication*	*Carotid arteries*	*TIA (%)*	*Minor stroke (%)*	*Major stroke (%)*	*Any stroke (%)*
Dietrich [12]	1996	116	5	5	2	7
Eckert [11]	1996	61	8	2	1	3
Gil-Peralta [10]	1996	85	3	0	4	4
Kachel [9]	1996	71	1	0	1	1
Roubin [13]	1996	147	-	7	2	9
Criado [14]	1997	33	0	0	0	0
Smedema [15]	1997	33	0	0	1	1
Yadav [16]	1997	74	-	5	2	7
Gaines [18]	1998	187	23	12	5	17
Naylor [19]	1998	7	-	2	3	5
Teitelbaum [20]	1998	25	-	-	-	5
Waigand [21]	1998	56	3	1	1	2
Bergeron [17] *	1999	96	4	1	0	1
Gross [22]	1999	88	-	3	2	5
Mathias [28]	1999	799	-	4	2	6
Gupta [23]	2000	100	5	0	1	1
Henry [24]	2000	314	4	4	5	9
Qureshi [25]	2000	111	-	-	-	14
Shawl [26]	2000	190	-	4	1	5
Wholey [8] **	2000	5 210	134	129	112	241
Yoon [27]	2000	48	-	1	1	2
Total		**7 851**	**190 (3)**	**180 (2.3)**	**146 (1.9)**	**345 (4.4)**

TIA: transient ischemic attack
* European Cast I Study including 7 European surgical centers
** Multicenter study including 36 centers

possible to advance the occlusion balloon across the stenosis and this patient developed a transient ischemic attack during subsequent angioplasty. All other procedures were successful without any complications. Despite the theoretical advantages, cerebral protection has gained little enthusiasm in the past. In a survey of 24 carotid stent investigative sites around the world, Wholey et al. [44] found that only two centers used cerebral protection before 1997. Currently there are several more sophisticated devices (both of the occlusive and filter type) under investigation. Last year, Henry et al. reported their first experience with the *PercuSurge Guardwire system*, an occlusive-type protection device [45]. They presented 48 patients who underwent 53 carotid angioplasties. Immediate technical success was achieved in all patients. One patient with a contralateral internal carotid artery occlusion did not tolerate the occlusion technique, losing consciousness 30 seconds after inflation of the occluded balloon. The balloon was deflated and stenting was performed successfully without cerebral protection. Another patient developed transient amaurosis due to stent thrombosis during placement. Otherwise there were no complications. More recently, Parodi et al. [46] used three different protection devices in 25 patients. All procedures were successful and there were no neurological events, compared to one transient ischemic attack and one minor stroke observed in 21 patients treated without cerebral protection. These differences were not statistically significant. They concluded fairly that cerebral protection during carotid angioplasty and stenting is technically feasible. Cerebral protection appears to be effective in preventing procedure-related neurologic complications, but further investigation is warranted.

RECURRENT STENOSIS

Carotid angioplasty has also been recommended as a better alternative to operative management in case of carotid restenosis after endarterectomy. In 1996, Bergeron et al. published a series of 15 patients with carotid restenosis, who underwent 17 balloon angioplasties in 3 common carotid and 14 internal carotid arteries [47]. The neurological complication rate was 33%, while 3 lesions required immediate stenting because of postdilation complications. They concluded that balloon angioplasty alone appears too risky for treating recurrent carotid disease and that stents may offer a safer alternative, particularly when primarily implanted. This conclusion was confirmed by Hobson et al., who presented a series of

16 patients, undergoing 17 carotid artery stentings for carotid restenosis [48].

During the 30-day periprocedural period, no neurological complications occurred. The mean follow-up was 11 months and restenosis was identified in only one patient. These results were compared to 16 conventional surgical procedures for carotid restenosis. In these series there were also no strokes or deaths but one patient (6.2%) developed a recurrent laryngeal nerve palsy. Hobson et al. concluded that the periprocedural complication rates of conventional surgery and carotid stenting are comparable and that carotid stenting may become the preferred procedure. Once again, this conclusion might be too easy, certainly when looking at the report of Raithel et al. [49]. They compared their past experience of 66 operative reconstructions for carotid restenosis with a recent series of 60 patients who underwent intra-operative balloon dilatation and stenting. After conventional surgery two patients (3.1%) suffered from a permanent neurological deficit and one patient developed a TIA (1.5%). After dilatation and stenting eight patients (13.3%) suffered from a stroke. They therefore concluded that balloon angioplasty and stenting cannot be recommended as routine therapy for carotid restenosis. The nature of the plaque is certainly an important factor in this regard, since the best results are reported in early hyperplastic restenoses with smooth, nonulcerated surfaces [48].

Finally a large range of different stents has been used by different authors. The balloon-expandable Palmaz stent was, certainly in vascular surgical centers, most popular in the beginning of carotid angioplasty. Indeed, the Palmaz stent was the only stent used in European CAST I study [17]. However, over the years the Palmaz stent lost much of its importance in favor of self-expandable stents, with the Wallstent as prototype. In their recent review of 5 210 carotid artery angioplasties, Wholey et al. pointed out that 56% of the procedures were performed with a Wallstent, whereas the Palmaz stent was used in 34% of the cases [8]. As for now, it does not seem likely that the early results are influenced by the type of stent used.

NON NEUROLOGIC COMPLICATIONS

Non neurologic procedure related complications have received only minor attention in most publications. As shown by Jordan et al. [50], these complications are certainly not trivial. These authors described a retrospective series of 268 patients who underwent a total of 293 carotid angioplasties with stenting. One hundred sixteen non neurologic complications were seen in 114 patients (43%) (Table III). Hypotension and bradycardia were the most common (87 patients) and as a result of these events, 94 patients (35%) required additional cardiopulmonary monitoring. Transient cardiovascular effects were also mentioned by Gil-Peralta et al. in over 50% of their procedures [10]. Hemodynamic instability as the most common periprocedural complication of carotid angioplasty and stenting was confirmed in another study by Qureshi et al. [51]. They presented a series of 51 patients, both with primary stenosis or restenosis after carotid artery surgery. Postprocedural hypotension was noted in 22% of the cases, hypertension in 39% and bradycardia in 27%. All complications were significantly associated with intraprocedural hemodynamic instability. In addition, postprocedural hypotension was independently predicted by previous myocardial infarction and postprocedural hypertension by previous

ipsilateral carotid endarterectomy. All events in these series resolved spontaneously, but they required an additional mean intensive care unit period of 25.7 hours (range 18 to 43 hours). The conclusion of this study was that patients with hemodynamic instability during the procedure are at the highest risk for postprocedural complications and that carotid artery stenting should be performed in environment settings suited for cardiopulmonary monitoring and management of cardiovascular emergencies.

Medium-term and late complications

Since carotid artery angioplasty is a relatively new and evolving technique, it may be no surprise that there are only few data on long-term results. Szilagyi in 1962 already stated: *"Critical surveys of well-observed and carefully followed angioplastic operations are sorely needed. I am afraid that in the past too much stress has been placed on the reporting of brilliant early results, the observation of which often seemed to have stopped in the recovery room or at the discharge office."* This statement seems to apply for the field of carotid angioplasty also. Follow-up is frequently rather incomplete and limited to patency (with no uniform definition of restenosis!) while no indications are given on the clinical evolution of the patients. Kachel [9] mentioned in this regard no instances of restenoses in a series of 65 patients with a mean observation period of 70 months. Mathias et al. [28] reported a 5-year patency rate of 91.6%, which is somewhat lower than the 4-year patency rate of 96% reported by Henry et al. [24]. Criado et al. [14] described a series of 33 patients with a mean follow-up of 8 months. All patients remained asymptomatic. Stent patency was 100% but there was one instance of intrastent stenosis.

The mean follow-up in the European CAST I study (99 patients) [17] was 13 months (range 1 to 24 months). There were no neurological events and two nonprocedural-related late deaths. In the first year there were 3 asymptomatic non-flow-limiting (smaller than 60%) stenoses. The patency rate at 1 year was 98%, with patency defined as preservation of adequate flow through the stented area.

In their review of 4 757 patients Wholey et al. [8] found a restenosis rate of 3.46% at 1 year, restenosis defined as residual stenosis greater than 50%. Eighty-four percent of the patients were followed for

Table III	Non neurologic complications as described by Jordan et al. [50] in a series of 293 carotid angioplasties		
Complications		Number	%
Hypotension		68	23
Bradycardia		19	6.5
Hematoma*		8	2.7
Increased creatinine of >0.5		6	2
Urinary tract infection		6	2
GI bleeding		3	1
Hypertension		1	0.3
Anemia		1	0.3
Myocardial infarction		1	0.3
Pulmonary edema		1	0.3
Lower extremity ischemia		1	0.3
Acute renal failure		1	0.3

* 2 requiring transfusion and prolonged cardiopulmonary monitoring

12 months and in that period there were 56 new neurologic events (TIAs and stroke). With 3 924 patients at follow-up, the neurologic-related death rate at 1 year was 1.39%. These results might look excellent, but the authors themselves state that one of the limitations of their study is the reliance on accurate follow-up and that it is unlikely that 100% follow-up could be obtained.

Although the early results seem to be independent on the type of stent used, the balloon-expandable Palmaz stent does seem to perform less well at longer term. Wholey et al. [8] reported indeed 45 cases of stent deformation (50% or more narrowing or compression) occurring exclusively with the Palmaz stent. For a total of 1 804 Palmaz stents used in their study, the rate of deformation at 6 months was 2.5%. Additional cases of such crush deformation have been reported by Gross et al. [22] and Waigand et al. [21]. As of now no neurological related problems have been reported, but this phenomenon has never been observed with self-expandable stents.

Is carotid angioplasty an alternative to carotid endarterectomy?

It took over forty years and several international randomized studies for carotid endarterectomy to become the gold standard in the treatment of significant symptomatic carotid artery stenosis. Even nowadays there is still discussion about the best treatment for asymptomatic patients. With regard to carotid angioplasty, only one randomized trial has been published yet [19]. Naylor et al. [52] started a prospective randomized trial comparing carotid endarterectomy and carotid angioplasty. This trial was stopped after 17 patients, since 5 of the 7 patients who underwent carotid angioplasty developed a periprocedural stroke. In contrast, there were no complications in 10 patients who were allocated to carotid endarterectomy. Although the results seem clear, this trial has, probably correctly, been criticized because of the small number of patients which may result in a type II error.

A second randomized trial, the *Carotid and Vertebral Artery Transluminal Angioplasty Study* (CAVATAS), has been finished but is not published yet. The data have nevertheless been presented in abstract form and suggest a relatively high but equivalent stroke and mortality rate of around 10% for angioplasty and endarterectomy [53]. This trial has been criticized for its methods of patient selection. Nevertheless, and despite the lack of objective evidence, some interventionalists have already concluded that carotid angioplasty is an effective alternative for cartid endarterectomy. In their review, Wholey et al. [8] concluded that the risks of carotid angioplasty are comparable to the *American Heart Association* guidelines for carotid endarterectomy: less than 6% for patients with TIAs and less than 7% for patients after stroke [54]. The surgical answer is expressed in the meta-analysis presented by Golledge et al. [55]. These authors analyzed the 30-day outcome of carotid angioplasty and carotid andarterectomy for symptomatic carotid artery disease in 33 single-center studies published since 1990. On the basis of 714 angioplasties and 6 970 endarterectomies, they documented a 30-day stroke or death rate of 7.8% for angioplasty versus 4% for endarterectomy. Their conclusion is that carotid angioplasty cannot be recommended for the majority of patients with symptomatic carotid artery disease. Certainly, this debate will continue as long as we do not have objective evidence from large randomized controlled trials. Such studies are currently under evaluation both in Europe and the United States and results may be expected within some years.

REFERENCES

1 Eastcott HHG, Pickering GW, Rob CG. Reconstruction of internal carotid artery in a patient with intermittent attacks of hemiplegia. *Lancet* 1954; II: 994-996.

2 Bockenheimer SAM, Mathias K. Percutaneous transluminal angioplasty in arteriosclerotic internal carotid artery stenosis. *AJNR Am J Neuroradiol* 1983; 4: 791-792.

3 Wiggli U, Gratzl O. Transluminal angioplasty of stenotic carotid arteries: case reports and protocol. *AJNR Am J Neuroradiol* 1983; 4: 793-795.

4 Freitag G, Freitag J, Koch RD et al. Percutaneous angioplasty of carotid artery stenoses. *Neuroradiology* 1986; 28: 126-127.

5 Brown MM. Balloon angioplasty for cerebrovascular disease. *Neurol Res* 1992; 14 (Suppl): 159-163.

6 Wilms GE, Smits J, Baert AL et al. Percutaneous transluminal angioplasty in fibromuscular dysplasia of the internal carotid artery: one year clinical and morphological follow-up. *Cardiovasc Intervent Radiol* 1985; 8: 20-23.

7 Lacroix H, Beets G, Nevelsteen A et al. Occlusion de l'artère carotide interne contralatérale comme facteur de risque en chirurgie carotidienne. *J Mal Vasc* 1993; 18: 76.

8 Wholey MH, Wholey M, Mathias K et al. Global experience in cervical carotid artery stent placement. *Catheter Cardiovasc Intervent* 2000; 50: 160-167.

9 Kachel R. Results of balloon angioplasty in the carotid arteries. *J Endovasc Surg* 1996; 3: 22-30.

10 Gil-Peralta A, Mayol A, Marcos JR et al. Percutaneous transluminal angioplasty of the symptomatic atherosclerotic carotid arteries. Results, complications, follow-up. *Stroke* 1996; 27: 2271-2273.

11 Eckert B, Zanella FE, Thie A et al. Angioplasty of the internal carotid artery: results, complications and follow-up in 61 cases. *Cerebrovasc Dis* 1996; 6: 97-105.

12 Dietrich EB, Ndiaye M, Reid DB. Stenting in the carotid artery: initial experience in 110 patients. *J Endovasc Surg* 1996; 3: 42-62.

13 Roubin GS, Yadav S, Iyer SS et al. Carotid stent-supported angioplasty: a neurovascular intervention to prevent stroke. *Am J Cardiol* 1996; 78: 8-12.

14 Criado FJ, Wellons E, Clark NS. Evolving indications for and early results of carotid stenting. *Am J Surg* 1997; 174: 111-114.

15 Smedema JP, Saaiman A. Carotid stent-assisted angioplasty. *S Afr Med J* 1997; 87 Supp ll: C9-14.

16 Yadav JS, Roubin S, Iyer S et al. Elective stenting of the extracranial carotid arteries. *Circulation* 1997; 95: 376-381.

17 Bergeron P, Becquemin JP, Jausseran JM et al. Percutaneous stenting of the internal carotid artery: the European CAST I Study. *J Endovasc Surg* 1999; 6: 155-159.

18 Gaines P, Cleveland T, Sivaguru A et al. Endovascular carotid intervention: a single centre audit. *Cardiovasc Intervent radiol* 1998; 21 (suppl 1): S 86: abstract.

19 Naylor AR, Bolia A, Abbott R et al. Randomized study of carotid angioplasty and stenting versus carotid endarterectomy: a stopped trial. *J Vasc Surg* 1998; 28: 326-334.

20 Teitelbaum GP, Lefkowitz MA, Giannotta SL. Carotid angioplasty and stenting in high-risk patients. *Surg Neurol* 1998; 50: 300-312.

21 Waigand J, Gross CM, Uhlich F et al. Elective stenting of carotid artery stenosis in patients with severe coronary artery disease. *Eur Heart J* 1998; 19: 1365-1370.

22 Gross CM, Kramer J, Uhlich F et al. Treatment of carotid artery stenosis by elective stent placement instead of carotid endarterectomy in patients with severe coronary artery diseases. *Thromb Haemost* 1999; 82 Suppl 1: 176-180.

23 Gupta A, Bathia A, Ahuja A et al. Carotid stenting in patients older than 65 years with inoperable carotid artery disease: a single center experience. *Catheter Cardiovasc Interv* 2000; 50: 1-8.

24 Henry M, Amor M, Klonaris C et al. Angioplasty and stenting of the extracranial carotid arteries. *Tex Heart Inst J* 2000; 27: 150-158.

25 Qureshi AI, Luft AR, Janardhan V et al. Identification of patients at risk for periprocedural neurological deficits associated with carotid angioplasty and stenting. *Stroke* 2000; 31: 376-382.

26 Shawl F, Kadro W, Domanski MJ et al. Safety and efficacy of elective carotid artery stenting in high-risk patients. *J Am Coll Cardiol* 2000; 35: 1721-1728.

27 Yoon YS, Shim WH, Kim SM et al. Carotid artery stenting in patients with symptomatic coronary disease. *Yonsei Med J* 2000; 41: 89-97.

28 Mathias K, Jager H, Sahl H et al. Interventional treatment of arteriosclerotic carotid stenosis. *Radiology* 1999; 39: 125-134.

29 Mathur A, Roubin GS, Iyer SS et al. Predictors of stroke complicating carotid artery stenting. *Circulation* 1998; 97: 1239-1245.

30 Chastain HD 2nd, Gomez CR, Iyer S et al. Influence of age upon complications of carotid artery stenting. *J Endovasc Surg* 1999; 6: 217-222.

31 Ohki T, Marin ML, Lyon RT et al. Ex vivo human carotid artery bifurcation stenting: correlation of lesion characteristics with embolic potential. *J Vasc Surg* 1998; 27: 463-471.

32 Riles TS, Imparato AM, Jacobowitz GR et al. The cause of perioperative stroke after carotid endarterectomy. *J Vasc Surg* 1994; 19: 206-216.

33 McCleary AJ, Nelson M, Dearden NM et al. Cerebral haemodynamics and embolization during carotid angioplasty in high-risk patients. *Br J Surg* 1998; 85: 771-774.

34 Coggia M, Goeau-Brissonniere O, Duval JL et al. Embolic risk of the different stages of carotid bifurcation angioplasty: an experimental study. *J Vasc Surg* 2000; 31: 550-557.

35 Manninen HI, Rasanen HT, Vanninne RL et al. Stent placement versus percutaneous transluminal angioplasty of human carotid arteries in cadavers in situ: distal embolization and findings at intravascular US, MR imaging and histopathologic analysis. *Radiology* 1999; 212: 483-492.

36 Jordan WD Jr, Voellinger DC, Doblar DD et al. Microemboli detected by transcranial Doppler monitoring in patients during carotid angioplasty versus carotid endarterectomy. *Cardiovasc Surg* 1999; 7: 33-38.

37 AbuRahma AF, Covelli MA, Robinson PA et al. The role of carotid duplex ultrasound in evaluating plaque morphology: potential use in selecting patients for carotid stenting. *J Endovasc Surg* 1999; 6: 59-65.

38 Biasi GM, Mingazzini PM, Baronio L et al. Carotid plaque characterization using digital image processing and its potential in future studies of carotid endarterectomy and angioplasty. *J Endovasc Surg* 1998; 5: 240-246.

39 Holdsworth RJ, McCollum PT, Bryce JS et al. Symptoms, stenosis and plaque morphology. Is plaque morphology relevant? *J Vasc Endovasc Surg* 1995; 9: 80-85.

40 Carr SC, Cheanvechai V, Virmani R et al. Histology and clinical significance of the carotid atherosclerotic plaque: implications for endovascular treatment. *J Endovasc Surg* 1997; 4: 321-325.

41 Théron J, Courtheoux P, Alachkar F et al. New triple coaxial catheter system for carotid angioplasty with cerebral protection. *AJNR Am J Neuroradiol* 1990; 11: 869-877.

42 Théron JG, Payelle GG, Coskun O et al. Carotid artery stenosis: treatment with protected balloon angioplasty and stent placement. *Radiology* 1996; 201: 627-636.

43 Albuquerque FC, Teitelbaum GP, Lavine SD et al. Balloon protected carotid angioplasty. *Neurosurgery* 2000; 46: 918-921.

44 Wholey MH, Wholey M, Bergeron P et al. Current global status of carotid artery stent placement. *Cathet Cardiovasc Diagn* 1998; 44: 1-6.

45 Henry M, Amor M, Henry I et al. Carotid stenting with cerebral protection: first clinical experience using the PercuSurge GuardWire system. *J Endovasc Surg* 1999: 6: 321-331.

46 Parodi JC, La Mura R, Ferreira LM et al. Initial evaluation of carotid angioplasty and stenting with three different cerebral protection devices. *J Vasc Surg* 2000; 32: 1127-1136.

47 Bergeron P, Chambran P, Benichou H et al. Recurrent carotid disease: will stents be an alternative to surgery? *J Endovasc Surg* 1996; 3: 76-79.

48 Hobson RW 2nd, Goldstein JE, Jamil Z et al. Carotid restenosis: operative and endovascular management. *J Vasc Surg* 1999; 29: 228-238.

49 Raithel D, Schunn C, Hetzel G et al. Treatment of carotid restenosis. *Zentralbl Chir* 2000; 125: 270-274.

50 Jordan WD Jr, Voellinger DC, Fisher WS et al. A comparison of carotid angioplasty with stenting versus endarterectomy with regional anesthesia. *J Vasc Surg* 1998; 28: 397-403.

51 Qureshi AI, Luft AR, Janardhan V et al. Frequency and determinants of postprocedural hemodynamic instability after carotid angioplasty and stenting. *Stroke* 1999; 30: 2086-2093.

52 Naylor AR, London NJ, Bell PR. Carotid endarterectomy versus carotid angioplasty. *Lancet* 1997; 349: 203-204.

53 Brown MM. Vascular Surgical Society of Britain and Ireland: results of the carotid and vertebral artery transluminal angioplasty study. *Br J Surg* 1999; 86: 710-711.

54 Moore WS, Barnett HJ, Beebe HG et al. Guidelines for carotid endarterectomy: a multidisciplinary consensus statement from the ad hoc committee, American Heart association. *Stroke* 1995; 26: 188-201.

55 Golledge J, Mitchell A, Greenhalgh RM et al. Systematic comparison of the early outcome of angioplasty and endarterectomy for symptomatic carotid artery disease. *Stroke* 2000; 31: 1439-1443.

18

19

COMPLICATIONS OF SUPRA-AORTIC ARTERIAL ENDOVASCULAR INTERVENTIONS

PETER A GAINES

Chronic occlusive disease in the upper limb is different in many ways than lower limb disease. It is less frequent than lower limb disease, has a left sided dominance and tends to be focal and ostial. The age and sex distribution is similar to aorto-iliac disease rather than infra-inguinal atherosclerosis.

The majority of endovascular interventions in the upper limb is undertaken for chronic occlusive disease rather than aneurysmal disease and was first described just twenty years ago. Since then there have been many publications on the use of angioplasty and stents, which are now regarded by many vascular units as the initial treatment of choice for upper limb chronic arterial disease. While these therapies are well described in the literature the vast majority is related to intervention in the subclavian artery. Data on complications of upper limb intervention is very sparse. Any sort of data is even more rare for individual lesions e.g. brachiocephalic and left common carotid intervention. Furthermore there is virtually no sensible high quality data on outcome and complications of treating upper limb aneurysmal disease.

Chronic upper limb ischemia

PROCEDURAL DEATH AND LONG-TERM PATENCY

Surgery has a mortality rate of 0%-3% for extra-thoracic procedures and 6%-19% for intra-thoracic procedures [1,2]. Endovascular intervention in the upper limbs appears to be largely without procedural death, making it ideal for a disease pattern that has a good long-term prognosis [1,2]. The long-term patency of angioplasty, however, is not as good as surgery. The 2-5 year patency for angioplasty of stenoses is 54%-97% compared to 83%-95% for surgery. The primary success of treating occlusions by simple angioplasty is not as high as stenoses and ranges between 15%-88%; the patency at one year is 50%-80% [1,2].

What is unclear is how reocclusion affects the patient clinically and whether re-intervention is a similarly benign and successful procedure.

Stents have recently been introduced into upper limb practice ostensibly to increase the primary success and outcome but numbers are small, many have been placed for simple stenoses, and the majority of papers do not report the technical success rate on an intention to treat basis or the long-term patency.

OTHER PROCEDURAL COMPLICATIONS

A review of the recent literature [3-15] focused upon large series or potentially high-risk patients indicate a wide spread in the reported incidence of complications from 0%-21%. Although it is recognized that the majority of complications are related to the access site there are up to 13% of patients who have a major complication defined as one that requires surgical intervention, delays discharge or results in a deterioration in ischemia or ischemia to another territory (e.g., stroke/TIA). It is clear that the risk of complications is related to the complexity of the procedure. Thus simple angioplasty of subclavian stenoses is successful in 95%-100% of cases and has a very low complication rate. However, branch vessel occlusions have a primary failure rate of up to 54% (range 0%-54%) [2-8] and because these are usually approached from the arm, have a significant complication rate relating to the brachial approach, and some risk of embolization because of the bulky nature of the disease (Fig. 1).

This section will describe significant complications and ways to reduce the risk of occurrence.

ACCESS SITE COMPLICATIONS

Access for upper limb intervention is usually from the femoral artery, and no precautions particular to upper limb intervention are then required.

Where a brachial approach is required then there appears to be a significant morbidity associated with this. Sullivan et al. [5] recorded that 5 of their 18 complications were at the brachial access site and 2 required surgical intervention. All the major complications in our own series dealing with the *blue digit syndrome* were related to the brachial arteriotomy [9]. Percutaneous access is difficult where the brachial artery is collapsed and impalpable because of proximal disease. To minimize damage to the

vessel we initially preferred an arteriotomy. However, in small vessels this appears to have its own complication rate, so that we now prefer to:

1 - puncture the vessel guided by ultrasound,
2 - limit the brachial sheath size by limiting intervention to low profile balloon angioplasty where possible,
3 - approach from the arm, bring the wire out through the femoral artery and stent from the groin when the brachial artery is small (usually in elderly women),
4 - using liberal doses of antispasmodics through the brachial sheath,
5 - use adequate amounts of heparin (at least 5 000 units as a bolus) throughout the procedure.

PROTECTING THE VERTEBRAL ARTERY

Embolization does occur to the vertebral artery, albeit rarely. In the situation where subclavian artery disease produces distal embolization (blue digit syn-

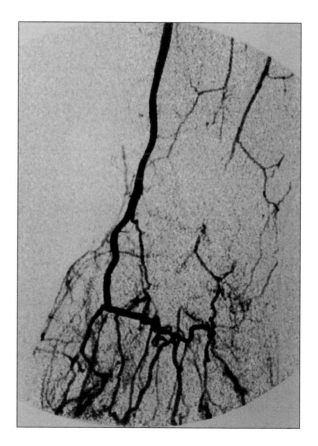

FIG. 1 Following angioplasty and subsequent stent placement, there is an embolus in the ulnar artery.

drome) there is often normal antegrade flow in the vertebral artery. In this situation there is a potential risk that emboli may enter the vertebro-basilar system, resulting in significant permanent morbidity. It is prudent to consider protecting the vertebral artery by placing an occlusion balloon in the vessel prior to subclavian dilatation. This can best be achieved from the arm prior to crossing the lesion from either the arm or leg.

When the subclavian lesion encroaches upon the ostium of the vertebral artery there is a risk of spreading the plaque and subsequently occluding the vessel. Although this may not be of importance in many patients, those who are being treated because of a subclavian steal often suffer from carotid or contralateral vertebral artery disease, or may have a contralateral vertebral artery ending in the posterior cerebellar artery. In this situation it may be catastrophic to lose the vertebral artery. If there is retrograde flow in the vertebral artery, protection against embolization is not required and it is our practice to place a fine wire into the vertebral artery, usually from the arm, prior to treating the stenosis. In this way if plaque does occlude the vessel then access is already present to the vertebral artery and a balloon can be used to open the ostium.

LIMITING CAROTID EMBOLIZATION

Embolization is the most significant complication affecting supra-aortic endovascular intervention. It complicates both stenoses and occlusions and appears to be as common with stent placement as angioplasty. Clearly the principal concern is where there is antegrade flow in the vertebral artery (discussed above) and when proximal carotid or brachiocephalic disease is being treated.

For ostial carotid artery disease there are major technical difficulties treating these from the groin so that we prefer to use a carotid artery cut-down and treat these from above. In this way the vessel can be flushed and the internal carotid artery occluded during intervention.

Brachiocephalic disease is challenging to treat because of the risks of carotid embolization. We take measures to ensure the carotid artery is protected at all times by preferably placing a cerebral protection device (occlusion balloon or filter) from the arm (Fig. 2), or manually compressing the carotid artery if this is not possible. The lesion can then be approached from either the arm or groin.

STENT PROBLEMS

Because much of the atherosclerotic disease affecting the upper limb vessels is ostial, many practitioners choose balloon expandable stents rather than their self-expanding cousins because of their perceived greater crush resistance and easier precise placement. However, balloon mounted stents have an unpleasant tendency to come off the balloon. Usually this results in the stent being displaced down the shaft of the balloon catheter. If the stent is being placed from the groin, hopefully it can be coaxed back onto the balloon, perhaps with the help of the sheath. If this is the case it is unlikely that the stent can then be retrieved through the sheath and it is wise to deposit the stent somewhere harmless, either the common or external iliac artery according to the size of balloon. If the balloon cannot be coaxed back into the stent then one faces a big problem because neither the balloon, nor the stent can be retrieved. Our solution has been to bring the balloon out through the contralateral femoral artery by snaring the wire, using a large

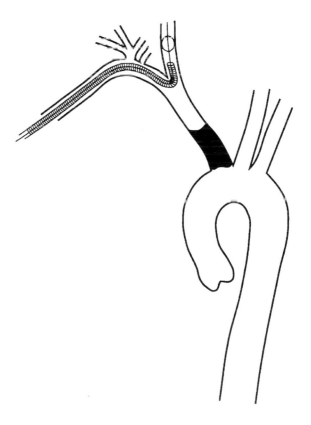

FIG. 2 Protection balloon placed in the light common carotid artery prior to dilatation of the brachiocephalic lesion.

sheath and cutting off the back of the balloon catheter. By using a 4 Fr catheter it is then possible to feed a fine wire and low profile balloon inside the stent, dilate up the stent, and finally use a suitable sized balloon to deposit the stent in the iliac artery.

If the stent is being placed from the arm then again it should be placed in a non-crushable part of the artery.

Whilst many practitioners choose the balloon expandable stent for the reasons given above, the author knows of at least two cases where the stent has subsequently crushed in the brachiocephalic artery (Fig. 3). The mechanism of this remains obscure. Covered stents in the upper limbs have been used to treat aneurysms and trauma. Few complications have been reported. We have witnessed early stent graft thrombosis and because these devices are small and potentially more thrombogenic than uncovered stents it makes sense to use anticoagulation or aggressive antiplatelet therapy. Many devices are difficult to place from the leg and because the deployment systems are of large diameter, and many upper limb access site vessels are small, we have also witnessed aggressive restenosis along the brachial artery six months after using this vessel to place a subclavian covered stent. The

author is also aware of an arterial self-expanding covered stent being crushed underneath the clavicle. This is of concern and presumably a similar fate could happen to an uncovered conventional stent.

ACUTE LIMB ISCHEMIA

The majority of acute limb ischemia in the upper limbs is due to emboli and therefore the experience of using endovascular techniques is limited. There are few references to the use of thrombolytic therapy [16-19] and these document remarkably few of the complications common to the use of fibrinolytics generally. However, there are some specific problems. Vasospasm may occur because the arm vessels are small and prone to vasoconstriction. This may be treated by antispasmodics. Of more concern is the report of at least two cases in the literature of peri-catheter thrombosis causing cerebral embolization. The author is aware of a similar case whereby either peri-catheter thrombus embolized to the brain or thrombus was dislodged to the carotid artery during a forceful injection of contrast. For this reason it is strongly recommended that catheters are placed directly into the upper limb vessels, particularly on the right side.

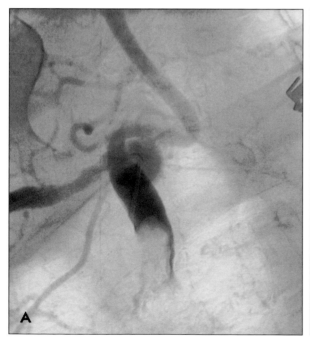
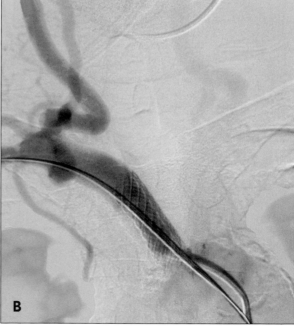

FIG. 3   A - Brachiocephalic stenosis demonstrated from a catheter placed from the right arm.   B - Balloon expandable stent, well placed.

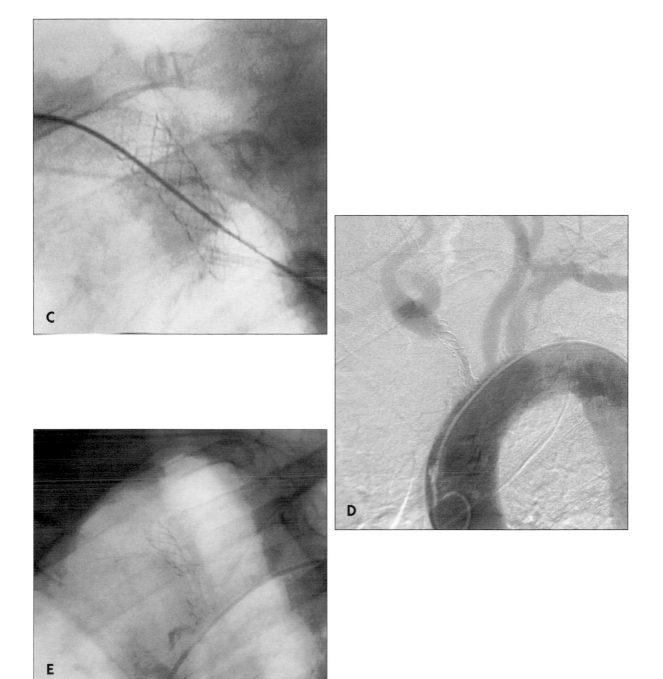

FIG. 3   C - Radiograph of the stent at the time of placement. D - Three months later the patient is symptomatic from a crushed brachiocephalic stent. E - Plain radiograph of the stent.

REFERENCES

1 Brunkwall J, Bergentz S-E. Long-term results of arterial reconstruction of the upper extremity. In: James ST Yao & William H Pearce (eds). *The ischemic extremity advances in treatment.* Appleton & Lange, Stamford, Connecticut 1995: pp 211-228.

2 Kessel DO, Robertson I, Scott DJ. The treatment of upper limb ischemia. *Intervention* 2000; 3: 99-104.

3 Whitbread T, Cleveland TJ, Beard JD et al. A combined approach to the treatment of proximal arterial occlusions of the upper limb with endovascular stents. *Eur J Vasc Endovasc Surg* 1998; 15: 29-35.

4 Queral LA, Criado FJ. The treatment of focal aortic arch branch lesions with Palmaz stents. *J Vasc Surg* 1996; 23: 368-375.

5 Sullivan TM, Gray BH, Bacharach JM et al. Angioplasty and primary stenting of the subclavian, innominate, and common carotid arteries in 83 patients. *J Vasc Surg* 1998; 28: 1059-1065.

6 Kumar K, Dorros G, Bates MC, et al. Primary stent deployment in occlusive subclavian artery disease. *Cathet Cardiovasc Diagn* 1995; 34: 281-285.

7 Martinez R, Rodriguez-Lopez J, Torruella L et al. Stenting for occlusion of the subclavian arteries. Technical aspects and follow-up results. *Tex Heart Inst J* 1997; 24: 23-27.

8 Criado FJ, Queral LA. The role of angioplasty and stenting in the treatment of occlusive lesions of supra-aortic trunks. *J Mal Vasc* 1996; 21 (Suppl A): 132-138.

9 Gaines PA, Swarbrick MJ, Lopez AJ et al. The endovascular management of blue finger syndrome. *Eur J Vasc Endovasc Surg* 1999; 17: 106-110.

10 Romanowski CA, Fairlie NC, Procter AE et al. Percutaneous transluminal angioplasty of the subclavian and axillary arteries: initial results and long-term follow-up. *Clin Radiol* 1992; 46: 104-107.

11 Burke DR, Gordon RL, Mishkin JD et al. Percutaneous transluminal angioplasty of subclavian arteries. *Radiology* 1987; 164: 699-704.

12 Mathias KD, Luth I, Haarmann P. Percutaneous transluminal angioplasty of proximal subclavian artery occlusions. *Cardiovasc Intervent Radiol* 1993; 16: 214-218.

13 Duber C, Klose KJ, Kopp H et al. Percutaneous transluminal angioplasty for occlusion of the subclavian artery: short- and long-term results. *Cardiovasc Intervent Radiol* 1992; 15: 205-210.

14 Motarjeme A. Percutaneous transluminal angioplasty of supra-aortic vessels. *J Endovasc Surg* 1996; 3: 171-181.

15 Hebrang A, Maskovic J, Tomac B. Percutaneous transluminal angioplasty of the subclavian arteries: long-term results in 52 patients. *Am J Roentgenol* 1991; 156: 1091-1094.

16 Johnson SP, Durham JD, Subber SW et al. Acute arterial occlusions of the small vessels of the hand and forearm: treatment with regional urokinase therapy. *J Vasc Interv Radiol* 1999; 10: 869-876.

17 Baguneid M, Dodd D, Fulford P et al. Management of acute nontraumatic upper limb ischemia. *Angiology* 1999; 50: 715-720.

18 Lambiase RE, Paolella LP, Haas RA et al. Extensive thromboembolic disease of the hand and forearm: treatment with thrombolytic therapy. *J Vasc Interv Radiol* 1991; 2: 201-208.

19 Coulon M, Goffette P, Dondelinger RF. Local thrombolytic infusion in arterial ischemia of the upper limb: mid-term results. *Cardiovasc Intervent Radiol* 1994; 17: 81-86.

20

COMPLICATIONS OF STENT-GRAFT PLACEMENT IN THE THORACIC AORTA

TIM C REHDERS, CHRISTOPH A NIENABER

Thoracic aortic aneurysms represent a major health problem. Like abdominal aortic aneurysms, most thoracic aortic aneurysms are asymptomatic and are diagnosed incidentally. Although less common than abdominal aortic aneurysms, aneurysms of the thoracic aorta are associated with an even more unfavorable outcome [1-3]. Following diagnosis, untreated patients with thoracic aortic aneurysms greater than 5.5 centimeters have a 2-year survival rate of less than 30%, with half of all deaths occurring as a result of aneurysm rupture [2]. This poor rate is significantly improved by an operative intervention [4]. However, surgical repair of an aneurysm may itself be associated with considerable morbidity and mortality.

Mortality and morbidity

Although most recently mortalities of about 10% have been achieved [5-8], the incidence of postoperative paraplegia may still amount to 25% [9,10]. Another serious complication is renal failure, which is encountered in up to 20% of patients undergoing surgical repair [9,10]. In addition, many of these patients have comorbid medical conditions, such as advanced coronary artery disease or chronic obstructive lung disease, which place them at risk for peri-operative complications. In such high-risk patients with thoracic aortic aneurysms, the risk associated with surgical repair may actually outweigh potential benefits derived from treatment.

Similarly, acute aortic dissection is a life-threatening scenario associated with a high early mortality as basically the most catastrophic event to affect the aorta. There are 10 to 20 cases per million per year in the normal population [11,12], and if the condition is left untreated in the proximal aorta, 36% to 72% of patients die within 48 hours of diagnosis, while 62% to 91% die within one week [13]. The number of deaths from aortic dissection is reported to exceed the number of deaths from rupture of an abdominal aortic aneurysm [14]. During the past two decades, a consensus has evolved and guidelines for treatment of patients with acute aortic dissection have been developed; however, despite recent advances in medical, surgical and endovascular treatment concepts, acute aortic diseases remain a therapeutic challenge.

For patients with acute Stanford type A dissections (involving the ascending aorta), surgical intervention is performed immediately after diagnosis to avert the high risk of death from complications, such as cardiac tamponade, aortic regurgitation, and myocardial infarction [15]. In contrast, the preferred treatment for most patients with Stanford type B dissections (without involvement of the ascending aorta) is medical treatment with antihypertensive drugs and betablockers. Surgical treatment is reserved for specific cases complicated by progression of dissection, impending rupture, refractory systemic hypertension, localized false aneurysm, continued pain, or end-organ ischemia from compromised aortic branches [16]. The current mortality rate among patients under medical therapy for type B dissection remains about 20% [17,18] whereas mortality rates of patients subjected to emergency surgical repair of acute type A and B dissections are currently about 19% to 35% [19,20]. In acute dissection complicated by end-organ ischemia, surgical mortality rate may amount to 50% [21,22].

Endovascular treatment

Recently, interventional placement of endovascular stent-grafts has emerged as an alternative concept to surgical graft placement for patients with diseases of the descending thoracic aorta. Both efficacy and safety have been reported for various entities such as thoracic aortic aneurysms and pseudo-aneurysms, abdominal aortic aneurysms, and peripheral arterial aneurysms [23-29]. Recently, two studies showed for the first time stent-grafts to be useful to cover the primary aortic intimal tear and thereby obliterate the false lumen of the aorta in patients with acute and subacute aortic dissections [30,31]. This less traumatic interventional approach seems to offer the potential to decrease morbidity and mortality associated with surgery to the descending thoracic aorta, particularly in patients with multiple comorbidities and considered at high risk. In this chapter, we meta-analyze the clinical experience of four centers with balloon and self-expanding endovascular grafts used in the treatment of thoracic aortic aneurysms and type B dissections, with focus on early complications [30-34].

Endovascular techniques

The meta-analysis concerning early complications after treatment of thoracic aortic aneurysms and pseudo-aneurysms by endovascular stent-grafting includes the data of three studies, which represent the experience at *Stanford University, University of Vienna*, and at the *Mount Sinaï Medical Center* in New York [32-34]. In addition, we reviewed the medical records of patients who had undergone the same treatment in our institution. Combining the results of four medical centers, a total of 174 patients underwent endovascular stent-graft repair of the descending thoracic aorta between July 1992 and October 2000 (Table I). The majority of patients in this meta-analysis was treated at *Stanford University*, where in comparison with the other three centers, a *home-brew*, non-self-expanding first-generation device was used. Grabenwöger et al. and Temudom et al. used mainly and Nienaber et al. used exclusively self-expanding devices.

Before stent-graft placement all candidates were evaluated by both conventional angiography and either a high-resolution dynamic computed tomography (CT) scan or three-dimensional magnetic resonance angiography (MRA) with intravenous contrast.

Endovascular stent-grafting procedures were performed either in the operating room or angiographic suite with the patient under general or regional anesthesia. Vascular access sites included the femoral artery, iliac artery, and infrarenal aorta (the native aorta was used as well as a previously implanted abdominal aortic tube graft or a commitantly inserted aortic graft in three instances). The access site was surgically exposed and punctured with a needle, followed by the placement of a sheath, guide wire, and pigtail catheter directed into the ascending aorta. After aortography with road mapping, the pigtail catheter was exchanged for a super stiff guide wire. Arteriotomy (or a small aortotomy if access to the iliofemoral artery was not possible) was performed at the puncture site. Under fluoroscopic guidance the stent-graft device was inserted into the aorta and deployed after the mean arterial pressure was lowered to 30-50 mmHg using various combinations of short-acting intravenous antihypertensives. Repeat aortography was performed intra-operatively to assess the adequacy of aneurysm exclusion, to rule out an early stent-graft endoleak, and to document sealing of proximal

Table I   COMPLICATIONS OF STENTING FOR THORACIC AORTIC ANEURYSMS

Authors **Total number of treated patients** Time period of treatment time point Stent graft systems	Dake et al. **103** 7/92-10/97 Stanford "home-brew"	Grabenwöger et al. **21** 11/96-2/99 Palmaz/Vanguard Excluder	Temudom et al. **14** 2/97-6/98 Talent/Prograft	Nienaber et al. **36** 2/98-10/00 Talent	Meta-analysis **174** 7/92-10/00
Early complication types	Number (%)	Number (%)	Number (%)	Number (%)	Number (%)
Early death (hospital mortality)	9 (9)	2 (10)	2 (14)	2 (6)	15 (9)
Stroke	7 (7)	0	0	0	7 (4)
Paraplegia/paraparesis	3 (3)	0	0	0	3 (2)
Transient neurological deficit	0	0	1 (7)	1 (3)	2 (1)
Myocardial infarction	2 (2)	0	0	0	2 (1)
Pulmonary insufficiency (±tracheostomy)	12 (12)	1 (5)	0	0	13 (8)
New aortic dissection (proximal)	1 (1)	1 (5)	0	0	2 (1)
Hemorrhage (local)	5 (5)	0	1 (7)	1 (3)	7 (4)
Hemorrhage (systemic/coagulopathy)	2 (2)	0	0	0	2 (1)
Wound infection	3 (3)	0	0	0	3 (2)
Lymph fistula of the groin	0	0	1 (7)	0	1 (1)
Stent graft maldeployment	3 (3)	0	1 (7)	1 (3)	5 (3)
Extension (additional stent grafts)	0	15 (72)	0	1 (3)	16 (9)
Occlusion of left subclavian artery	8 (8)	9 (43)	0	2 (6)	19 (11)
Left subclavian-carotid transposition/ left carotid-to-subclavian bypass	3 (3)/5(5)	9 (43)/0	0	1(3)/0	18 (10)
Initial stent graft endoleak	25 (24)	3 (15)	2 (14)	2 (6)	32 (19)

Malperfusion post stenting (a. + b. + c.)
  a. Gut ischemia/infarction
  b. Acute renal failure (±dialysis)
  c. Distal arterial thromboembolism
	8 (8)
	1 (1)
	5 (5)
	2 (2)
		1 (5)
		1 (5)
		0
		0
			1 (7)
			0
			0
			1 (7)
				0
				0
				0
				0
					10 (6)
					2 (1)
					5 (3)
					3 (2)

Injury of access femoral artery (a. + b.)
  a. Patch/reconstruction
  b. Interposition
	0
	0
	0
		1 (5)
		0
		1 (5)
			0
			0
			0
				2 (6)
				1 (3)
				1 (3)
					3 (2)
					1 (1)
					2 (1)

Peripheral intervention (PTA, stents) for access preparation	4 (4)	0	3 (21)	0	7 (4)
Peripheral operation for access preparation	1 (1)	0	4 (28)	0	5 (3)
Conversion to retroperitoneal access/open surgical repair	0/0	0/0	0/1 (7)	3 (9)/0	3 (2)
Deep vein thrombosis/ venous injury	1 (1)	0	0	0	1 (1)

entries in case of dissection. Early follow-up CT or MRA scans were performed at day 5 to 7 of the post-surgical period.

Results

This meta-analysis reveals that the in-hospital mortality rate for endovascular stent-grafting of descending thoracic aortic aneurysms was 9%. Early major procedural complications included stroke in 4%, paraplegia or paraparesis in 2%, and pulmonary insufficiency in 8% of patients. Myocardial infarction, new aortic dissection and transient neurological deficits each were observed in 1% of treated patients similarly, and systemic hemorrhage, like rupture of the treated aneurysms, occurred also in 1% of patients. Minor procedural complications included local hemorrhage in 4%, wound infection in 2%, and development of a lymph fistula of the groin in 1% of patients.

Of major concern with the stent-grafting of thoracic aortic aneurysms was a leak around the stent-graft into the aneurym sac, or *endoleak*. Early endoleak was documented by angiography or CT scanning in 19% of patients. Stent-graft maldeployment occurred in 3% of patients and the use of more than one stent-graft was necessary in 9% of patients. In 11% of patients, the proximal neck between the left subclavian artery and the aneurysm was considered inadequate to allow an adequate exclusion of the aneurysm; thus, in 11% of patients the left subclavian artery was occluded as a result of overstenting the artery and 10% of patients underwent either left subclavian to carotid transposition or left carotid-to-subclavian artery bypass to create a longer proximal stent-graft landing zone. Malperfusion of abdominal endorgans or distal arterial thrombo-embolism directly related to stent-graft placement occurred in 6% of patients.

Difficulty attaining femoral access was encountered in 7% of patients who had either marked iliac tortuosity and/or severe iliac occlusive disease. These patients were treated either by preprocedural balloon angioplasty (in some cases in combination with stent placement) or vascular surgical techniques. Injury of the access femoral artery occurred in 2% of patients; these injuries were repaired by reconstruction, patch, or graft interposition. For details, see Table I.

In comparison to the clinical experience with endovascular grafts and the treatment of thoracic aortic aneurysms and pseudo-aneurysms, there is little data available regarding the use of stent-grafts to cover the primary aortic intimal tear and thereby obliterate the aortic false lumen in patients with Stanford type B-dissections. For this meta-analysis we pooled the published data [30,31] and the currently unpublished data of another group of 84 patients treated with stent-grafts at our institution until October 2000 (Table II).

Interestingly, the incidence of initially incomplete occlusion of the entry tear was 12% and reduced to 3% at 3-month follow-up.

Altogether, 113 patients underwent stent-graft placement and in this setting the hospital mortality rate was only 3%. Dake et al. reported no late death rate for 19 treated patients (follow-up range: 4-28 months), however, they encountered three early or per-interventional casualties [32]. Our own data reveal also a 100% survival rate for 94 treated patients, with follow-up ranging from 3 to 36 months. The incidence of almost each type of early complications was lower than the incidence in treatment of thoracic aortic aneurysms and pseudo-aneurysms. Especially the rates of stroke, paraplegia/paraparesis, myocardial infarction, pulmonary insufficiency, wound infection, stent-graft maldeployment, necessity for additional stent-grafts, malperfusion of abdominal organs post stenting, overstenting of left subclavian artery, and surgical interventions for the left subclavian artery were markedly lower when treating dissection compared with data documented for treatment of thoracic aortic aneurysms.

Discussion

During the last six years of clinical use of endovascular aortic prostheses, typical side effects and complications of this new method have been encountered. Whereas in the initial phase of using endovascular aortic prostheses access problems, migration of the stent or misplacement within the aorta had been the most prevalent problems, we have observed a constant decline in the incidence of complications after stent-graft placement from the initial days of *homebrew* stents to the currently available commercial hardware. The refinement in manufacturing endovascular stent-grafts have led to better material (nitinol with wraps of dacron or teflon), smaller dimensions of the stent-graft introducer and, most importantly, much more flexible stent-grafts.

Table II   COMPLICATIONS OF STENTING FOR THORACIC AORTIC DISSECTION

Authors	Dake et al.	Nienaber et al.	Meta-analysis
Total number of treated patients	**19**	**94**	**113**
Treatment time-period	10/96-10/98	10/97-10/00	10/96-10/00
Stent graft systems	Stanford "home-brew"	Talent	
Early complication types	Number (%)	Number (%)	Number (%)
Early death (hospital mortality)	3 (16)	0	3 (3)
Late death	0 (follow-up: 4-28 months)	0 (after one year)	0
Aortic rupture with hematoma peri-aortically	2 (10)	0	2 (2)
Stroke	0	1 (1)	1 (1)
Paraplegia/paraparesis	0	0	0
Transient neurological deficit	0	1 (1)	1 (1)
Myocardial infarction	0	0	0
Pulmonary insufficiency (±tracheostomy)	1 (5)	0	1 (1)
Hemorrhage (local)	0	3 (3)	3 (3)
Wound infection	0	1 (1)	1 (1)
Stent graft maldeployment	0	0	0
Extension (additional stent grafts)	2 (10)	2 (2)	4 (4)
Overstenting of left subclavian artery	0	3 (3)	3 (3)
Left subclavian-carotid transposition /left carotid-to-subclavian bypass	0	0	0
Initial incomplete occlusion of entry tear	3 (16)	10 (11)	13 (12)
Incomplete occlusion of entry tear at 3 months	1 (5)	2 (2)	3 (3)
Malperfusion post stenting (a. + b. + c.)	2 (10)	0	2 (2)
a. Gut ischemia/infarction	1 (5)	0	1 (1)
b. Acute renal failure (±dialysis)	1 (5)	0	1 (1)
c. Distal arterial thrombo-embolism	0	0	0
Additional stenting of collapsed true lumen	5 (26) infrarenal aorta, iliac arteries	2 (2) renal	7 (7)
Injury of access femoral artery (a. + b.)	0	3 (3)	3 (3)
a. Patch/reconstruction	0	2 (2)	2 (2)
b. Interposition	0	1 (1)	1 (1)
Peripheral intervention (PTA, stents) for access preparation	0	1 (1)	1 (1)
Conversion to retroperitoneal access / open surgical repair	0	0	0

In the near future technology development should aim for less vascular trauma, fewer cardiovascular accidents, and less need for extensive repair at the access site. Eventually, by reducing the size of stent-grafts, further percutaneous access to the groin vessels by direct puncture using the Seldinger technique is likely to be established. With sleeker stent-grafts and higher flexibility, difficulty to attain primary access should decrease from 7% at present to less than 3% in the near future. Moreover, since access problems constitute a major portion of all complications, stents with a smaller diameter and easier vascular access will eventually shorten both implantation and fluoroscopy time and possibly also avoid the need for general anesthesia; a lower conversion rate to open surgery is also likely to occur.

A second relatively frequently occurring problem is the need to occlude sidebranches either accidentally or intuitively when placing an endovascular stent-graft prosthesis in thoracic aortic aneurysm or dissection. With a tailor-made stent for a given anatomy this problem could be reduced to the minimum by, for instance, using bare spring segments of a stent to cross the ostium of a relevant sidebranch. The concept of endovascular therapy should not just limit itself to the aorta, but should also infer the option of stenting sidebranches such as renal arteries and iliac arteries if necessary (for instance to reestablish flow when the dissecting lamella obstructs an ostium of a sidebranch). As a rule endovascular therapy implies life-long surveillance of a given patient in order to follow his or her disease and to repair other segments of the arterial tree in the light of a progressive disease. Clinical surveillance should also implement regular imaging by MR-angiography or CT-angiography in suitable intervals together with carefully monitored antihypertensive medication.

Thirdly and conversely, however, even with further technical refinement in the manufacturing and miniaturization of stent-grafts, the incomplete exclusion of an aneurysm or incomplete sealing of a dissecting communication may remain a vexing problem. Endoleakages of any kind need to be treated if not spontaneously resolved within two or three months. One way to make sure that endoleakage is completely abolished in a higher percentage of patients is to use customized stents and stent-grafts to better conform the peculiarities of a given individual aorta; another way is the post-hoc correction of endoleakage by insertion of appropriate coils, by thrombin injection into the endoleak space, or by clipping of feeder vessels.

Finally, besides all technological improvement, accepted guidelines for selecting patients for endovascular treatment strategies need to be established and fundamental agreement on pre- and postinterventional medical care and follow-up measures are desperately needed. All interested and participating fields of medicine are called upon to work together under the umbrella of a vascular center for diagnosing and treating aortic and any kind of vascular disease by the endovascular approach. This implies the presence of a vascular or thoracic surgeon in the center as well as the close interaction between the diagnostic fields of radiology and ultrasound, together with interventional radiology or cardiology. Only in a well balanced team are the further decline of side effects and better short- and long-term results likely to be witnessed.

REFERENCES

1 Bickerstaff LK, Pairolero PC, Hollier LH et al. Thoracic aortic aneurysms: a population-based study. *Surgery* 1982; 92: 1103-1108.
2 Crawford ES, DeNatale RW. Thoraco-abdominal aortic aneurysm: observations regarding the natural course of disease. *J Vasc Surg* 1986; 3: 578-582.
3 Svensson LG. Natural history of aneurysms of the descending and thoraco-abdominal aorta. *J Card Surg* 1997; 12 (Suppl): 279-284.
4 Crawford ES, Crawford JL, Safi JH et al. Thoraco-abdominal aortic aneurysms: preoperative and intra-operative factors determining immediate and long-term results of operations in 605 patients. *J Vasc Surg* 1986; 3: 389-404.

5 Hollier LH, Symmonds JB, Pairolero PC et al. Thoraco-abdominal aortic aneurysm repair: analysis of postoperative morbidity. *Arch Surg* 1988; 123: 871-875.
6 Golden MA, Donaldson MC, Whittemore AD et al. Evolving experience with thoraco-abdominal aortic aneurysm repair at a single institution. *J Vasc Surg* 1991; 13: 792-797.
7 Svensson LG, Crawford ES, Hess KR et al. Experience with 1509 patients undergoing thoraco-abdominal aortic operations. *J Vasc Surg* 1993; 17: 357-370.
8 Schepens MA, Defauw JJ, Hamerlijnck RP et al. Surgical treatment of thoraco-abdominal aortic aneurysms by simple crossclamping. Risk factors and late results. *J Thorac Cardiovasc Surg* 1994; 107: 134-142.

9 Panneton JM, Hollier LH. Nondissecting thoraco-abdominal aortic aneurysms: Part I. *Ann Vasc Surg* 1995; 9: 503-514.

10 Panneton JM, Hollier LH. Dissecting descending thoracic and thoraco-abdominal aorticaneurysms: Part II. *Ann Vasc Surg* 1995; 9: 596-605.

14 Sorenson HR, Olsen H. Ruptured and dissecting aneurysms of the aorta incidence and prospects of surgery. *Acta Chir Scand* 1964; 128 : 644-650.

12 Pate JW, Richardson RJ, Eastridge CE. Acute aortic dissections. *Ann Surg* 1976; 42: 395-404.

13 Anagnostopoulos CE, Prabhakar MJS, Kittle CF. Aortic dissections and dissecting aneurysms. *Am J Cardiol* 1972; 30: 263-273.

14 Kochoukos NT, Dougenis D. Surgery of the thoracic aorta. *N Engl J Med* 1997; 336: 1876-1888.

15 Miller DC, Stinson EB, Oyer PE et al. Operative treatment of aortic dissections: experience with 125 patients over a sixteen-year period. *J Thorac Cardiovasc Surg* 1979; 78: 365-382.

16 Fann JI, Miller DC. Aortic dissection. *Ann Vasc Surg* 1995; 9: 311-323.

17 Wheat MW. Current status of medical therapy of acute dissecting aneurysms of the aorta. *World J Surg* 1980; 4: 563-569.

18 Elefteriades JA, Hartleroad J, Gusberg RJ et al. Long-term experience with descending aortic dissection: the complication-specific approach. *Ann Thorac Surg* 1992; 53: 11-21.

19 Ergin MA, Phillips RA, Galla JD et al. Significance of distal false lumen after type A dissection repair. *Ann Thorac Surg* 1994; 57: 820-825.

20 Crawford ES, Svensson LG, Coselli JS et al. Aortic dissection and dissecting aortic aneurysms. *Ann Surg* 1988; 208: 254-273.

21 Miller DC, Mitchell RS, Oyer PE et al. Independent determinants of operative mortality for patients with aortic dissection. *Circulation* 1984; 70: Suppl I: I 153-164.

22 Cambria RP, Brewster DC, Gertler J et al. Vascular complications associated with spontaneous aortic dissection. *J Vasc Surg* 1988; 7: 199-209.

23 Parodi JC, Palmaz JC, Barone HD. Transfemoral intraluminal graft implantation for abdominal aortic aneurysms. *Ann Vasc Surg* 1991; 5: 491-499.

24 Blum U, Voshage G, Lammer J et al. Endoluminal stent-grafts for infrarenal abdominal aortic aneurysms. *N Engl J Med* 1997; 336: 13-20.

25 Razavi MK, Dake MD, Semba CP et al. Percutaneous endoluminal placement of stent-grafts for the treatment of isolated iliac artery aneurysms. *Radiology* 1995; 197: 801-804.

26 Dake MD, Miller DC, Semba CP et al. Transluminal placement of endovascular stent-grafts for the treatment of descending thoracic aortic aneurysms. *N Engl J Med* 1994; 331: 1729-1734.

27 Mitchell RS, Miller DC, Dake MD. Stent-graft repair of thoracic aortic aneurysms. *Semin Vasc Surg* 1997; 10: 257-271.

28 Mitchell RS, Dake MD, Semba CP et al. Endovascular stent-graft repair of thoracic aortic aneurysms. *J Thorac Cardiovasc Surg* 1996; 111: 1054-1062.

29 Perreault P, Soula P, Rousseau H et al. Acute traumatic rupture of the thoracic aorta: delayed treatment with endoluminal covered stent. A report of two cases. *J Vasc Surg* 1998; 27: 538-544.

30 Nienaber CA, Fattori R, Lund G et al. Nonsurgical reconstruction of thoracic aortic dissection by stent-graft placement. *N Engl J Med* 1999; 340: 1539-1545.

31 Dake MD, Kato N, Mitchell RS et al. Endovascular stent-graft placement for the treatment of acute aortic dissection. *N Engl J Med* 1999; 340: 1546-1552.

32 Dake MD, Miller DC, Mitchell RS et al. The "first generation" of endovascular stent-grafts for patients with aneurysms of the descending thoracic aorta. *J Thorac Cardiovasc Surg* 1998; 116: 689-704.

33 Temudom T, D'Ayala M, Marin ML et al. Endovascular grafts in the treatment of thoracic aortic aneurysms and pseudo-aneurysms. *Ann Vasc Surg* 2000; 14: 230-238.

34 Grabenwöger M, Hutschala D, Ehrlich MP et al. Thoracic aortic aneurysms: treatment with endovascular self-expandable stent grafts *Ann Thorac Surg* 2000; 69: 441-445.

21

COMPLICATIONS OF OPEN SURGERY OF THE AORTIC ARCH

ROLAND HETZER, MIRALEM PASIC

Surgery of the aortic arch encompasses several procedures performed for different pathological entities. From the surgical point of view, it can be divided into combined surgery for ascending aorta and aortic arch, isolated arch surgery (non-A, non-B dissection, isolated atherosclerotic or mycotic arch aneurysm), or combined surgery for arch and descending thoracic aorta (true aneurysm, type B dissection). Aortic dissection and atherosclerotic aneurysms are commonly observed in these patients. In recent years, open surgery of the aortic arch has also been performed with increasing frequency to treat complications following endovascular treatment of aortic diseases. The possible complications of this type of surgery are multiple with severe sequela. The aim of this chapter is to identify and discuss the complications of open surgery of the aortic arch, including prevention and treatment.

21
193

Aortic arch surgery

Surgical treatment of lesions of the aortic arch offers one of the most formidable challenges in cardiovascular surgery. Arch aneurysms can be caused by syphilis, atherosclerosis, cystic medionecrosis, trauma or congenital connective tissue disease. Aortic dissection involving the ascending and/or complete arch also requires surgical repair, facing potential intra- and postoperative complications. For aneurysms involving the transverse arch proximal to the ligamentum arteriosum the best approach is through a median sternotomy. This

access allows control of the distal thoracic aorta with performance of the distal anastomosis through the anterior approach. In lesions involving not only the transverse arch but also a segment of the descending thoracic aorta, a different approach might be necessary like a transverse bilateral thoracotomy.

The most widely used procedure applied for surgery of the aortic arch is replacement of the ascending aorta associated with partial or complete arch replacement for acute type A aortic dissection [1] or atherosclerotic aneurysm. In a case of an isolated saccular aneurysm, we prefer patch repair if possible (Figs. 1 A and 1 B). In some rare cases of isolated

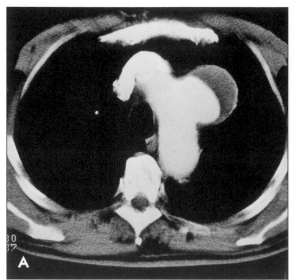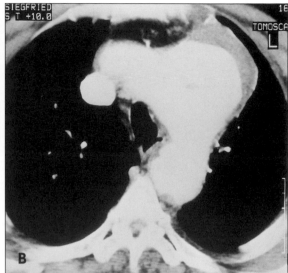

FIG. 1 CT showing an isolated small (A) and a huge (B) saccular aneurysm of the aortic arch. In both instances, the arch was repaired with a dacron patch during a short period of circulatory arrest and deep hypothermia.

dissection of the aortic arch (type non-A, non-B dissection) (Figs. 2 A and 2 B) [2] the arch can be repaired either with a glue or with tailoring plasty of the arch without using prosthetic material (Fig. 2 C). In almost all instances, surgery of the aortic arch needs cardiopulmonary bypass with some type of cerebral protection. Rarely, aortic arch reconstruction is possible without cardiopulmonary bypass in patients with a small saccular atherosclerotic aneurysm of the arch (Fig. 3).

COMPLICATIONS

Cerebral injury following repair of transverse aortic arch aneurysms is one of the most feared complications and major cause of severe morbidity. Cerebral damage mainly results from peripheral embolization, prolonged ischemia and malperfusion through a dissected aorta.

In general, complications of open surgery of the aortic arch can be divided into early and late complications. Besides the listed complications in the Table, ischemic problems can also be caused by an unrecognized variation of vascular anatomy (e.g. abberant origin of the arch branches) (Fig. 4) and peripheral embolism with particles of glue (such as gelatin-resorcin-formol glue) used for obliteration of the false lumen of acute aortic dissection [3].

The late complications include pseudo-aneurysm formation at an anastomotic line on the proximal or distal anastomosis or suture line of a patch plasty, late operation on the aorta because of progression of a pathological process (such as in patients with Marfan syndrome) or new formation of an atherosclerotic or chronic dissecting aneurysm in a remote place, development of an aortobronchial fistula, late prosthetic infection, and late neurologic complications.

Open surgery of the aortic arch bears a certain risk of intra-operative or postoperative death with an early mortality of about 10% with a range from 5% to 30% [4-7]. It depends on the type and extension of surgery, the localization of the pathological process, and the degree of urgency for surgery. Surgery for acute aortic dissection or simultaneous repair of arch and descending thoracic or thoraco-abdominal aneurysm carries a higher risk than surgery of an isolated aortic arch aneurysm. Furthermore, the early mortality is significantly higher in patients who develop postoperative complications than in those without postoperative problems. Independent risk factors for early mortality are age, pump time, emergency surgery, postoperative renal failure and repeat thoracotomy for bleeding [4,6]. The type of cerebral protection may have an influence on the rate of postoperative complications and, therefore, indirectly on the rate of early mortality. Coselli and LeMaire reported a lower mortality rate (7.9% vs. 8.8%) in patients with profound

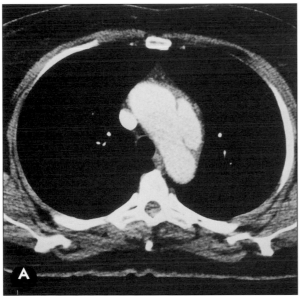

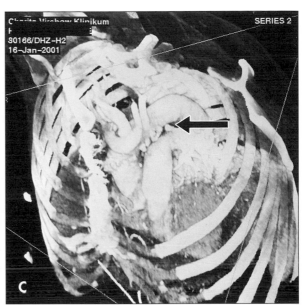

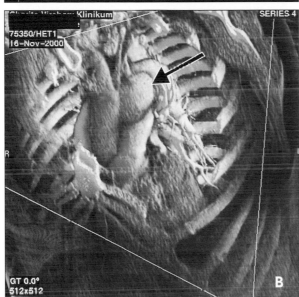

FIG. 2   A-B - Preoperative CT scan of isolated dissection of the aortic arch (type non-A, non-B dissection). C - The arch was repaired with tailoring plasty of the arch without using prosthetic material.

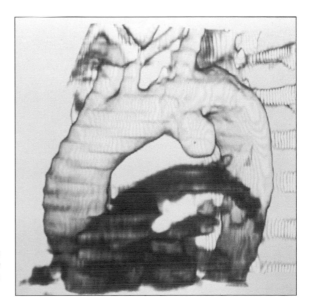

FIG. 3   CT scan showing a small saccular aneurysm of the aortic arch. The arch was reconstructed without cardiopulmonary bypass using several polypropilene mattress sutures supported with teflon pledgetes.

Table	COMPLICATIONS (INTRA- AND POSTOPERATIVE) OF AORTIC ARCH SURGERY	
Early complications		*Late complications*
➤ Cerebral ischemia/embolization		➤ Cerebral embolization
➤ Injury *Vagus nerve*		➤ Myocardial infarction
Phrenic nerve		➤ Respiratory failure
Recurrent laryngeal nerve		➤ Renal failure
Left pulmonary artery		➤ Graft infection
Left lung		➤ Pseudo-aneurysm
➤ Left sided hemotothorax		➤ New, remote aneurysm
➤ Pneumothorax		➤ Aortobronchial fistula
➤ Subcutaneous emphysema		➤ Supraaortic graft occlusion
➤ Cardiac events		
➤ Ischemia *Kidneys*		
Viscera		
Extremities		
Spinal cord		

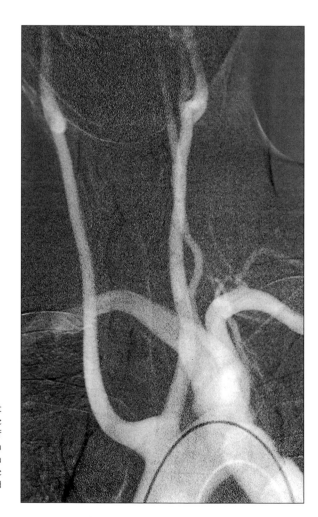

FIG. 4 Aberrant origin of the right subclavian artery arising from the aneurysmatically changed distal part of the aortic arch. This patient with Marfan syndrome was operated on because of a huge chronic dissecting aneurysm of the distal part of the aortic arch and descending thoracic aorta.

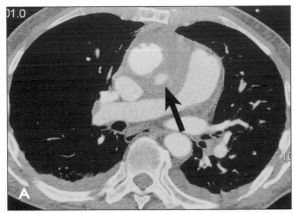

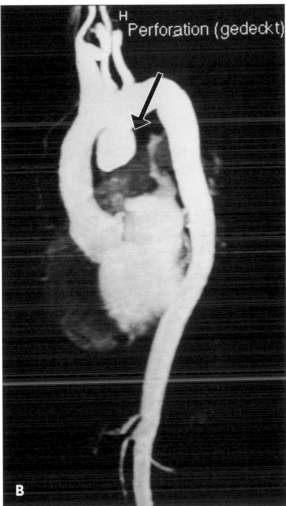

FIG. 5   A rare case of early postoperative prosthetic graft infection with a pseudo-aneurysm of the distal anastomosis *(arrow)* (A and B) after replacement of the ascending aorta and aortic arch with a tube graft because of an atherosclerotic aneurysm. The infected grafts were removed and replaced with a new prosthetic graft and the graft was wrapped with the greater omentum, and prolonged antibiotic therapy.

hypothermia and circulatory arrest with retrograde cerebral perfusion in comparison to patients operated on with profound circulatory arrest but without retrograde cerebral perfusion [8]. In contrast, Takano et al. [9] reported that the rate of early mortality comparing the three different methods of cerebral protection (deep hypothermia, antegrade cerebral perfusion with moderate hypothermia, antegrade hypothermic cerebral perfusion) was not statistically different (21.4% for deep hypothermia, 11.8% for antegrade cerebral perfusion with moderate hypothermia, and 7.1% for antegrade hypothermic cerebral perfusion) [9].

Postoperative bleeding and the need for blood products are associated with the type of intra-operative cerebral protection. Bleeding complications are increased in patients with deep hypothermia in comparison to patients with only moderate hypothermia [9]. Aortobronchial fistula is an extremely rare late complication after aortic arch surgery. It can be caused not only by an anastomotic stitch that injures the tracheobronchial tree but also by a remnant of a side branch used for temporary bypass, which is used by some surgeons for antegrade perfusion after completion of the distal anastomosis [10].

Early or late prosthetic graft infection is rare. However, when it occurs, it needs urgent re-operation. The infected graft should be removed and all infected tissue should be excised [11]. The infected graft should preferably be replaced with a homograft [11,12]. An alternative is replacement of the infected graft with a new prosthetic graft, transposition of the greater omentum and wrapping of the prosthetic graft with the omentum, and prolonged antibiotic therapy (Fig. 5) [12,13].

NEUROLOGIC DEFICITS

Postoperative neurological deficits are serious complications of open surgery of the aortic arch. They can occur as embolic complications caused by air or atheromatous debris or as a consequence of global brain ischemia during prolonged clamp time or arrest. Furthermore, it can be caused by insufficient cooling, or by prolonged ischemia beyond tolerable limits, even with deep hypothermia. The incidence of neurological complications caused by air or atheromatous debris embolization can be prevented or reduced by the use of retrograde cerebral perfusion. Probably, its main effect is mechanical wash-out of all particles from the brain vessels. Furthermore, insufflation of carbon dioxide into the operative field may reduce the risk of air embolization, because of its high solubility in blood in comparison to air. The embolization of the brain by atheromatous debris is mostly due to turbulence and subsequent dislodgement of the debris from the descending thoracic aorta during retrograde perfusion while on femoro-femoral bypass. It can be prevented by choosing an axillary artery acces for arterial cannulation [14]. In case of a combined arch and descending aortic aneurysm, antegrade perfusion can be established primarily via the arch itself (by direct cannulation) followed by perfusion through the implanted graft after a period of circulatory arrest.

The neurological complications are manifested as transient neurological disturbances or permanent deficit. Transient neurological disturbances include delayed awakening, convulsion, delirium or double vision. In contrast to patients with permanent neurological deficit, these patients mostly have no substrate on CT scan [14]. Patients with permanent neurological deficits have stroke or signs of global cerebral dysfunction. Paraplegia or paraparesis are complications that only occur in conjunction with simultaneous operation of the aortic arch and thoracic or thoracoabdominal aneurysm. However, they are possible theoretical complications in patients with isolated arch repair/replacement using selective antegrade perfusion and moderate hypothermia. Although extremely rare, paraplegia or paraparesis can occur in acute dissection during retrograde perfusion via the femoral vessels with subsequent malperfusion of the intercostal arteries.

Cognitive dysfunction after deep hypothermia is not clearly distinguished from that after general use of cardiopulmonary bypass. A surprisingly high prevalence of early and late depression of cognitive functions has recently been reported [15], however, it has remained a solitary finding. The authors observed a relatively high prevalence (53% at discharge) and persistence (24% at 6 months) of cognitive decline after use of cardiopulmonary bypass, like in patients after coronary bypass grafting [15]. Following a pattern of early improvement, it was followed by a later decline (42% at 5 years) that was predicted by the presence of early postoperative cognitive decline [15]. Reich et al. [16] showed that late memory and fine motor deficits are associated with advanced age and deep hypothermic circulatory arrest of 25 minutes or longer.

There are several methods commonly used for brain protection:

1 - deep hypothermic circulatory arrest without retrograde or antegrade cerebral perfusion,
2 - deep hypothermic circulatory arrest with retrograde cerebral perfusion,
3 - deep hypothermic circulatory arrest with selective antegrade cerebral perfusion,
4 - selective antegrade cerebral perfusion with moderate hypothermia,
5 - selective antegrade hypothermic cerebral perfusion in conjunction with mild hypothermic visceral perfusion, so-called *cool head - warm body perfusion.*

Deep hypothermia with circulatory arrest is the most common technique but has a limited safe period for circulatory arrest. Ergin et al. [17] demonstrated an incidence of 19% of temporary neurological disturbances and a stroke rate of 11% in 183 patients with hypothermic circulatory arrest. Coselli and LeMaire showed that if retrograde cerebral perfusion was added to profound hypothermic circulatory arrest, the stroke rate decreased from 6.5% to 2.4% [8]. Ehrlich et al. [18] compared the neurological complications in a group of 109 patients undergoing aortic arch operation with and without the use of retrograde cerebral perfusion. They showed that the incidence of permanent neurologic complications was higher (9% vs. 27%) in a group of patients without retrograde cerebral perfusion. However, retrograde cerebral perfusion did not reduce the prevalence of temporary neurologic dysfunction (17% vs, 18%) [18]. Okita et al. [5] reported delirium in 25% of patients, with stroke in 4% of 148 patients undergoing arch repair using hypothermic circulatory arrest with retrograde cerebral perfusion. Therefore, selective antegrade perfusion with direct cannulation of the brachiocephalic trunk or selective cannulation of the branches has been introduced to prolong this safe period and to enable prolonged reconstruction of the aortic arch. Some authors reported no permanent neurologic deficits using selective cerebral perfusion [6,7] and only 5.3% of transient neurological dysfunction [6]. However, the incidence of neurologic complications reported in some articles is still high despite selective cerebral perfusion techniques [4]. Ueda et al. [4] showed in a series of 113 consecutive patients with different aortic procedures combined with aortic arch repair and selective cerebral perfusion that 25% of patients had some cerebral complications with a rate of 9% of permanent neurological disability [4]. Takano et al. [9] reported that the rate of stroke was not statistically different between the methods of cerebral perfusion: 7.1% for deep hypothermia, 6.3% for antegrade cerebral perfusion with moderate hypothermia, and 3.6% for antegrade hypothermic cerebral perfusion [9].

The independent risk factors for cerebral complications are a history of cerebrovascular disease, perioperative shock, distal anastomosis below the left pulmonary artery, malperfusion of extremities, age over 60 years, and extended atherosclerosis of the descending thoracic aorta [4,16]. No use of retrograde cerebral perfusion during deep hypothermic circulatory arrest has been recognized as a statistically significant independent risk factor for permanent neurologic dysfunction [18]. Di Bartolomeo et al. [6] showed that postoperative cardiac complications were the only independent predictor for transient neurologic dysfunction [6]. Some authors observed that the occurrence of cerebral complications was not related to the duration of selective cerebral perfusion [4]. Furthermore, total aortic arch replacement in comparison to partial replacement is not a risk factor for cerebral complications [4,5,17]. Similarly to the early mortality rate, a risk of neurologic complications is lower for surgery of isolated aortic arch aneurysm in comparison to surgery for acute aortic dissection or simultaneous repair of arch and descending thoracic or thoracoabdominal aneurysm. Shiiya et al. [19] reported that 1.9% of 52 patients with atherosclerotic arch aneurysms and selective cerebral perfusion developed permanent focal neurologic deficit and 11.5% of them had temporary brain complications.

Personal experience

Between 1986 and 2000, a total of 208 patients underwent open surgery of the aortic arch. Combined surgery for ascending aorta and aortic arch was performed in 156 patients (group I) (aneurysm, n = 54; type A dissection, n = 102), isolated arch surgery in 18 patients (group II) (localized dissection of the arch [non-A, non-B dissection], n = 1; isolated atherosclerotic arch aneurysm, n = 17), and combined surgery for distal arch and descending thoracic aorta was performed in 34 patients (group III) (aneurysm, n = 19; chronic type B dissection, n = 15). Methods we commonly use for brain protection were deep hypothermic circulatory arrest with or without retrograde cerebral perfusion. Selective antegrade cerebral perfusion

with moderate hypothermia or selective antegrade hypothermic cerebral perfusion in conjunction with mild hypothermic visceral perfusion, so-called *cool head-warm body perfusion*, were not applied in this group of patients.

The early mortality rates were 16% for group I (aneurysm 9.2%; acute dissection, 19.6%), 0% for group II and 11.7% for group III. The stroke rates were 7.0% for group I (aneurysm, 5.5%; dissection, 7.8%), 0% for group II and 2.9%% for group III. Deep hypothermia was associated with increased mortality and complication rate if the operation was performed on an emergency base and in patients with advanced age. Furthermore, prolonged ventilatory support was required in most patients and early tracheostomy was applied in a liberal manor. Most postoperative complications were not related to the surgical procedure itself, but rather by secondary organ failure (heart, kidneys, lungs). Prosthetic infection was seen in two patients with combined ascending aorta and partial arch replacement. In both patients, the infected grafts were removed and replaced with a new prosthetic graft and the graft was wrapped with the greater omentum, and prolonged antibiotic therapy, was administered.

Conclusion

Increasing experience and progress in the field of aortic surgery during the last decade have led to a significant reduction in operative mortality and morbidity. However, although the complications are rare, the specific complications of this type of surgery are mostly serious with transient or permanent brain damage. Advanced age is a risk factor for developing neurologic complications. A prolonged period of circulatory arrest is rarely needed for surgery of the aortic arch. In these instances, such as complex reoperative procedures with reimplantation of particular branches of the aortic arch, antegrade cerebral perfusion with deep hypothermia is recommended.

REFERENCES

1 Daily PO, Trueblood HW, Stinson EB et al. Management of acute aortic dissections. *Ann Thorac Surg* 1970; 10: 237-247.
2 Pasic M, Knollman F, Hetzer R. Isolated non-A, non-B dissection of the aortic arch. *N Engl J Med* 1999; 341 (23): 1775.

3 Carrel T, Maurer M, Tkebuchava T et al. Embolization of biologic glue during repair of aortic dissection. *Ann Thorac Surg* 1995; 60: 1118-1120.

4 Ueda T, Shimizu H, Ito T et al. Cerebral complications associated with selective perfusion of the arch vessels. *Ann Thorac Surg* 2000; 70: 1472-1477.

5 Okita Y, Takamoto S, Ando M et al. Mortality and cerebral outcome in patients who underwent aortic arch operations using deep hypothermic circulatory arrest with retrograde cerebral perfusion: no relation of early death, stroke, and delirium to the duration of circulatory arrest. *J Thorac Cardiovasc Surg* 1998; 115: 129-138.

6 Di Bartolomeo R, Pacini D, Di Eusanio M, Pierangeli A. Antegrade selective cerebral perfusion during operations on the thoracic aorta: our experience. *Ann Thorac Surg* 2000; 70: 10-16.

7 Hirotani T, Kameda T, Kumamoto T, Shirota S. Results of a total aortic arch replacement for an acute aortic arch dissection. *J Thorac Cardiovasc Surg* 2000; 120: 686-691.

8 Coselli JS, LeMaire SA. Experience with retrograde cerebral perfusion during proximal aortic surgery in 290 patients. *J Card Surg* 1997; 12 (Suppl 2): 322-325.

9 Takano H, Sakakibara T, Matsuwaka R et al. The safety and usefulness of cool head-warm body perfusion in aortic surgery. *Eur J Cardiothorac Surg* 2000; 18: 262-269.

10 Ono M, Takamoto S, Kawauchi M et al. Aortobronchial fistula late after transverse arch replacement. *Ann Thorac Surg* 2000; 70: 964-966.

11 Pasic M. Mycotic aneurysm of the aorta: evolving surgical concept. *Ann Thorac Surg* 1996; 61: 1053-1054.

12 Knosalla C, Weng Y, Yankah AC et al. Using aortic allograft material to treat mycotic aneurysms of the thoracic aorta. *Ann Thorac Surg* 1996; 61: 1146-1152.

13 Krabatsch T, Hetzer R. Infected ascending aortic prosthesis: successful treatment by thoracic transposition of the greater omentum. *Eur J Cardiothorac Surg* 1995; 9: 223-225.

14 Whitlark JD, Goldman SM, Sutter FP. Axillary artery cannulation in acute ascending aortic dissections. *Ann Thorac Surg* 2000; 69: 1127-1129.

15 Newman MF, Kirchner JL, Phillips-Bute B et al. Longitudinal assesment of neurocognitive function after coronary-artery bypass surgery. *N Engl J Med* 2001; 344: 395-402.

16 Reich DL, Uysal S, Sliwinski M et al. Neuropsychologic outcome after deep hypothermic circulatory arrest in adults. *J Thorac Cardiovasc Surg* 1999; 117: 156-163.

17 Ergin MA, Galla JD, Lansman SL et al. Hypothermic circulatory arrest in operations on the thoracic aorta. Determinants of operative mortality and neurologic outcome. *J Thorac Cardiovasc Surg* 1994; 107: 788-799.

18 Ehrlich MP, Fang WC, Grabenwoger M et al. Impact of retrograde cerebral perfusion on aortic arch aneurysm repair. *J Thorac Cardiovasc Surg* 1999; 118: 1026-1032.

19 Shiiya N, Kunihara T, Imamura M et al. Surgical management of atherosclerotic aortic arch aneurysms using selective cerebral perfusion: 7-year experience in 52 patients. *Eur J Cardiothorac Surg* 2000; 17: 266-271.

22

COMPLICATIONS OF DESCENDING THORACIC AORTIC SURGERY

MICHAEL JACOBS, TED ELENBAAS
GEERT-WILLEM SCHURINK, BAS DE MOL, BAS MOCHTAR

The most common diseases of the descending thoracic aorta comprise acute and chronic dissection, aneurysm formation, injury and coarctation. Although endovascular modalities are increasingly applied to various thoracic aortic disorders, open repair remains the therapy of choice in complex pathologic conditions. Morbidity- and mortality rates are dependent on many pre-, intra- and postoperative variables, which have progressively been identified during the last decades. This chapter addresses the main complications of surgical descending thoracic aortic repair.

Stroke

Patients with thoracic aortic aneurysms suffer from generalized atherosclerotic disease. If the aneurysm is restricted to the descending thoracic aorta, the ascending aorta and aortic arch might appear with a normal diameter on a preoperative CT-scan. However, these parts of the aorta contain atheroma which are potential sources for embolization to the brain, especially after crossclamping the proximal descending aorta, initiating turbulence, and dislodging of debris. Royse et al. screened the thoracic aorta for atheroma by means of manual palpation, transesophageal- and epi-aortic ultrasonograhpy [1]. The thoracic aorta was divided into six zones: proximal, mid and distal ascending aorta,

proximal and distal arch, and proximal descending aorta. The frequency of atheroma was age-related, with the youngest at 55 years. Of 68 patients with adequate imaging of all zones, 36 had moderate or severe disease in the distal arch and proximal descending aorta (53%), indicating the high incidence of atheroma in this region of non-aneurysmal thoracic aortas. Meissner et al. [2] performed a prospective population-based study, randomly selecting a cohort of 1 475 residents aged 45 years or older, of whom 588 agreed to participate. The study was designed to identify risk factors for stroke and cardiovascular disease using transesophageal echocardiography and carotid ultrasonography. The prevalence of aortic atherosclerosis increased with age and was most common and extensive in the descending thoracic aorta, again emphasizing the important role as an embolic source in endovascular and surgical manipulations.

No exact data on stroke rate following thoracic aortic repair arc available. Furthermore, the intra-operative contribution of carotid artery disease to neurologic complications is also unclear. However, it is evident that a mid-thoracic aortic aneurysm, requiring crossclamping far distal to the subclavian artery, will hardly cause cerebral embolization. In contrast, proximal descending thoracic aneurysms which demand clamping at the left subclavian artery or between the subclavian and carotid arteries are prone for turbulence in the aortic arch with subsequent dislodging of atherosclerotic debris. It becomes even more catastrophic if the distal aortic arch is involved. In these cases a non-clamping technique by means of profound hypothermic circulatory arrest could be a solution, however, encephalopathy and stroke seem unavoidable and occur in up to 50% of patients [3]. In our own experience with thoracic aortic aneurysms repair the only strokes we encountered occurred in patients with a combined distal aortic arch aneurysm.

Our current technique in patients undergoing combined distal arch and descending aortic repair through a left thoracotomy is moderate hypothermia and selective, antegrade perfusion to the brain, allowing an open anastomosis and adequate repair of the supra-aortic arteries. Following the proximal anastomosis, the patient is rewarmed and the rest of the reconstruction is performed.

Paraplegia

Postoperative paraplegia is a devastating complication following thoracic aortic surgery. The incidence of postoperative paraplegia greatly depends on the existence of an (acute) aortic dissection. Furthermore, the extent of the diseased aortic segment determines the extent of the aortic repair and subsequent risk of spinal cord ischemia.

AORTIC DISSECTION

For the sake of clarity the Stanford classification distinguishes the type A which involves the ascending aorta and type B when the ascending aorta is not involved. The type B dissection can therefore originate at the left subclavian artery and extent along the thoracic and/or abdominal aorta, even involv-

ing the iliac and femoral arteries. In the DeBakey classification a type III also refers to a dissection not involving the ascending aorta or aortic arch, however, the subtype IIIa describes the dissecting process limited to the descending thoracic aorta and subtype IIIb extending below the diaphragm. The mechanism of a descending aortic dissection is complex. Besides the typical acute pain in the back and between the shoulders, acute paraplegia rarely occurs (1%-8%) [4]. If neurologic symptoms appear they most often improve spontaneously. This relatively mild side effect of acute dissection is probably the consequence of time and false lumen perfusion, supplying blood to intercostal arteries which originate from both channels.

The incidence of paraplegia increases significantly after emergency surgery for acute dissections. The indications for surgical repair in type B dissections are aortic rupture, hemothorax, visceral, renal and/or lower limb ischemia. The main cause of increased paraplegia rate is the extremely bad aortic wall quality, not allowing adequate reattachment of intercostal arteries with subsequent spinal cord ischemia, leading to neurologic deficit in 16%-56% [4]. Elefteriades et al. recently published their management and results of 100 consecutive patients with acute dissection of the descending aorta [5]. Nine patients died and 31 patients had a course complicated by rupture (8), vascular occlusion (17), early expansion or extension (12), and continued pain (4). Forty-two patients were treated surgically and six patients (14%) died and six patients suffered from paraplegia (14%).

Chronic descending aortic dissection is treated according to the same and general guidelines as for descending aortic aneurysms. The indications for surgery in atherosclerotic patients are similar (pain, aneurysm diameter greater than 6 centimeters) and results with respect to neurologic deficit are comparable. In patients with chronic aortic dissection and congenital diseases (Marfan, Ehlers-Danlos) surgery is indicated if the enlargement reaches 4-5 centimeters.

THORACIC AORTIC ANEURYSM

The extent of the diseased aortic segment determines the risk of paraplegia following surgical and also endovascular repair. Therefore, it is mandatory to describe the extent and level of the aneurysm in detail in order to interpret the results in the literature and compare the individual series [6]. In healthy persons, the arteria radicularis magna or

Adamkiewicz artery originates between T8 and T12 in approximately 80% and between T5 and T8 in 15% [7]. In patients with atherosclerotic aortic aneurysms, however, most intercostal arteries are occluded and spinal cord perfusion is provided by collaterals.

As stated before, the extent of the aneurysm is rarely described in detail. The Crawford classification distinguishes type I, II, III and IV for thoraco-abdominal aortic aneurysms, in which the most extensive form (type II) carries the highest risk of paraplegia. In thoracic aortic aneurysms there is no classification available. One might debate whether such a classification is necessary because the surgical results are excellent: Safi et al. reported a neurologic deficit of less than 1% in patients undergoing descending aortic aneurysm repair [8]. It should be emphasized that all patients were operated with left heart bypass, spinal fluid drainage, and passive hypothermia. Despite these excellent results it would be desirable to distinguish limited, saccular aneurysms from extensive aneurysms involving the complete descending thoracic aorta from the subclavian artery to the celiac axis. It is evident that the latter group carries a significantly higher paraplegia risk, not only in open surgery but also after endovascular treatment [6,8]. Besides the extent of the aneurysm, other factors influence the neurologic outcome of open aortic repair. There is substantial evidence and general consensus that distal aortic perfusion during thoracic aortic cross-clamping reduces neurologic deficits significantly [8]. Several techniques to provide distal aortic perfusion can be applied, including the Gott shunt, extracorporeal circulation, and left heart bypass. Table I summarizes the neurologic outcome following thoracic aortic aneurysm repair. Verdant et al. [9] used a 9 millimeter Gott shunt in 366 patients with a descending thoracic aortic aneurysm, not providing details on the longitudinal extent of the aneurysm. They encountered no paraparesis or paraplegia. Borst et al. used the left heart bypass technique in 132 patients undergoing replacement of the descending aorta: six patients (4.5%) developed spinal cord ischemia, three of whom were permanent [10].

Neurologic deficit following thoraco-abdominal aortic aneurysm repair reflects a different entity. Especially in type I and II aneurysms the incidence of paraplegia rises to 30% without adjunctive procedures, but has been reduced to 10%-15% with distal aortic perfusion and spinal fluid drainage [12,13]. The disturbed anatomy in type I and II aneurysms of the intercostal and lumbar arteries has a major impact on spinal cord blood supply. In our experience, the mean number of patent segmental arteries along the entire thoracic and abdominal aorta was only 3 in type I and 7 in type II aneurysms indicating that in the absence of the arteria radicularis magna or other radiculomedullary arteries, collateral circulation is extremely important in feeding the anterior spinal artery [14]. Monitoring motor evoked potentials showed evidence that a substantial part of this collateral blood supply was provided by the iliac arteries and lumbar arteries between L3 and L5. These crucial networks are not involved in

Table I	NEUROLOGIC COMPLICATIONS FOLLOWING THORACIC AORTIC ANEURYSM REPAIR USING DISTAL AORTIC PERFUSION		
1st author [ref.]	*Number of patients*	*Technique*	*Neurologic deficit (%)*
Verdant [9]	366	9 mm Gott shunt	0 (0)
Borst [10]	132	Left heart bypass	6 (4.5) 3 permanent (2.3)
Safi [8]	131	Left heart bypass Spinal fluid drainage	1 (0.7)
Mercier [11]	123	Extra corporeal circulation	3 (2)

thoracic aortic aneurysms and they are all perfused during distal aortic perfusion, explaining the significant lower rate of neurologic complications after descending thoracic aortic repair.

Renal failure

The main determinants of the operative risks and major postoperative complications after thoracic and thoraco-abdominal aortic aneurysm repair are paraplegia, renal failure, and visceral ischemia.

The incidence of renal failure has extensively been reported in patients undergoing thoraco-abdominal aortic aneurysm repair but to a much lesser extent after thoracic aortic aneurysm exclusion. The main difference between both entities is the potential ischemic time during crossclamping. In thoracic aortic aneurysms, the clamp time is depending on the time required for the proximal and distal anastomosis and, if necessary, for reattachment of intercostal arteries. In thoraco-abdominal aortic repair, the clamp time is significantly prolonged because the visceral and renal arteries have to be reattached or reconstructed. Evidently, renal failure occurs more commonly after thoraco-abdominal than after thoracic aortic repair (Table II). Renal failure is a significant risk factor for early and late postoperative mortality. In Safi's experience the mortality rate for patients with acute renal failure was 49% [16]. Preoperative renal insufficiency is an absolute risk factor for postoperative renal failure with odds ratios exceeding 10 [16]. This means that patients with a thoracic aortic aneurysm requiring surgical repair with preoperative renal insufficiency not only envisage an increased risk on hemodialysis but also a significantly higher mortality rate (up to 50%).

What should be the surgical strategy in thoracic aortic aneurysm repair? Based on the data in the literature the surgical scenario mainly depends on the preoperative function of the kidneys. Furthermore, ischemic clamp times should not exceed 30 minutes, indicating the need for experienced and skilled surgeons. In patients with normal kidney function undergoing an uncomplicated aneurysm resection, the clamp-and-sew technique without

Table II	RENAL FAILURE FOLLOWING THORACO-ABDOMINAL AORTIC ANEURYSM (TAAA) AND THORACIC AORTIC ANEURYSM (TAA) REPAIR			
1st author [ref.]	*Number of patients*	*Technique*	*Renal failure %*	*Dialysis %*
TAAA				
Svensson [15]	1 509	Clamp-sew	18	9
Safi [16]	234	Distal aortic perfusion + selective perfusion	17.5	15
Cambria [17]	160	Clamp-sew	10	2.5
Jacobs [18]	73	Distal aortic perfusion + selective perfusion	8	7
TAA				
Cooley [19]	132	Clamp-sew	6.8	6.8
Verdant [9]	366	Passive shunt	2.4	0.2
Mercier [11]	123	Extracorporeal circulation	1.1	1
Personal experience	54	Distal aortic perfusion	2	0

adjunctive procedures will lead to an uneventful outcome. In patients with renal insufficiency (creatinine greater than 200 μmol/L) the clamp-and-sew technique, irrespective the ischemic clamp time, will lead to temporary or permanent renal failure. Distal aortic perfusion by means of left atrium or pulmonary vein to femoral artery bypass is a simple technique, allowing continuous perfusion distal to the clamp. Potential complications like embolization or dislodged atheroma rarely occur. The mean arterial pressure of the distal aortic perfusion should be at least 60 mmHg. However, many patients with thoracic aneurysms suffer from hypertension and their kidneys are used to elevated mean perfusion pressures which might even be as high as 100 mmHg [18]. Especially in patients with preoperative renal insufficiency and hypertension it is mandatory during crossclamping to increase the distal aortic pressure to the patient's individual requirements. The easiest way to assess adequate perfusion pressure is to monitor urine output continuously. Decreased output or anuria following crossclamping should immediately be corrected by increasing the distal aortic pressure. Using this simple strategy we have successfully treated patients with preoperative renal failure undergoing thoracic aneurysm repair [18].

Visceral ischemia

The incidence of gastro-intestinal, hepatopancreatic, and biliary ischemia following extensive thoraco-abdominal aortic aneurysm repair is limited [15], but probably underestimated. The immune responses of the visceral ischemia-reperfusion injury and the subsequent impact on multiple organ failure are currently under extensive investigation.

In thoracic aortic aneurysm repair, visceral ischemia appears to be irrelevant because few studies report on its occurrence or do not even mention it as a clinical problem. Nevertheless, the advantage of distal aortic perfusion is, besides renal perfusion, prevention of visceral ischemia.

Lower limb ischemia

Lower limb ischemia can be caused by aortic dissection, distal embolization during aneurysm repair,

or preoperative severe occlusive disease in the leg. Fann et al. [20] described the incidence of peripheral vascular complications in 272 patients with aortic dissection. Eighty-five patients (31%) sustained one or more peripheral vascular complications: 7 (3%) had a stroke, 9 (3%) had paraplegia, 22 (8%) had impaired renal perfusion, 14 (5%) suffered from compromised visceral perfusion, and 66 (24%) sustained loss of a peripheral pulse with leg ischemia. Aortic repair or fenestration usually restores blood flow to the leg but amputation rate, notably in patients with preexistent occlusive disease, remains high.

Leg ischemia after thoracic or thoraco-abdominal aneurysm repair has been noted in up to 5% of patients [21] and is due to peripheral vascular disease or distal embolization.

Pulmonary complications

Respiratory failure is the most common complication after descending thoracic aortic repair. The incidence of pulmonary complications is depending on many pre-, intra-, and postoperative variables. In a prospective study, Svensson et al. [22] evaluated 1 414 patients. Independent predictors for respiratory failure, defined as ventilatory support exceeding 48 hours, were chronic pulmonary disease, history of smoking, cardiac and renal complications. Pulmonary complications requiring respiratory support with tracheostomy were observed in 112 patients (8%) and 40% of these patients died. Money et al. [23] encountered 21% respiratory failure following thoracic aortic repair with a mortality rate of 42%. In patients who did not develop respiratory failure, mortality rate was 6%. They identified age, type of aneurysm, excessive intra-operative blood transfusions, elevated creatinine and postoperative pneumonia as independent variables affecting respiratory failure. The mean number of days of intubation was 5.8. It should be emphasized that the studies of Svensson et al. and Money et al. mainly comprised patients with thoraco-abdominal aortic aneurysms. Few studies focus on respiratory failure following thoracic aneurysm repair, but it is evident that pulmonary complications occur less frequently than after thoraco-abdominal aortic surgery. The main reason for this difference is transection of the diaphragm. Leaving the diaphragm intact significantly improves respiratory outcome, especially

22

205

in type II aneurysms. In our own experience we reduced the incidence of respiratory failure from 61% to 45% by only transecting the first 5 centimeters of the diaphragm instead of complete transection, in patients with type II aneurysms.

The left lung should be handled with utmost care. Direct surgical trauma causing air leaks, subcutaneous emphysema, atelectasis, or bleeding will provoke respiratory failure. For several years now we leave the left lung ventilated, even during the thoracic part of the procedure. We feel that a continuously ventilated lung improves clinical outcome, however, not collapsing the lung increases the risk of damage (air leak, bleeding) by pushing or retracting.

Pulmonary function can also be impaired by cytokine-induced multiple organ dysfunction as part of a systemic inflammatory response reaction to ischemia-reperfusion or intra-operative factors like blood transfusion or the application of circulatory assist techniques [24]. Additional increased endotoxin release from the gastro-intestinal tract can also contribute to organ dysfunction and respiratory failure [25].

Descending thoracic aortic aneurysm repair can be performed by means of several techniques: crossclamp without adjunctive procedures, left heart bypass, or deep hypothermic circulatory arrest. Pulmonary complications occur more frequently when extracorporeal circulation is used [3] as compared to single cross clamp techniques [19].

Cardiac complications

Preoperative evaluation of patients undergoing major vascular surgery is essential and determines short- and long-term outcome of thoracic aortic surgery [26]. Operative mortality is greatly influenced by cardiac causes, ranging between 20% and 67% [4], comprising myocardial infarction, heart failure and arrhythmias. Therefore, preoperative assessment of significant risk factors like diminished left ventricular function, aortic valve insufficiency or coronary artery disease is crucial and valve repair or revascularization has to be considered, if necessary.

Descending thoracic aortic aneurysm can be treated by means of cross-clamp techniques or adjunctive procedures like left-heart bypass, femoro-femoral cannulation with oxygenator, or profound hypothermia and circulatory arrest. The main advantage of left heart-bypass is unloading the heart and subsequent cardiac support during and after crossclamping.

Myocardial contractility may be depressed by surgical injury, hypothermic damage, anesthetic agents, deterioration of cardiopulmonary bypass functions or infarction. Surgical injury also includes manipulation of the left atrium, which can cause atrium fibrillation with subsequent hemodynamic instability and decreased organ perfusion during and after the procedure. Not only left heart failure but also right heart failure is a serious problem which can occur during thoracic aortic surgery due to previous cardiac surgery, coronary artery disease or right ventricular hypertrophy. Right ventricular dysfunction should be treated with reduction of right ventricular afterload, reduction of pulmonary vasoconstriction, and maintenance of myocardial contractility.

Aorto-esophageal fistula

Gastro-intestinal hemorrhage after descending thoracic aortic surgery is a disastrous complication if caused by an aorto-esophageal fistula (AEF). The patient rapidly develops hypovolemic shock with profound hematemesis and ultimate death. Fortunately this complication rarely occurs, but surgical repair has a high mortality. The exact incidence of postoperative aorto-esophageal fistulas is unknown, however, surgical techniques can be adjusted in order to prevent this complication. At the proximal descending thoracic aorta, the inlay-technique of the anastomosis can easily lead to a prolene suture injury of the esophagus, especially at the medial, posterior wall of the aorta thereby introducing the AVF. Therefore it is recommended to completely separate the aorta from the esophagus, allowing an anastomosis without attaching or even touching the esophagus. Also the distal anastomosis is susceptible for suture injury of the esophagus, especially in large thoracic aneurysms which cross the spine and push the esophagus to the right side. During surgery the esophagus can easily be identified by palpating the nasogastric tube, subsequently allowing secure dissection from the aneurysm.

Thoracic aortic injury

The majority of traumatic aortic injuries are the result of penetrating causes like stab wounds, gunshots, fractured rib puncture, and therapeutic iatrogenic misadventures. Blunt aortic injury occurs as the result of rapid deceleration, however, seemingly innocuous mechanisms, including low speed motor vehicle accidents, can also cause traumatic aortic ruptures. The distribution of blunt aortic injury most often involves the proximal descending thoracic aorta or aortic isthmus (85%), followed by the ascending and transverse arch (10%-14%), and the mid- or distal descending thoracic aorta (12%) [27]. The mechanism for blunt aortic rupture can be attributed to the shear forces applied to the aorta at a point that is fixed, compression of the vessels between bony structures like the spine and sternum, and excessive intraluminal hypertension during a severe traumatic event. In the nomenclature it is important to distinguish blunt aortic rupture or transection and blunt aortic injury: rupture or transection applies to the complete full thickness separation of the aorta and blunt aortic injury refers to a lesion less than a complete circumferential disruption. True traumatic aortic dissection involving the entire aorta longitudinally rarely occurs. After initial evaluation, patients who maintain adequate vital signs will require further diagnostic examinations, like catheter arteriography, computed tomography or transesophageal echocardiography. Catheter aortography remains the gold standard [27].

Though urgent operative repair of confirmed aortic injuries is recommended, delayed repair may be considered in selected patients with severe head injury, risk factors for infection (major burns, sepsis, contaminated wounds), and severe multi-system trauma with poor physiologic reserve. Indications for urgent operative repair include hemodynamic instability, increasing hemorrhage from the chest tubes, and radiographic evidence of an expanding hematoma. Surgical exposure depends on the anatomic location of the injury, including median sternotomy (ascending aorta, transverse arch, innominate and left carotid artery, pulmonary artery) and left thoracotomy (descending thoracic aorta, left subclavian artery).

Survival rates for patients with ascending aortic, aortic arch, or innominate artery injury may approach 50% [27]. Injuries to the descending thoracic aorta are associated with a pre-hospital mortality of 85% and in-hospital mortality of 1% per hour for the initial 48 hours.

PARAPLEGIA FOLLOWING DESCENDING AORTIC INJURY REPAIR

Paraplegia is the most dreadful complication of surgical repair for descending aortic injury, occurring in 5%-19% of patients. The standard operative approach has always been aortic clamping and direct reconstruction and excellent results have been reported [28]. The risk of spinal cord damage, however, increases exponentially if cross-clamp times exceed 30 minutes. Attar et al. [29] showed a significant correlation between longer cross-clamp times and paraplegia. They also demonstrated a significant reduction of paraplegia when using distal aortic perfusion. It should be emphasized that this study had a retrospective design. The use of protective adjuncts like distal aortic perfusion still elicits considerable debate. Razzouk et al. [30] retrospectively compared 83 patients operated according to the clamp and sew technique with 32 patients surgically treated with additional distal perfusion. Paraplegia was 6% in both groups and they concluded that simple aortic cross-clamping is feasible in the majority of patients. Fabian et al. [31] conducted a prospective multicenter trial involving 50 trauma centers in North America. There were 274 blunt aortic injury cases, of which 81% caused by automobile crashes. Two-hundred-seven patients underwent aortic repair: clamp and sew technique was used in 73 patients (35%) and bypass techniques in 134 patients (65%). Overall mortality was 31% and was not affected by the method of repair. Paraplegia occurred significantly more in the clamp and sew group and aortic clamp times over 30 minutes were associated with paraplegia.

Von Oppell et al. [32] performed a meta-analysis of articles concerning the surgical management of acute traumatic rupture of the descending thoracic aorta published in the English language literature between 1972 and 1992. The overall mortality of 1 742 patients who arrived at the hospital alive, was 32%. Paraplegia was observed prior to surgery in 2.6% and overall paraplegia complicated the surgical procedure in 9.9% of 1 492 patients. Simple aortic cross-clamping in 443 patients was associated with a hospital mortality of 16% and paraplegia rate of 19.2%. Passive perfusion shunts in 424 patients had a mortality of 12.3% and paraplegia rate of 11.1% whereas partial left heart bypass was associated with a mortality of 15% and paraplegia rate of

2.3%. The authors therefore advocated the use of partial left heart bypass.

The determinants of postoperative paraplegia are multifactorial, and especially in multitrauma patients not one single factor is attributable in any individual patient. In the absence of prospective randomized trials the surgical technique should be customized to the individual patient and is directed by the complexity of the injury, the estimated clamp time and the local experience of the surgical team.

Coarctation

Infant aortic coarctation is a congenital disease, often associated with other intracardiac lesions like ventricular septal defect. The surgical strategy for coarctation changed from subclavian flap aorto- plasty to resection with extended end-to-end anasto- mosis. Balloon angioplasty is also a therapeutic option, but not successful in all patients.

The incidence of spinal cord ischemia following aortic coarctation repair is low. Keen performed an inquiry into the clinical practice and paraplegia rate associated with operations for coarctation con- ducted by surgeons in the United Kingdom and Ireland. Paraplegia occurred in 16 patients in a total of 5 492 operations, an incidence of 0.3%, or once in 343 operations [33]. However, paraplegia follow- ing coarctation repair does occur [34] and the gen- eral recommendation is to perform an extended end-to-end anastomosis or, in adults, an interposi- tion graft with any adjunctive technique providing distal aortic perfusion during crossclamping. The overall mortality rate is low (less than 2%) and recoarctation rate is acceptable (3%) [35].

R E F E R E N C E S

1 Royse C, Royse A, Blake D et al. Screening the thoracic aorta for atheroma: a comparison of manual palpation, transesophageal and epi-aortic ultrasonography. *Ann Thor Cardiovasc Surg* 1998; 4: 347-350.

2 Meissner I, Whisnant JP, Khanderia BK et al. Prevalence of potential risk factors for stroke assessed by transesophageal echocardiography and carotid ultrasonography: the SPARC study. Stroke prevention: assessment of risk in a community. *Mayo Clin Proc* 1999; 74: 862-869.

3 Safi HJ, Miller CC 3rd, Subramaniam MH et al. Thoracic and thoraco-abdominal aortic aneurysm repair using cardiopul- monary bypass, profound hypothermia, and circulatory arrest via left side of the chest incision. *J Vasc Surg* 1998; 28: 591-598.

4 Panneton JM, Hollier LH. Dissecting descending thoracic and thoraco-abdominal aortic aneurysms: Part II. *Ann Vasc Surg* 1995; 9: 596-605.

5 Elefteriades JA, Lovoulos CJ, Coady MA et al. Management of descending aortic dissection. *Ann Thor Surg* 1999; 67: 2002-2005.

6 Balm R, Reekers JA, Jacobs M. Classification of endovascular procedures for thoracic aortic aneurysms. In: Branchereau A, Jacobs M (eds.). *Surgical and endovascular treatment of aortic aneurysms.* Futura Publishing Company, Inc. 2000; pp 19-26.

7 Fann JI, Miller DL. Descending thoracic aortic aneurysms. In: Barre AE, Geha AS, Hammond GL, Laks H, Nannheim KS (eds.). *Glenn's thoracic and cardiovascular surgery,* 6th edition Stanford Conn: Appleton and Lange, 1996; pp 2255-2272.

8 Safi HJ, Subramaniam MH, Miller CC et al. Progress in the management of type I thoraco-abdominal and descending thoracic aortic aneurysms. *Ann Vasc Surg* 1999; 13: 457-462.

9 Verdant A, Cossette R, Page A et al. Aneurysms of the descending thoracic aorta: three hundred sixty-six consecutive cases resected without paraplegia. *J Vasc Surg* 1995; 21: 385-390.

10 Borst HG, Jurmann M, Buhner B et al. Risk of replacement of descending aorta with a standardized left heart bypass. *J Thor Cardiovasc Surg* 1994; 107: 126-132.

11 Mercier F, Fabiani JN. Chirurgie des anévrysmes de l'aorte descendante: traitement chirurgical moderne et résultats. *J Cardiovasc Surg* 1998; 39 (suppl.1): 11-14.

12 Schepens MA, Vermeulen FE, Morshuis WJ et al. Impact of left heart bypass on the results of thoraco-abdominal aortic aneurysm repair. *Ann Thor Surg* 1999; 67: 1963-1967.

13 Coselli JS, LeMaire SA, Koksoy C et al. Cerebrospinal fluid drainage reduces paraplegia following thoraco-abdominal aortic aneurysm repair: results of a prospective randomized trial. *J Vasc Surg,* in press.

14 Jacobs MJHM, Meylaerts SA, de Haan P et al. Strategies to prevent neurologic deficit based on motor-evoked potentials in type I and II thoraco-abdominal aortic aneurysm repair. *J Vasc Surg* 1999; 29: 48-59.

15 Svensson LG, Crawford ES, Hess KR et al. Experience with 1509 patients undergoing thoraco-abdominal aortic operations. *J Vasc Surg* 1993; 17: 357-370.

16 Safi HJ, Harlin SA, Miller CC et al. Predictive factors for acute renal failure in thoracic and thoraco-abdominal aortic aneurysm surgery. *J Vasc Surg* 1998; 24: 338-345.

17 Cambria RP, Davison JK, Zanetti S et al. Thoraco-abdominal aneurysm repair: perspectives over a decade with the clamp-and- sew technique. *Ann Surg* 1997; 226: 294-303.

18 Jacobs MJ, Eijsman L, Meylaerts SA et al. Reduced renal failure following thoraco-abdominal aortic aneurysm repair by selective perfusion. *Eur J Cardiothorac Surg* 1998; 14: 201-205.

19 Cooley DA, Golino A, Frazier OH. Single-clamp technique for aneurysms of the descending thoracic aorta: report of 132 consecutive cases. *Eur J Cardiothorac Surg* 2000; 18: 162-167.

20 Fann JI, Sarris GE, Mitchell RS et al. Treatment of patients with aortic dissection presenting with peripheral vascular complications. *Ann Surg* 1990; 212: 705-713.

21 Schwartz LB, Belkin M, Donaldson MC et al. Improvement in results of repair of type IV thoraco-abdominal aortic aneurysms. *J Vasc Surg* 1996; 24: 74-81.

22 Svensson LG, Hess KR, Coselli JS et al. A prospective study of respiratory failure after high risk surgery on the thoraco-abdominal aorta. *J Vasc Surg* 1991; 14: 271-282.

23 Money SR, Rice K, Crockett D et al. Risk of respiratory failure after repair of thoraco-abdominal aortic aneurysms. *Am J Surg* 1994; 168: 152-155.

24 Franssen EJ, Maessen JG, Dentener MA et al. Impact of blood transfusions on inflammatory mediater release in patients undergoing cardiac surgery. *Chest* 1999; 116: 1233-1239.

25 Landow L, Andersen LW. Splanchnic ischaemia and its role in multiple organ failure. *Acta Anaesthesiol Scan* 1994: 38: 626-639.

26 Fleisher LA, Beattie C. Current practice in the preoperative evaluation of patients undergoing major vascular surgery: a survey of cardiovascular anesthesiologists. *J Cardiothorac Vasc Anesth* 1993; 7: 650-654.

27 Esterra A, Mattox KL, Wall MJ. Thoracic aortic injury. *Sem Vasc Surg* 2000; 13: 345-352.

28 Sweeney M, Young D, Frazier O et al. Traumatic aortic transections: eight-year experience with the *clamp-sew* technique. *Ann Thorac Surg* 1997; 64: 384-387.

29 Attar S, Cardarelli MG, Downing SW et al. Traumatic aortic rupture: recent outcome with regard to neurologic deficit. *Ann Thorac Surg* 1999; 67: 959-965.

30 Razzouk AJ, Gundry SR, Wang N et al. Repair of traumatic aortic rupture: a 25-year experience. *Arch Surg* 2000; 135: 913-919.

31 Fabian TC, Richardson JD, Croce MA et al. Prospective study of blunt aortic injury: multicenter trial of the American Association for the surgery of trauma. *J Trauma* 1997; 42: 374-380.

32 Von Oppell UO, Dunne TT, De Groot MK et al. Traumatic aortic rupture: twenty-year meta-analysis of mortality and risk of paraplegia. *Ann Thorac Surg* 1994; 58: 585-593.

33 Keen G. Spinal cord damage and operations for coarctation of the aorta: aetiology, practice, and prospects. *Thorax* 1987; 42: 11-18.

34 Vanhulle C, Durand I, Tron P. Paraplegia due to medullary ischemia after repair of coarctation of the aorta in an infant. *Arch Pediatr* 1998; 5: 633-636.

35 Backer CL, Mavroudis C, Zias EA et al. Repair of coarctation with resection and extended end-to-end anastomosis. *Ann Thorac Surg* 1998; 66: 1365-1370.

23

POSTOPERATIVE STROKE ASSOCIATED WITH NON-CEREBROVASCULAR SURGERY

MARC AAM SCHEPENS, WIM-JAN VAN BOVEN

Stroke, related to surgery or not, remains a devastating event for the patient and the family. The costs related to stroke are high due to the necessity of long-term care facilities.

Theoretically any kind of surgery can cause neurologic problems but in particular interventions on the heart or major vessels carrying blood to the brain are prone to central neurologic complications.

It is the responsibility of the surgeon to try to identify the risk factors of these vulnerable patients in order to take precautions and protective measures in the complete peri-operative period.

We will restrict ourselves to the topic of stroke related to non-cerebrovascular interventions.

Which kind of interventions are we dealing with?

The different interventions related to stroke are listed in Table I. Excluded are the interventions on the cerebripetal vessels (carotid and vertebral arteries). However, one should not forget the high incidence of carotid artery stenosis in patients scheduled for coronary artery bypass grafting (CABG); our treatment protocol in these circumstances has been described extensively [1].

As can be learned from Table I, most operations are related to surgery of the heart and great vessels although other kind of interventions, vascular or nonvascular, may also carry a risk of stroke. Fracture of long bones e.g. in multitrauma patients may cause fat emboli which usually give multiple cerebral hemorrhages.

Table I	TYPES OF SURGICAL INTERVENTIONS THAT CAN BE RELATED TO STROKE (REPAIR OF CEREBRIPETAL VESSELS EXCLUDED)

Cardiac
  Coronary artery revascularization
  Left ventricular aneurysm repair
  Valve repair or replacement
  Intracardiac tumours
  Endocarditis of the cardiac valves
  Complex intracardiac congenital or adult repair
  Combinations

  Aortic
  Root replacement
  Ascending aorta replacement
  Arch replacement
  Descending aorta replacement
  Thoracoabdominal aorta replacement
  Abdominal aortic aneurysm repair

Peripheral vascular interventions

Endovascular procedures

Angiography

Pathophysiologic mechanisms of stroke associated with non-cerebrovascular surgery

One of the mechanisms of cerebral infarction during or after surgery is embolization. These emboli can be small, such as an aggregate of bacteria, or huge, such as a dislodgement of a fragment of an atherosclerotic plaque during side-clamping of the aorta or clamp manipulation. Theoretically emboli can be heart-borne, aorta-borne or related to the extra-corporeal circulation (ECC). An overview of all potential sources is given in Table II.

Systemic embolization of fragments of a left atrial thrombus in case of chronic atrial fibrillation, of infected material on a native or prosthetic left-sided cardiac valve and of tumor fragments of an intracardiac neoplasm mostly occur spontaneously; this means not related to surgical manipulation or intervention. Nevertheless, the surgeon should be very carefull when operating on these patients in these particular circumstances. Paradoxic embolism can occur when an abnormal communication exists between the right and left sides of the heart; embolic material arising in the veins of the lower extremity or anywhere in the systemic venous tree may bypass the pulmonary circulation and reach the cerebral vessels. Septic emboli from vegetations on

Table II	ETIOLOGY OF STROKE RELATED TO NON-CEREBROVASCULAR SURGERY

Emboli (macro or micro)
  1. *Atherosclerotic debris:* from valves, from ascending aorta or aortic arch, from proximal arch vessels
  2. *Clot/thrombus:* in case of chronic atrial fibrillation and insufficient anticoagulation, left ventricular aneurysms (postinfarction)
  3. *Infected material vegetations:* dislodgement of infected thrombus from left ventricle *mycotic aneurysm,* vegetations from the aortic or mitral valve
  4. *Tumor particles:* left atrial myxoma or other cardiac tumors
  5. *Gas:* air after open cardiac procedures, from ECC, due to the Venturi-effect, due to physical properties governing the solubility of gas in a fluid
  6. *ECC-particles:* fat or cellular aggregates

Perfusion-related
  1. *Hypoperfusion:* due to resuscitative hypotension in hypovolemic (eg serious bleeding in AAA, TAA, TAAA surgery) or cardiogenic (eg cardiac tamponade) shock
  2. *Malperfusion:* in acute aortic dissections
  3. *Hyperperfusion*

ECC: extra-corporeal circulation

valves or on clot as well as embolization of tumor fragments usually causes multiple brain infarction. On the contrary, air-borne emboli are most frequently related to surgery or catheter interventions. Air embolism can occur during intra-arterial manipulations of catheters in the heart or in the aortic segment proximal to the left subclavian artery, whether it is diagnostic (angiography) or therapeutic (balloon dilatations, placement of endografts). During valve and other intra-cardiac surgery, the surgeon should be aware that air is one of the great enemies to defeat. On the other hand surgeons are well aware of the fact that it is almost imposssible to de-air the heart completely after these procedures; this can be nicely demonstrated by transesophageal echocardiography, for example at the end of mitral valve plasty (Fig. 1). Fortunately, this almost never has serious neurologic consequences.

A special attention deserves the air which can enter into the arterial system due to the Venturi-effect and to the physical properties of solubility of gases in a fluid, e.g. during cooling and rewarming of the blood when deep hypothermic circulatory arrest is used.

Another very important mechanism that can explain peri-operative stroke is hypoperfusion of certain vascular territories of the brain. This is mostly related to hypotension due to serious bleeding during or after vascular interventions or hemodynamic instability during or shortly after weaning from bypass. Certain areas of the brain, the so-called *watershed* areas (the boundaries between areas of distribution of different cerebral arteries) are particular vulnerable to this kind of ischemic damage. Malperfusion of the brain in acute aortic dissection deserves special attention (see below). Hyperperfusion may also play a very important role in postoperative stroke; it can result in unilateral hypertensive encephalopathy leading to intracranial hemorrhage.

Cerebral ischemia whether it is air-borne, ECC-borne, aortic-borne or related to hypoperfusion can be worsened due to metabolic circumstances.

Continuously elevated glycemia for example is a negative factor in the progressive destruction of neural tissue once an injury has occurred. Because an ischemic area of the brain is partially perfused with a high glucose level, this enables anerobic glycolysis to continue with the inevitable accumulation of lactic acid. Cerebral outcome can also be influenced by ECC-protocols like pH- and alfa-stat. Finally, interactions between the patients blood and the artificial surfaces of the ECC circuit are believed to induce humoral and cellular activation, leading to a systemic inflammatory response. Features of this syndrome include adhesion, aggregation and subsequently micro-embolism formation of neutrophils and other blood cellular elements. Although this potential mechanism for protruding brain injury remains speculative, it would be consistent with the consequences of the systemic inflammatory response of other body systems. Magnetic

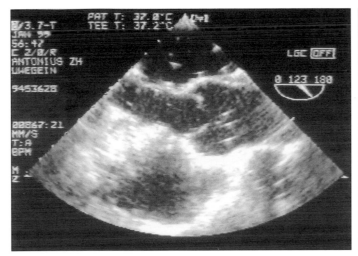 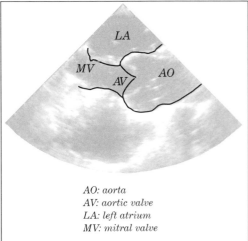

AO: aorta
AV: aortic valve
LA: left atrium
MV: mitral valve

FIG. 1   Air in the heart after mitral valve reconstruction.

resonance imaging of the brain within 60 minutes of the end of coronary surgical procedures show substantial diffuse brain swelling with loss of normal appearance of the sulci and gyri.

Incidence of stroke related to the type of surgery

Coronary artery bypass surgery is associated with stroke in 1% to 3% of patients between 51 and 60 years; this incidence rises to 9% in patients older than 80 years. When neurologic baselines are measured prospectively, the incidence of neurologic injury increases up to 33%. However, neuropsychological dysfunction is reported to occur in 20% to 60% of patients and include often very subtle defects such as mood, memory, concentration and changes in personality. These minor deficits are still present after one year in 25% to 30% of the patients [2].

Which patients are especially at risk for stroke after cardiac surgery? After CABG, older age (odds ratio 1.9 per decade, 95% confidence interval [CI] 1.73-2.09, p = 0.00001), previous TIA (odds ratio 2.2, 95% CI, 1.32-3.68, p = 0.002) and carotid bruits (odds ratio 1.9, 95% CI, 1.29-2.84, p = 0.0009) show a strong correlation with stroke after multivariate regression analysis [3].

Since advanced age, tobacco abuse, left main coronary stenosis, extensive peripheral vascular disease and a history of previous cerebrovascular accidents or TIA are all correlates to carotid disease, it it important to explore and examine these risk factors preoperatively.

Those who undergo combined intracardiac and revascularization procedures (given that more than 200 000 patients worldwide undergo open-chamber cardiac procedures annually, of which approximately 100 000 are combined with CABG), it is estimated that annually 15 000 to 30 000 patients will suffer from stroke [4].

When using antegrade selective cerebral perfusion (ASCP) in total aortic arch repair, recent studies of Kazui et al. [5] and Dossche et al. [6] have shown excellent results with regard to the stroke rate. In 220 [5] and 106 [6] consecutive arch replacements using this technique of brain protection, the reported incidence of postoperative temporary neurologic dysfunction was 6% (95% CI, 2.8% to 9.3%) [5] and 3.8% (70% CI, 2.0% to 5.6%) [6],

respectively. Independent predictors for temporary neurologic dysfunction after multivariate analysis were cerebral ischemia caused by acute aortic dissection and an old cerebral infarct [5] and preoperative hemodynamic instability and perioperative technical problems [6]. Permanent neurologic dysfunction occurred in 3.3% (95% CI, 1.3% to 10.7%) [5] and 5.4% (70% CI, 3.2% to 7.6%) [6] respectively. Factors influencing this in the series of Kazui et al. [5] were a prolonged ECC time of more than 300 minutes and an old cerebral infarction, whereas in the series of Dossche et al. [6] preoperative hemodynamic instability and a left thoracotomy approach had a negative impact on permanent neurologic outcome. Anyhow, the reported incidence of 25% mortality in aortic arch surgery of which 80% was due to stroke, is no longer acceptable [7].

In descending thoracic and thoracoabdominal aortic repair the proximal clamping site is very often on the aortic arch, more precisely between the left common carotid and left subclavian artery. This manoeuver certainly can cause embolization to the brain in case the arch or origin of the brachiocephalic vessels are diseased or calcified. Sometimes it is even necessary to put the clamp more proximal to the left common carotid artery. In these circumstances intraoperative EEG control can be very helpfull as well as a preoperative assessment of the completeness of the circle of Willis. When one uses the left heart bypass air can enter the left atrium at the moment of cannulation of the left atrial appendage or left pulmonary vein. One has also to be very carefull with de-airing of the vascular prosthesis after completion of the proximal anastomosis when using sequential clamping. The incidence of postoperative stroke after descending aorta replacement is identical to that after thoracoabdominal repair. In the early series of Crawford, the incidence of postoperative stroke was unclear; anyhow, it contributed substantially to hospital mortality. In the larger series (1509 patients) from the same group described by Svensson et al. [8], stroke complicated TAAA repair in 2.5%. Of these patients 33% died during their hospital stay. After multivariate analysis of 30-day mortality the odds ratio for stroke was 6.17 (95% CI, 2.57 to 14.8, p = 0.0001) [8].

The problem of the "bad" aorta during cardiac surgery

(Synonyms: unclampable or untouchable aorta, porcelain aorta)

Since the early days of cardiac surgery, cardiac surgeons have been well aware of the high stroke rates among patients with severely atheromatous aortae. Roughly 50% of patients with coronary artery disease have some degree of atheroma in the ascending aorta. Only in half of them the existence of atheromas can be diagnosed by finger palpation. Most patients with this kind of aortas are in their late seventies or eighties: at necropsy aortic atheroma is found in 80% over the age of 75 years. As the number of elderly patients undergoing CABG has increased, the decline in overall mortality and morbidity has been largely obscured by the increasing neurologic complication rate. It is without any doubt the most problematic issue to deal with in CABG operations and a safer outcome is to be expected when adequate information about the ascending aorta would be available. Although large numbers of emboli enter the cerebral circulation during cardiac surgery only a fraction appear to be symptomatic. The impact of such embolization may depend on particle size, the constitution of emboli, total embolic volume, the collateral arterial supply of the affected brain region, and the quality of the pre-existing parenchymal brain function.

Aortic knob calcification on chest X-ray can give an uncertain indication of severe disease. At coronary angiography, the plain supravalvular image of the aorta can also reveal the porcelain aorta. Visual inspection of the ascending aorta is of little value. Most cardiac surgeons assess the aorta intraoperatively using manual palpation. This means proper tactile examination of the entire aortic wall (total ascending aorta, distal to the pericardial reflection and the aortic root) with the index finger or between the index finger and the thumb; it is the traditional and most used method for intraoperative assessment of aortic atheroma. It underestimates the plaque by at least 50% compared to TEE [9], it can be a cause of embolization in itself and 30% to 70% of the plaques are not discovered by palpation alone. However, it is easy to perform, unmistakable, cost-free and can be universally applied.

Undisputable, the technique of choice for intraoperative evaluation of the aorta is ultrasonography; one can choose between transesophageal echocardiography (TEE) or epiaortic echography. In TEE it must be remembered that the ascending aorta and the junction with the arch is the most difficult segment of the aorta to visualize due to the interposition of the right main bronchus between the esophagus and the aorta, preventing transmission of ultrasound. This is a major drawback of TEE. Direct epiaortic ultrasonography is much more sensitive than palpation and allows evaluation of the complete ascending aorta and arch. It should precede aortic manipulation. Therefore a hand-held probe of 5 or 7.5 Mhz can be used. Both techniques (epiaortic ultrasound and TEE) can be complementary for the assessment of atherosclerosis of the thoracic aorta [10]. The severity of the lesions should be classified and quantified (Table III) for example according to Montgomery et al. [11]. Transcranial doppler ultrasonography (TCD) can detect emboli passing by through both middle cerebral arteries. Flurries of emboli are frequently seen at the inception of bypass, cannulation of the aorta, after releasing the site clamps. However, only a fraction of the emboli entering the cerebral circulation are detected.

The ascending aorta is the least atheromatous segment of the thoracic aorta. Most mobile plaques are found in the descending thoracic aorta and the aortic arch is intermediate. The bulk of disease in the ascending aorta is in its upper part and more specific at the junction with the aortic arch.

Table III	ECHOCARDIOGRAPHIC CLASSIFICATION OF ATHEROSCLEROTIC LESIONS	
Lesion grade	Description	
1	Normal	
2	Intimal thickening > 2 mm, ± calcifications	
3	Atheroma < 4 mm, ± calcifications	
4	Atheroma ≥ 4 mm, ± calcifications	
5	Any mobile or ulcerated lesion, ± calcifications	

Soft plaques in which cholesterol debris gushes through the aortotomy opening, are even more threatening to the patient than calcified lesions because they are impossible to detect by finger palpation. These non-calcified, *cheesy* soft lesions contain more loose necrotic material with a higher probability of embolization.

Possible surgical measures related to the bad aorta

A lot of surgical measures and precautions can be taken to avoid stroke in patients with a *bad* aorta (Table IV). However, none of these surgical modifications has been validated. Attempts to avoid dislodging aortic atheroma include the no touch, no clamp, no cannulation, no proximal hooking of grafts on a *bad* aorta, avoidance of repetitive cross-clamping or side clamping, prevention of direct penetration of aortic atheroma by cannulas or clamps. If this strategy is followed, the risk of complications of any kind should be no higher than in other patients having CABG! Special attention must be given to the endoballoons, the one-shot device for proximal anastomoses and off-pump CABG. The first endoclamps or endoballoons were developed for minimal access or port-access cardiac surgery. Initially there were some thoughts that this aortic occlusion technique might be less emboligenic, later, however, this opinion was abandonned. Endoballoons can migrate and they can give rise to embolization as can the catheter on its own. In the heavily calcified or porcelain aorta the endoballoon can occlude the aortic lumen while other clamp techniques cannot. Intra-aortic filter devices are developed. These polyester mesh filters can extract particulate emboli from the circulation while unclamping the aorta. Histological examinations of the filters show indeed atheroma's, platelet aggregates and other components (Fig.2). Initial clinical experience from a multi-centre prospective study using these filters reports a very low stroke rate.

Another potential improvement is the *one shot* device for the proximal anastomosis on the ascending aorta. This allows to perform the anastomosis without clamping. The application of this device together with epiaortic ultrasound might have some theoretical advantages.

In off-pump CABG the negative effects of the ECC on the brain are avoided. Particulate or air emboli generated by the heart-lung machine are absent as well as the induced inflammatory response. When total arterial revascularization is performed without proximal anastomoses on the ascending aorta, the desired no-touch technique can be reached. Another potential hazardous effect of the heart-lung machine is hypoperfusion and non-pulsatile flow. This is subject of discussion since organ perfu-

Table IV	SURGICAL MEASURES THAT CAN BE TAKEN DURING CARDIAC INTERVENTIONS TO AVOID CEREBRAL DAMAGE
Description of the aorta	*Possible solution*
Normal (flexible, soft)	No surgical modification
Focal atheroma	Change in positioning of the arterial cannulation, the crossclamp site or proximal venous graft anastomoses, or both
	Use arterial cannula with filter
Extensive scattered atheromas, no safe crossclamp site	Femoral or subclavian artery cannulation. Work on fibrillating heart (with lower temperatures) or use endoaortic occlusion balloon.
Very extensive atheroma	Use as much as possible in situ IMA's or construct Y-grafts (eg with radial artery), connect vein grafts to innominate artery or IMA's, connect venous grafts to other venous grafts.
Porcelain aorta	Consider partial ascending replacement under profound hypothermic circulatory arrest

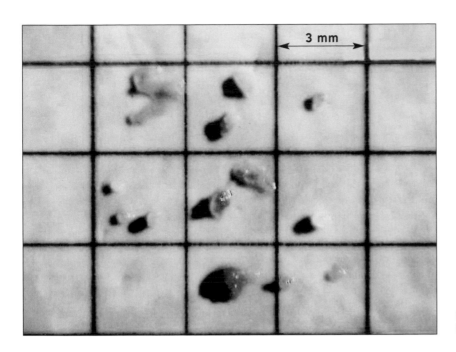

FIG. 2 Elements removed from intra-aortic filter.

sion can also be reduced in off-pump CABG proce dures during the tilting of the heart. Cerebral perfusion, however, can be monitored adequately during these procedures with EEG or TCD. Up to now only a few publications showed reduced stroke rate in off-pump surgery [12,13]. Recent studies show that cognitive deficits after cardiac surgery seem to be associated to cardiopulmonary bypass and the occurrence of micro-emboli [14].

Malperfusion during surgery for acute type A aortic dissection

Hypoperfusion or malperfusion of certain vascular beds downstream the aortic valve can be explained by the mechanism of the dissection itself (Fig.3). Expansion and pressurization of the false channel, and the intimal flap itself can narrow or occlude aortic side branches. This creates ischemia or infarction. Potentially all vessels originating from the aorta are at risk. This explains why patients with an acute type A aortic dissection might develop acute myocardial infarction (coronary artery occlusion), stroke (cerebral vessel occlusion), paraplegia (intercostal artery occlusion), mesenterial infarc-

tion (occlusion of the celiac trunk and/or superior mesenteric artery), renal failure (renal artery occlusion), claudication or peripheral ischemia (lower abdominal aorta and/or iliac artery occlusion). These phenomenon can be induced, aggravated or reversed by surgical manoeuvres. The preoperative central neurologic status of the patient should be analyzed scrutinously because very often the ischemic stroke is irreversible in contrast to e.g. renal insufficiency which can be changed after restoring blood flow through the true lumen.

Adequate intraoperative neuromonitoring and careful surgical neuroprotective measures are the cornerstones to success. As long as the heart is beating and sufficient output is made, retrograde arterial perfusion via the femoral artery, which is more or less the standard approach, can do little harm but when the heart fibrillates due to the cooling or the aortic clamp is put on the ascending aorta, retrograde perfusion might expand and pressurize the false lumen so that antegrade cerebral perfusion is at least compromised or even can be blocked completely. This can be prevented by avoiding to clamp the aorta and monitor both radial artery pressures, TCD- and TEE-monitoring and electroencephalography (EEG) intra-operatively. With all these adjuncts and not clamping the aorta, the critical moments related to cerebral perfusion in this particular surgery should give optimal results.

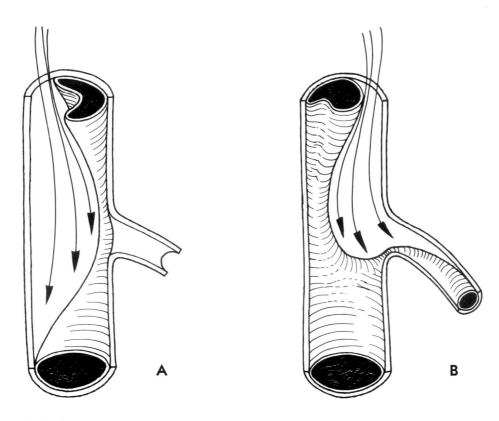

FIG. 3 Mechanisms of side branch malperfusion or occlusion in case of type A aortic dissection. In A the false lumen expands and obstructs the blood flow to the side branch; in B the dissection process extends into the side branch obstructing antegrade blood flow.

Cerebral protection during ascending aorta and aortic arch surgery

Surgery of the distal ascending aorta and aortic arch carries a great risk of central neurologic problems since manipulation in this particular region of the vascular tree involves directly the centripetal blood flow. Therefore errors and inaccuracies have serious consequences. The etiology of cerebral damage related to surgery of this aortic segment is not different from the rest: emboli, air, and hypoperfusion. Atherosclerotic plaques are not at all exceptional in the aortic arch or at the origin of the cerebral vessels. A special attention must be given to optimal protection of the brain because together with utmost conscientious technique; these two points form the key to success. When the total cerebral blood flow is interrupted for about 3 minutes

or longer at normothermia, irreversible neurologic damage will follow. Since it is impossible to perform any repair in less than 10 minutes, no matter how simple it may be (e.g. an open distal circular anastomosis), special attention must be taken te preserve cerebral function. This is even more obligatory when complex reconstructions are planned (e.g. total arch replacement plus elephant trunk). Deep hypothermic circulatory arrest (DHCA) in which the blood temperature is cooled down gradually untill 13 to 14 degrees Celsius is reached, corresponding to a nasopharyngeal and rectal temperature of about 18 degrees Celsius, is probably the oldest and still the most frequently used technique which allows surgeons to perform repair in this particular anatomical region. At this temperature oxygen-consumption is zero and the EEG is iso-electric. Because there are no prospective randomized studies, it is the comprehensive series of Svensson and Crawford [15] with 656 patients undergoing DHCA with a 10% mortality and 7% risk of neurologic deficit against which other brain protection techniques should be compared. In our opinion the safe time limit to perform the repair using DHCA is 30 minutes at most; when it is anticipated that the complexity of the repair will necessitate a longer arrest time, other protective measures should be taken. DHCA certainly has some advantages. In situations where the brachiocephalic arteries are diffusely calcified and atheromatous, it is preferable to avoid manipulation and cannulation. Also the operative field is completely empty making the repair simpler. Retrograde cerebral perfusion can be added to DHCA because it will extend somewhat the safe time limit of the arrest. One of the most important benefits of retrograde brain perfusion is the flushing out of air or embolic material. The *Mount Sinaï Group* has shown that the shorter the arrest times, the lower the adverse outcome and transient neurologic dysfunction [16]. Nevertheless, we will rely only on antegrade selective cerebral perfusion (ASCP) when the repair takes more than 30 minutes. This technique allows visual introduction of balloon-expandable perfusion catheters in the innominate artery and the left common carotid artery. Even in case of acute dissection or when the orifices of the cerebral vessels are heavily calcified, it is possible to introduce the catheters a vue into the true lumen or higher into a healthy part of the vessel. ASCP rather avoids cerebral embolization of debris although the opponents of this technique claim the contrary. We believe that complex repairs e.g. redo's or in Marfan patients only offers the best chances of success using ASCP [5,6].

Is retrograde aortic perfusion dangerous?

One of the alternative cannulation sites in case of serious atherosclerosis of the ascending aorta or arch is the femoral artery. Most surgeons will use it routinely for acute aortic dissection as they do in the case of left heart bypass for repair of thoracoabdominal or descending thoracic aortic aneurysms. Theoretically this could carry away atherosclerotic particles or debris upto the arch and into the cerebral vessels *retrograde embolization*, especially when we consider the bad aortas of all these vascular cripples.

We believe it was never proven that strokes in these particular cases were absolutely due to retrograde embolization [17].

Cannulation of the subclavian or axillary artery with interposition of a short piece of dacron prosthesis might be a very good alternative [18].

Prevalence of carotid artery stenosis prior to peripheral vascular surgery

Neurologic risks are not limited to cardiac surgery only. Peripheral vascular surgery also carries a postoperative risk on stroke, most often related to the presence of a tight carotid artery stenosis. The necessity to detect carotid artery stenosis and performing a prophylactic carotid endarterectomy prior to infrarenal abdominal aortic aneurysm (AAA) repair or peripheral bypass surgery depends on the degree and severity of these different lesions and the potential postoperative end/or long-term neurologic risks.

Patients undergoing infrarenal AAA repair or peripheral bypass surgery have an increased risk of carotid artery stenosis (Table V). Duplex scanning prior to infrainguinal bypass surgery demonstrates carotid artery stenosis of more than 50% in 17% to 28% of asymptomatic patients and up to 45% in patients with previous transient ischemic or stroke. In patients suffering from infrarenal occlusive aortic disease the prevalence of asymptomatic tight carotid artery stenosis is even higher than in patients with an AAA.

Cerebral vascular risk after peripheral vascular surgery

Despite the relatively high incidence of carotid stenosis among patients undergoing a peripheral vascular procedure, the occurrence of strokes after surgery is limited. Moneta et al. performed a literature search and reported a postoperative stroke rate of 0.5% following 2246 peripheral vascular interventions [23]. Harris et al. observed 13 neurologic events after 1390 non-carotid vascular interventions (0.2%), of which three patients died (0.2%) [24]. It comprised 12 vascular accidents in the carotid territory and one posterior stroke. In this study it is interesting to note that 8 of the 12 anterior neurologic events (67%) occurred after aortic surgery and that nine patients suffered from an ipsilateral carotid artery stenosis of 50% or more.

The postoperative neurologic risk following infrarenal abdominal aortic surgery varies between 0% and 3% (Table VI). Moneta et al. report a stroke rate of 1.3% after surgery for ruptured abdominal aneurysms [23]. The data and results of the differ-

ent studies can not be compared because some series only report on hemispheric accidents whereas others describe focal and non-focal accidents or even differentiate between transient ischemic attacks and strokes. The pathophysiologic mecha-

Table V	PREVALENCE OF CAROTID ARTERY DISEASE AS ASSESSED BY DUPLEX SCANNING BEFORE INFRARENAL OR PERIPHERAL VASCULAR SURGERY				
1st author [ref.]	Year of publication	Follow-up	Type of disease	Number of cases	Carotid stenosis 50-99 % N (%)
Alexandrova [19]	1996	2 years	PVD	373	121 (32)
Miralles [20]	1998	NA	AAA	58	12 (21)
			OAD	110	35 (32)
Cahan [21]	1999	1992-1998	AAA	139	24 (17)
			OAD	101	40 (40)
Pilcher [22]	2000	6 months	PVD	200	35 (17.5)

AAA: abdominal aortic aneurysm
OAD: occlusive aortic disease
PVD: peripheral vascular disease
NA: not available

Table VI	NEUROLOGIC COMPLICATIONS FOLLOWING INFRARENAL ABDOMINAL AORTIC SURGERY						
1st author [ref.]	Year of publication	Follow-up	Aortic disease	Number of cases	Neurologic events after aortic surgery		
					TIA N (%)	Lethal stroke N (%)	Stroke N (%)
Szilagyi [25]	1986	1954-1983	OAD	1647	NA	4 (0.24)	11 (0.7)
Johnston [26]	1989	1986	AAA	666	1 (0.15)	2 (0.3)	3 (0.45)
AURC [27]	1990	1989	AAA	780	5 (0.6)	2 (0.3)	6 (0.8)
Nevelsteen [28]	1991	1963-1987	OAD	869	NA	3 (0.4)	6 (0.7)
Poulias [29]	1992	1966-1990	OAD	1000	NA	5 (0.5)	30 (3)
Cahan [21]	1999	1992-1998	AAA + OAD	240	1 (0.4)	2 (0.8)	3 (1.2)
Bechtel [30]	2000	1994-1995	AAA + OAD	201	0	1 (0.5)	1 (0.5)

AAA: abdominal aortic aneurysm
OAD: occlusive aortic disease
TIA: transient ischemic attack
NA: not available

nisms of postoperative neurologic deficits following abdominal aortic surgery are rather unclear. The occurance of hypotensive periods due to intra-operative blood loss is often identified as one of the main causes of postoperative accidents.

The development of a stroke following aortailiac surgery most often occurs after a certain postoperative interval, whereas in cardiac surgery neurologic deficits develop during the procedure. [31,32].

Prophylactic carotid surgery prior to infrarenal aortic repair

Since the sixties, studies have been initiated in order to assess carotid artery disease in patients with other vascular indications for surgery and prophylactic carotid surgery was started. This surgical attitude was disputed and several studies have shown that the postoperative risk on stroke in the presence of a carotid stenosis did not differ with or without prophylactic surgery [32-34]. In contrast, three series have demonstrated an increased neurologic risk among patients with a carotid artery stenosis [35-37]. In a series of 374 asymptomatic patients, Gutierrez et al. observed a postoperative stroke rate of 3.2% in patients with a carotid lesion and no neurologic deficit in the absence of a carotid stenosis [36]. Gerraty et al. [37] performed carotid artery duplex scanning in 346 patients prior to cardiac or vascular surgery. They found 53 asymptomatic and 10 symptomatic carotid lesions. Prophylactic carotid endarterectomy was not performed and the postoperative outcome showed a stroke rate of 6.4% in patients with a tight stenosis and only 1% in patients with a normal duplex scan. Nevertheless, no stroke occurred in asymptomatic patients and therefore the authors concluded that prophylactic endarterectomy in these patients is not justified. From a practical point of view, the stroke rate following infrarenal aortic surgery has an important impact on the future of the patient. The late stroke rate after infrarenal aortic surgery, representing 7% to 11% of deaths, does not play a major role in survival but has a significant influence on the quality of life [25,29,38,39]. The objective of prophylactic carotid endarterectomy is to prevent a substantial number of these late strokes.

Methods of prophylactic surgery

As shown by the prevalence studies, the combined existence of a significant lesion in the carotid artery and abdominal aorta is not exceptional, requiring a strategic preoperative planning with respect to the different lesions. The first step evaluates the surgical risk for each lesion. For the carotid artery the risk depends on the degree of stenosis, the presence of contralateral disease, symptomatic versus asymptomatic and the presence of ischemic lesions at the preoperative CT-scan. Other factors should be considered as well, like the general status of the patient, life expectancy, and cardiopulmonary disease.

Except for emergency cases, carotid artery lesions are operated upon prior to the aortic repair. In case of a unilateral carotid stenosis the surgical scenario can either be sequential (carotid endarterectomy and aortic repair in two procedures) or simultaneous (both repairs in one procedure). The sequential strategy is basically the safest because both the surgical and anesthetic techniques are completely concentrated on the specific vascular procedure. The neurologic risk of sequential surgery is low and hardly differs from carotid surgery in general. Secondary aortic surgery also carries a minimal cerebral risk (Table VII). Bechtel et al. prospectively evaluated 201 aortic repairs (107 AAA, 94 occlusive aortic disease), performing 41 (20.4%) sequential procedures with an interval between the carotid and aortic repair of three to five days [30]. Carotid endarterectomy was always performed for stenosis greater than 70%; 18 symptomatic and 23 asymptomatic patients. No neurologic deficit occurred, neither after carotid endarterectomy nor following aortic repair. Overall mortality rate in 201 patients was 3.5% and one fatal stroke was observed in a patient with an occluded right internal carotid artery and a 50% stenosis of the left internal carotid artery. Despite the absence of a control group, the authors consider the sequential carotid-aortic strategy a safe procedure, respecting the classical indications for carotid endarterectomy.

Performing the carotid and aortic repair simultaneously captures several advantages, the most important of which is single anesthesia. Disadvantages comprise a prolonged operation time and the hemodynamic changes induced by the aortic procedure might cause thrombosis of the endarterectomized carotid artery during hypotension or hypovolumia. In contrast, periods of uncontrollable hypertension can cause bleeding at the reconstructed carotid artery and induce hemorrhagic cerebral infarction. During the postoperative phase, hemodynamic cardiac or pulmonary complications secondary to the aortic repair can have a negative impact on the carotid reconstruction. The combined surgical procedure, the results of which are presented in Table VIII, is less frequently performed than the sequential repair. Crawford et al. [40] only encountered one postoperative stroke (2.4%), whereas Ott et al. [43] reported three strokes (11%). In the latter study, however, patients underwent descending thoracic aortic aneurysm repair.

Cormier et al. [44] published a series of 50 patients, 15 of whom had bilateral carotid artery reconstruction, and observed three deaths, no stroke and one transient ischemic attack The neurologic complication rate (2%) did not differ from the experience with carotid artery surgery only. The authors considered that simultaneous repair could be recommended in case of unilateral carotid stenosis and aortic disease limited to the infrarenal aorta. It is obvious if one of the two lesions becomes urgent, that this requires surgical repair first: the treatment of a symptomatic or ruptured AAA in the presence of a tight carotid stenosis carries a higher vital risk than the potential risk of a postoperative stroke.

Table VII RESULTS OF SEQUENTAL SURGERY: CAROTID SURGERY FIRST, AORTIC REPAIR IN A SECOND PROCEDURE

1st author [ref.]	Year of publication	Follow-up	Number of cases	N*	Carotid surgery			N*	Aortic surgery	
					Mortality N (%)	Stroke N (%)	TIA N		Mortality N (%)	Stroke N (%)
Crawford [40]	1980	NA	40	46	0	0	1	40	2 (5)	0
Hertzer [41]	1984	1978-1982	54	63	1 (1.8)	1 (1.8)	0	NA	NA	0
Bower [42]	1993	1979-1989	99	99	0	0	NA	99	4 (4)	2 (2)●
Bechtel [30]	2000	1994-1995	41	46	0	0	NA	41	0	0

TIA: transient ischemic attack
NA: not available

* Number of carotid procedures
● An ipsilateral lethal stroke and a non-lethal contralateral stroke

Table VIII RESULTS OF COMBINED CAROTID AND AORTIC SURGERY

1st author [ref.]	Year of publication	Follow-up	Number of cases	Number of procedures	Mortality	Stroke	TIA
Crawford [40]	1980	NA	42	46	0	1	0
Ott [43]	1981	1977-1978	28	NA	4 *	3	0
Cormier [44]	1988	1983-1988	50	65	3 **	0	1

TIA: transient ischemic attack
NA: not available

* 2 strokes and 2 visceral ischemia
** 3 pulmonary complications

REFERENCES

1 Schepens MA, Vermeulen FE. Management of combined carotid and coronary artery disease. *Curr Opinion Cardiol* 1996; 11: 525-532.

2 Taylor KM. Brain damage during cardiopulmonary bypass. *Ann Thor Surg* 1998; 65: S20-26.

3 Puskas JD, Winston AD, Wright CE et al. Stroke after coronary artery operation: incidence, correlates, outcome and cost. *Ann Thorac Surg* 2000; 69: 1053-1056.

4 Wolman RL, Nussmeier NA, Aggarwal A et al. Cerebral injury after cardiac surgery. Identification of a group at extraordinary risk. *Stroke* 1999; 30: 514-522.

5 Kazui T, Washiyama N, Muhammad BA et al. Total arch replacement using aortic arch branched grafts with the aid of antegrade selective cerebral perfusion. *Ann Thorac Surg* 2000; 70: 3-9.

6 Dossche KM, Schepens MA, Morshuis WJ et al. Antegrade selective cerebral perfusion in operations on the proximal thoracic aorta. *Ann Thorac Surg* 1999; 67: 1904-1910.

7 Crawford ES, Saleh SA. Transverse aortic arch aneurysm: improved results of treatment employing new modifications of aortic reconstruction and hypothermic cerebral circulatory arrest. *Ann Surg* 1981; 194: 180-188.

8 Svensson LG, Crawford ES, Hess KR et al. Experience with 1509 patients undergoing thoracoabdominal aortic operations. *J Vasc Surg* 1993; 17: 357-370.

9 Barbut D, Gold JP. Aortic atheromatosis and risks of cerebral embolization. *J Cardiothor Vasc Anesthesia* 1996; 10: 24-30.

10 Dávila-Román VG, Phillips KJ, Daily BB et al. Intraoperative transesophageal echocardiography and epiaortic ultrasound for assessment of atherosclerosis of the thoracic aorta. *J Am Coll Cardiol* 1996; 28: 942-947.

11 Montgomery DH, Ververis JJ, McGorisk G et al. Natural history of severe atheromatous disease of the thoracic aorta: a transesophageal echocardiographic study. *J Am Coll Cardiol* 1996; 27: 95-101.

12 Murkin JM, Boyd WD, Ganapathy S et al. Beating heart surgery: why expect less central nervous system morbidity? *Ann Thorac Surg* 1999; 68: 1498-1501.

13 BhaskerRao B, VanHimbergen D, Edmonds Jr HL et al. Evidence for improved cerebral function after minimally invasive bypass surgery. *J Card Surg* 1998; 13: 27-31.

14 Diegeler A, Hirsch R, Schilling LO et al. Neuromonitoring and neurocognitive outcome in off-pump versus conventional coronary bypass operation. *Ann Thorac Surg* 2000; 69: 1162-1166.

15 Svensson LG, Crawford ES, Hess KR et al. Deep hypothermia with circulatory arrest: determinants of stroke and early mortality in 656 patients. *J Thorac Cardiovasc Surg* 1993; 106. 19-31.

16 Ehrlich MP, Ergin MA, McCullough J et al. Predictors of adverse outcome and transient neurological dysfunction after ascending aorta/hemiarch replacement. *Ann Thorac Surg* 2000; 69: 1755-1763.

17 MA Schepens. Discussion, session 2: Marfan's syndrome. *Ann Thorac Surg* 1999; 67: 1868-1870.

18 Sabik JF, Lytle BW, McCarthy PM et al. Axillary artery: an alternative site of arterial cannulation for patients with extensive aortic and peripheral vascular disease. *J Thorac Cardiovasc Surg* 1995; 109: 885-891.

19 Alexandrova NA, Gibson WC, Norris JW, Maggisano R. Carotid artery stenosis in peripheral vascular disease. *J Vasc Surg* 1996; 23: 645-649.

20 Miralles M, Corominas A, Cotillas J et al. Screening for carotid and renal artery stenoses in patients with aortoiliac disease. *Ann Vasc Surg* 1998; 12: 17-22.

21 Cahan MA, Killewich LA, Kolodner L et al. The prevalence of carotid artery stenosis in patients undergoing aortic reconstruction. *Am J Surg* 1999; 178: 194-196.

22 Pilcher JM, Danaher J, Khaw KT. The prevalence of asymptomatic carotid artery disease in patients with peripheral vascular disease. *Clin Radiol* 2000; 55: 56-61.

23 Moneta GL, DeFrang R, Porter JM. Stroke as a complication of noncerebrovascular surgery. In: Bernhard VM, Towne JB (eds). *Complications in vascular surgery*. Saint Louis, Quality Medical Publishing, Inc, 1991, pp 443-455.

24 Harris EJ Jr, Moneta GL, Yeager RA et al. Neurologic deficits following noncarotid vascular surgery. *Am J Surg* 1992; 163: 537-540.

25 Szilagyi DE, Elliott JP Jr, Smith RF et al. A thirty-year survey of the reconstructive surgical treatment of aortoiliac occlusive disease. *J Vasc Surg* 1986; 3: 421-436.

26 Johnston KW. Multicenter prospective study of nonruptured abdominal aortic aneurysm. Part II. Variables predicting morbidity and mortality. *J Vasc Surg* 1989; 9: 437-447.

27 L'AURC, Kieffer E, Koskas F, Dewailly J, P Gouny. Mortalité péri-opératoire de la chirurgie élective des anévrysmes de l'aorte abdominale: étude multicentrique de l'AURC. In: Kieffer E (ed). *Les anévrysmes de l'aorte abdominale sous-rénale*. Paris, AERCV, 1990, pp 235-243.

28 Nevelsteen A, Wouters L, Suy R. Aortofemoral dacron reconstruction for aorto-iliac occlusive disease: a 25-year survey. *Eur J Vasc Surg* 1991; 5: 179-186.

29 Poulias GE, Doundoulakis N, Prombonas E et al. Aorto-femoral bypass and determinants of early success and late favourable outcome. Experience with 1000 consecutive cases. *J Cardiovasc Surg* 1992; 33: 664-678.

30 Bechtel JF, Bartels C, Hopstein S, Horsch S. Carotid endarterectomy prior to major abdominal aortic surgery. *J Cardiovasc Surg* 2000; 41: 269-273.

31 Carney WI Jr, Stewart WB, DePinto DJ et al. Carotid bruit as a risk factor in aortoiliac reconstruction. *Surgery* 1977; 81: 567-570.

32 Barnes RW, Liebman PR, Marszalek PB et al. The natural history of asymptomatic carotid disease in patients undergoing cardiovascular surgery. *Surgery* 1981; 90: 1075-1083.

33 Treiman RL, Foran RF, Cohen JL et al. Carotid bruit: a follow-up report on its significance in patients undergoing an abdominal aortic operation. *Arch Surg* 1979; 114: 1138-1140.

34 Turnipseed WD, Berkoff HA, Belzer FO. Postoperative stroke in cardiac and peripheral vascular disease. *Ann Surg* 1980; 192: 365-368.

35 Kartchner MM, McRae LP. Carotid occlusive disease as a risk factor in major cardiovascular surgery. *Arch Surg* 1982; 117: 1086-1088.

36 Gutierrez IZ, Barone DL, Makula PA, Currier C. The risk of perioperative stroke in patients with asymptomatic carotid bruits undergoing peripheral vascular surgery. *Am Surg* 1987; 53: 487-489.

37 Gerraty RP, Gates PC, Doyle JC. Carotid stenosis and perioperative stroke risk in symptomatic and asymptomatic patients undergoing vascular or coronary surgery. *Stroke* 1993; 24: 1115-1118.

38 Van den Akker PJ, Van Schilfgaarde R, Brand R et al. Aortoiliac and aortofemoral reconstruction of obstructive disease. *Am J Surg* 1994; 167: 379-385.

39 Johnston KW. Nonruptured abdominal aortic aneurysm: six-year follow-up results from the multicenter prospective Canadian aneurysm study. Canadian Society for Vascular Surgery. Aneurysm Study Group. *J Vasc Surg* 1994; 20: 163-170.

40 Crawford ES, Palamara AE, Kasparian AS. Carotid and noncoronary operations: simultaneous, staged, and delayed. *Surgery* 1980; 87: 1-8.

41 Hertzer NR, Beven EG, Young JR et al. Incidental asymptomatic carotid bruits in patients scheduled for peripheral vascular reconstruction: results of cerebral and coronary angiography. *Surgery* 1984; 96: 535-544.

42 Bower TC, Merrell SW, Cherry KJ Jr et al. Advanced carotid disease in patients requiring aortic reconstruction. *Am J Surg* 1993; 166: 146-151.

43 Ott DA, Cooley DA, Chapa L, Coelho A. Carotid endarterectomy without temporary intraluminal shunt. Study of 309 consecutive operations. *Ann Surg* 1980; 191: 708-714.

44 Cormier F, Kieffer E. Chirurgie combinée carotidienne et aortique. In: Kieffer E, Bousser MG (eds). *Indications et résultats de la chirurgie carotidienne.* Paris, AERCV, 1988, pp 315-323.

24

COMPLICATIONS OF VASCULAR ACCESS FOR HEMODIALYSIS

JAN HM TORDOIR
FRANK VAN DE SANDE, KAREL ML LEUNISSEN

Vascular access complications are a major cause of morbidity and mortality in hemodialysis patients. It is estimated that 20% of native arteriovenous fistulas (AVFs) and 80% of prosthetic graft AVFs require revision interventions each year. The most common complication is thrombotic occlusion, due to low blood flow as a consequence of venous anastomotic stenoses. Clot removal, either by surgical or interventional techniques with additional revision of the stenotic lesion is the first option of treatment. At 1- and 2-year follow-up, outcomes after surgery or thrombolysis are similar with patencies of 70% and 50%, respectively.

Prosthetic graft infection is a potential dangerous complication of vascular access and may lead to sepsis and subsequently graft explantation. Due to the high blood flow and steal syndrome, patients with AVFs are at risk to develop hemodynamic complications like cardiac failure, upper extremity ischemia and venous hypertension. Flow-reducing operations and interventional methods serve to enhance distal perfusion and venous outflow, resulting in less morbidity.

Vascular access remains the lifeline for patients on hemodialysis treatment. Much effort by several disciplines is needed to create and maintain this access to the bloodstream.

The importance of AVFs

The increased number of patients on chronic hemodialysis, estimated over one million worldwide and more than 200 000 in Europe, the majority of whom are older than 65 years of age, tax the ingenuity of the surgeon in maintaining a route for vascular access. Hemodialysis is the most common treatment for chronic renal failure, and because of lack of available donors for renal transplants it is likely that hemodialysis will remain the mainstay for treatment of patients with renal failure.

Complications associated with vascular access are important causes of morbidity and mortality in dialysis patients. The complications leading to failure of the vascular access site are primarily thrombosis and infection. Hemodynamic and neurological complications do not jeopardize the vascular access but result in considerable discomfort and morbidity.

Before addressing treatment options of complications of vascular accesses, it is important to emphasize that native arteriovenous fistulas (AVF) have been demonstrated to be superior to the use of prosthetic grafts, especially regarding long-term patency and durability. Strategies to increase the percentage of native AVFs need to be implemented in order to diminish the number of complications and increase long-term patency. Because of these differences in performance, complications of native AVFs and prosthetic graft AVFs will be discussed separately.

Thrombosis

Certainly the foremost complication to be anticipated in constructing vascular access is clotting of the access site. The likelihood of thrombosis depends on multiple factors, including the anatomic configuration, site of arteriovenous anastomosis, the need to use artificial grafts and the adequacy of the veins and arteries. Thrombosis of AVFs may occur soon after operation or in the follow-up period. Early thrombosis, defined as occurring within the first month after placement, is often caused by technical factors, whereas late thrombosis is generally caused by venous run-off stenosis, continued trauma to the access site by needle puncture, external pressure on the graft or hypotension.

NATIVE AVFs

The radiocephalic AVF (Brescia/Cimino) is associated with a fairly high early failure rate of 10% to 15%. Failure may be caused by small diameter vessels, low blood pressure or venous outflow obstruction. It is recognized by the absence of a pulse and no palpable thrill. Thrombosis of the AVF is most frequently due to selection of an inadequate vein less than 2 mm and/or a poor radial artery. In some elderly patients and diabetics, the radial artery may be involved with arteriosclerotic disease with insufficient pressure to sustain the fistula. Preoperative vessel assessment by means of noninvasive ultra-

sound (duplex) investigation is indicated in all patients with poor superficial veins and suspicion of peripheral arterial disease [1]. Technical factors are also responsible for thrombosis of the newly created AVF. One must be careful not to narrow the lumen of the artery or vein during performance of the anastomosis and careful also not to incorporate the back wall of the vessels. Once successfully constructed, the radiocephalic AVF has an excellent long-term patency rate, varying from 45% to 72% at 3 years and from 30% to 55% at 5 years (Table I). Clotting of the AVF after the first 3 months of successful use is related to the repeated needle punctures with fibrosis and narrowing of the vein or to anastomotic intimal hyperplasia. A conservative estimate is that each year 10% of AVFs will fail, while 0.1 intervention per fistula/year is needed for maintenance.

ENDOVASCULAR TREATMENT OF STENOSED OR THROMBOSED NATIVE AVFs

Interventional radiological techniques are increasingly being used in the treatment of thrombosed vascular access. Pulse-spray catheters are introduced into the clotted segment and the thrombus is dissolved by infusion of urokinase or recombinant tissue plasminogen activator (rTPA). Mechanical methods of clot extraction have also been successful, however, the outcome depends on the dedication and experience of the radiologist. The primary and secondary patency rates of interventional treatment of thrombosed native AVFs may be as high as 49% and 81% after 1 year of follow-up, respectively [11]. Balloon catheter dilatation of stenotic areas in patients with AVFs may be successful in selected cases, when there is insufficient dialysis, insufficient inflow, difficulty in cannulation or poor maturation of the AVF.

SURGICAL TREATMENT OF STENOSED OR THROMBOSED NATIVE AVFs

Thrombotic occlusion due to stenotic lesions at the AV anastomosis is best managed by one of three methods depending on the extent of disease and adjacent venous anatomy:

1 - widening of the AV anastomosis with patch plasty,

2 - interposition of a short segment of prosthetic graft or

3 - construction of a more proximal AV anastomosis. (Fig. 1A and 1B).

Repetitive puncture of the fistula in the same area and extravasation of blood with local fibrosis may lead to extensive stenoses. In the worst case it is most expedient to convert the AVF to a bridge prosthetic graft or to create an elbow-or upper arm fistula.

PROSTHETIC GRAFT AVFs

Technical factors are often responsible for thrombosis of a newly placed graft. When placing a loop graft in the forearm, care must be taken to avoid a kink or twist in the distal portion of the loop. Inadequate hemostasis during the procedure or early puncture of the graft may result in extravasation of blood in the graft tunnel, requiring prolonged pressure for control. Thrombosis of grafts frequently occurs after hemodialysis. Undue pressure over the needle puncture site or application of compression dressing may result in thrombosis.

Table I	SECONDARY PATENCY RATES OF NATIVE AVFs (RADIOCEPHALIC FISTULAS)						
1st author [ref.]	Year	Number of grafts	1 year %	2 years %	3 years %	5 years %	
Reilly et al. [2]	1982	145	80	75	72	NA	
Tordoir et al. [3]	1983	129	80	74	71	NA	
Palder et al. [4]	1985	154	60	53	45	NA	
Kherlakian et al. [5]	1986	100	71	66	64	NA	
Simoni et al. [6]	1994	248	76	NA	NA	55	
Burger et al. [7]	1995	208	NA	79	NA	52	
Leapman et al. [8]	1996	150	56	NA	NA	30	
Enzler et al. [9]	1996	429	74	NA	64	NA	
Golledge et al. [10]	1999	107	75	63	NA	NA	

NA: not available

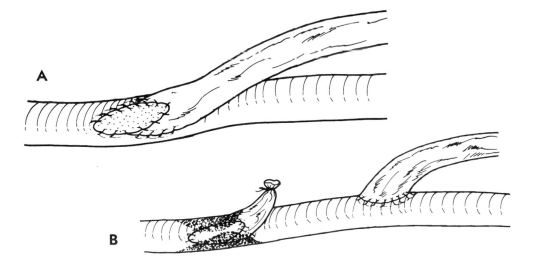

FIG. 1   A - Patch plasty at the site of the arteriovenous anastomosis of a radiocephalic fistula. B - New proximal radiocephalic anastomosis.

Although the patency rate of prosthetic AVFs tends to be higher initially, the patency at 1 and 3 years drops below that of native AVFs. Patency rates vary from 90% to 95% at 3 months, 58% to 95% at 1 year, 40% to 70% at 3 years and 40% to 47% at 5 years of follow-up (Table II).

Each year 20% of grafts will fail and 0.8 interventions per patient/year are needed to maintain patency. Late thrombosis of a prosthetic graft is usually due to obstruction at the site of the venous outflow. Development of stenosis at the site of the venous anastomosis may be recognized by a gradual increase in pressure within the grafts and a decrease in graft flow as measured by duplex ultrasound or in-line flow measurements. The combination of forceful pulsation throughout the graft and a loud bruit at the venous end suggests the existence of a stenosis. Anastomotic intimal hyperplasia causing stenoses has been attributed to mechanical endothelial damage, shear stress by the exaggerated blood flow and the high pressure pulsatile nature of arterial flow in the venous system.

ENDOVASCULAR TREATMENT OF STENOSED OR THROMBOSED PROSTHETIC GRAFT AVFs

Pharmacological thrombolysis

Thrombolysis plays no role in the treatment of early graft thrombosis. However, for the treatment of late-onset thrombosis it may be the first option for intervention. The technique of administering the thrombolytic agent has a major effect on success rates. Lysis of a thrombosed prosthetic graft must be performed differently from intraarterial lytic therapy. The reason for this is that: a) recent puncture sites may be points of potential hemorrhage; b) the stenoses are more resistant to dilatation and c) the arterial anastomosis is an embolic pathway for thrombus to be pushed in a retrograde direction. A crossed-catheter technique is often used to reestablish flow and elimination of the outflow stenosis. Concentrated urokinase (UK) is employed by a pulse-spray catheter through the entire length of the cloth. A total of 250 000 to 500 000 units of UK and 5 000 units of heparin are administered by pulse-spray. Balloon angioplasty is performed on any venous anastomotic or outflow stenosis.

Pharmacomechanical thrombectomy

Because of the time involved in thrombolysis, additional mechanical approaches have been studied in an attempt to decrease time and expense of declotting. Percutaneous balloon thrombectomy, using Fogarty catheters inserted through two sheaths results in an initial success of 93% and a primary patency rate of 42% at 3 months. Another option is manual thromboaspiration, which has been reported to have good patency rates. Pharmacomechanical declotting is faster, cheaper and as effective as thrombolysis alone.

Mechanical methods

Mechanical thrombolysis (MT) incorporates a combined approach consisting of angiography to visualize the graft and draining veins, mechanical

Table II	SECONDARY PATENCY RATES OF PROSTHETIC (PTFE) GRAFT AVFs						
1st author [ref.]	*Year*	*Number of grafts*	*1 year* %	*2 years* %	*3 years* %	*5 years* %
Munda et al. [12]	1983	67	67	50	NA	NA
Palder et al. [4]	1985	163	80	68	68	NA
Kherlakian et al. [5]	1986	100	75	61	50	NA
Tordoir et al. [13]	1988	100	74	59	59	47
Rizzuti et al. [14]	1988	189	76	NA	50	40
Puckett et al. [15]	1988	127	95	81	70	NA
Enzler et al. [9]	1996	69	58	NA	40	NA

NA : not available

clot maceration and angioplasty to dilate any stenosis. Balloon-assisted aspiration thrombectomy as well catheter-directed manual thromboaspiration have both been shown to have good results. Nowadays mechanical thrombectomy devices using motor-driven fragmentation cage or brushes or based on the Venturi effect by jet of saline at the catheter tip (Hydrolyzer) are available for percutaneous thrombectomy.

Percutaneous transluminal angioplasty (PTA) PTA of arterial and venous anastomotic and outflow stenoses is attractive, as it can be performed on an outpatient basis after dialysis. Guidewires and subsequent balloon catheters are inserted through the dialysis needles or by graft puncture with the needle directed to the venous anastomosis. Because of the nature of the stenosis, namely intimal hyperplasia, it can be very difficult to dilate it. Long inflation times (more than 30 min)

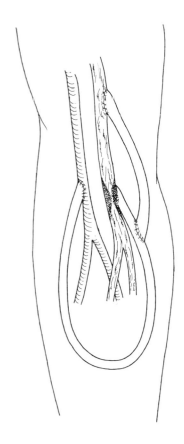

FIG. 2   Jump-graft of a stenosed venous anastomosis of forearm loop graft.

and high balloon pressures (up to 15-20 atm) may be required to achieve an acceptable result. Long-term results of PTA of prosthetic grafts are usually acceptable (initial success: 94%; 6 months patency 67%; 12 months patency 44%), but re-PTA is often necessary.

SURGICAL TREATMENT OF STENOSED OR THROMBOSED PROSTHETIC GRAFT AVFs

The traditional management of a thrombosed graft has been a thrombectomy with venous anastomosis revision, if indicated. These procedures are usually performed with the patient under general or regional anesthesia within some hours after clotting, although thrombectomies can be performed as late as two weeks after the event. A simple thrombectomy is performed via a small longitudinal incision close to the venous anastomosis. The clot is removed with a Fogarty balloon-tipped catheter. If a stenosis is present, patch plasty is performed by suturing a prosthetic patch in place, thereby widening the lumen of the venous anastomosis. After completion of the patch, intra-operative angiography is performed to confirm patency and to exclude residual stenoses. Placement of an interposition graft involves cutting the distal end of the prosthesis near the venous anastomosis (or an end-to-side anastomosis; Fig. 2) and suturing an additional graft to the original graft with an anastomosis to a suitable vein in the upper arm (either superficial or deep vein). Surgical therapy of stenoses in the axillary and subclavian veins is technically difficult and can best be treated by interventional means.

SURGICAL VERSUS INTERVENTIONAL TREATMENT

Comparative studies have reported different outcomes for interventional and surgical treatment of thrombosed grafts. Two studies favor surgical over catheter techniques of thrombosed grafts. Initial success was 83% to 94% for surgery versus 67% to 72% for thrombolysis. Thirty-six percent of grafts managed surgically remained functional at 6 months and 25% at 12 months. In the endovascular group, 11% and 9% were patent after 6 and 12 months, respectively. Compared to other studies the success rate of thrombolysis was rather low and recent series suggest shorter patency after surgical revision. Outcome data showed that results from thrombolysis combined with angioplasty were superior to surgical thrombectomy alone, and equivalent to surgical thrombectomy and patch plasty [16-19].

Infection

Dialysis patients carry a number of factors which increase the risk of vascular access infections. Uremia has a suppressive effect on immunity. Localization of infection to access sites is enhanced by increased bacterial access to tissues and grafts through repeated needle punctures. S. Aureus predominates as the causative organism in vascular access infection, being responsible for more than 90% of fistula infections.

NATIVE AVFs

Infection rates for native AVFs are very acceptable (2% to 3%) and because of this low potential for infection and a superior patency they remain the long-term access of choice. Native AVF infections are rare but superficial cellulitic wound infection following AVF creation may occur. Repeat needling may cause hematoma with secondary infection, which, if neglected, may proceed to abscess formation. If anastomotic infection develops, disruption of the anastomosis and pseudoaneurysm formation may occur.

TREATMENT OF NATIVE AVF INFECTION

Minor puncture and postoperative infections may respond to antibiotic therapy. Infected hematomas require incision and drainage. Deep wound infections and anastomotic infections are usually intractable problems requiring fistula ligation. Formation of a more proximal fistula through a clean operative field can provide early return of fistula function.

PROSTHETIC GRAFT AVFs

Reported infection rates for prosthetic grafts range from 11% to 35% [20]. Infections associated with graft implantation may be as high as 15%. The risk of graft infection is influenced by the site of implantation. Upper leg grafts have a high infection rate and significant incidence of life-threatening sepsis. Diabetes and advanced age may increase the incidence of infection. Needle puncture and other late causes of infection show erythema with local tenderness and occasionally skin breakdown exposing the graft. In graft-tunnel infection the cellulitic signs can extend along the length of the graft with development of abscesses. If the anastomoses are involved, anastomotic disruption, aneurysm formation and eventually hemorrhage may occur. In addition to local signs, many patients also have evidence of systemic infection with bacteremia or even sepsis.

TREATMENT OF PROSTHETIC GRAFT INFECTION

One of the greatest challenges in vascular access surgery is the treatment of infected prosthetic grafts. Graft excision is always a safe option, but graft salvage is ideal. Superficial cellulitic infections may respond to antibiotic therapy, but deeper infections require surgical treatment and if localized away from the anastomosis can be managed by either graft excision or segmental bypass. To perform a segmental bypass, the graft is exposed through clean wounds proximally and distally to the infected area and is divided at both sites. A new subcutaneous tunnel is created away from the infected area, and a new graft is interposed between the divided ends of the original graft (Fig. 3A to 3C). When infection involves most of the graft tunnel or the anastomoses, total graft excision is required.

Ischemia

Creation of a vascular access leads to significant hemodynamic changes of the upper extremity. Because of the low-resistance circuit through the AVF, absolute blood flow to the extremity is increased. However, the flow increase is usually less than fistula flow, resulting in a net reduction of flow to the hand. Although the decrease in hand blood flow is usually not of clinical significance, symptoms compatible with vascular impairment may develop. Diabetics and elderly patients with distal small vessel arteriosclerotic disease are at highest risk for ischemia.

NATIVE AVFs

The incidence of ischemic complications in radiocephalic AVFs is low compared to brachio cephalic or basilic fistulas in the elbow region. It is estimated that 0.2% to 2.0% of radiocephalic and up to 10%-25% of elbow fistulas will develop ischemia of the hand [21]. Reversal of flow in the radial artery beyond the anastomosis occurs in 70% of the patients and this radial steal actually diverts blood from the hand into the AVF. Radial artery steal is very frequent and often occurs even in patients without symptoms of hand ischemia. However, in the presence of central or distal arterial obstruction, such steal can be a critical factor in producing clinical signs of ischemia.

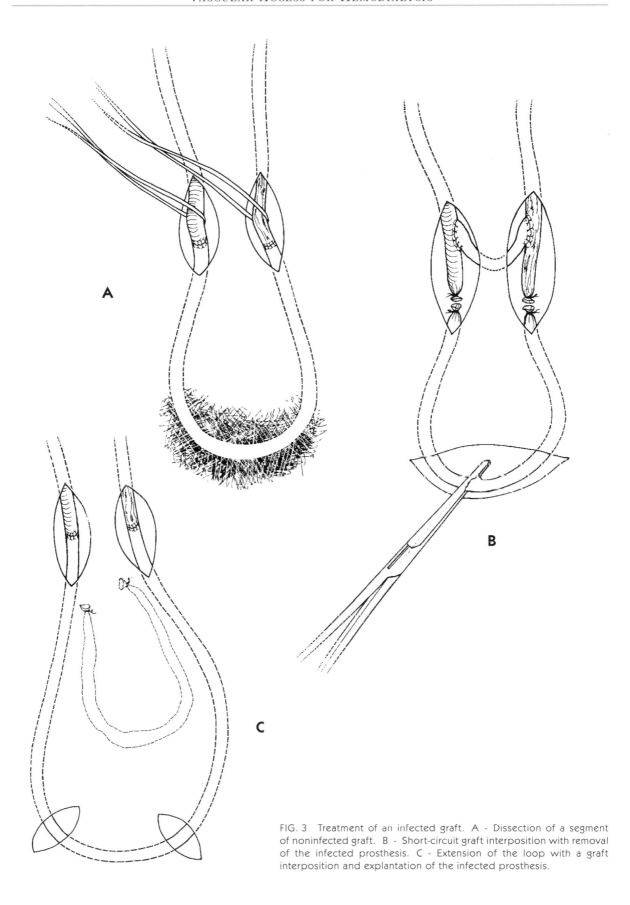

FIG. 3 Treatment of an infected graft. A - Dissection of a segment of noninfected graft. B - Short-circuit graft interposition with removal of the infected prosthesis. C - Extension of the loop with a graft interposition and explantation of the infected prosthesis.

PROSTHETIC GRAFT AVFS

In 2.7%-7% of prosthetic grafts with an anastomosis to the brachial artery, ischemia will occur [21]. Usually, the decrease in distal perfusion is related to the amount of blood flow which is shunted through the anastomosis. Thus the risk on ischemia is greater with a high flow through the graft.

TREATMENT OF ISCHEMIA

Symptomatic ischemic steal syndrome related to a functioning vascular access poses two challenges to the surgeon: preservation of the access and resolution of the distal ischemia. The treatment depends on the etiology of the ischemia, either a high flow fistula with significant steal or a normal flow fistula with peripheral arterial obstructive disease. Surgical correction of the steal phenomenon in the side-to-side Brescia/Cimino fistula may be accomplished by ligation of the radial artery immediately distal to the fistula. Flow-reducing operations are the first option in case of high-flow AVFs. This can be obtained by banding of the AVF or graft with a 2 cm width circular teflon patch or by applying a clip, just downstream the arterial anastomosis (Fig. 4). The flow must be reduced to at least 800 mL/min. An alternative method is the use of 4-7 mm prosthetic grafts or interposition of a segment of 4 mm graft, distal anastomosis being longer than proximal anastomosis (Fig. 5). A less familiar technique is a procedure which restores antegrade flow into the extremity distal to the access site, using a bypass which subsequently eliminates the pathway of steal through ligation of the artery between the access and the distal anastomosis (Fig. 6) [22]. In any patient where ischemia poses a limb threat, the AVF should be closed and the arterial patency restored.

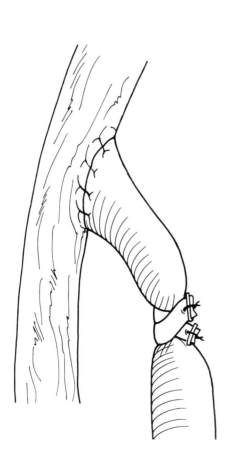

FIG. 4 Schematic drawing of bending the arterovenous fistula with a circular teflon strip.

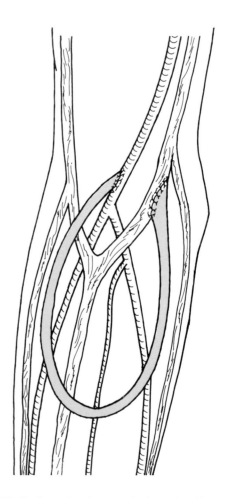

FIG. 5 Example of a prosthetic graft with a diameter of 4 cm at the arterial anastomosis, increasing to 7 cm at the venous anastomosis.

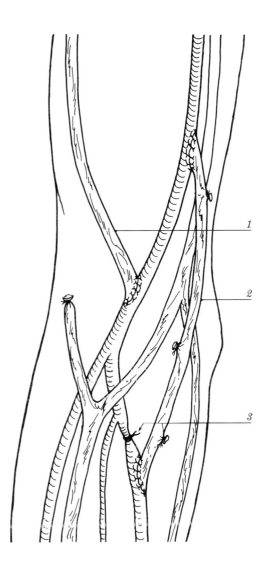

1. Cephalic vein anastomosed with the brachial artery
2. Venous bypass between the brachial and ulnar artery
3. Ligature on the ulnar artery

FIG. 6 Procedure to reduce steal by ligation of he ulnar artery (or even brachial artery) between the access and distal anastomosis with a bypass distal to the ligation.

Venous hypertension

Arterialization of the venous system may result in venous hypertension and, if the valves are incompetent, in retrograde venous flow. Remote outflow stenosis or occlusions have been identified with increasing frequency as the cause of venous hypertension. Usually, temporary dialysis catheters in the subclavian position cause the vast majority of these central venous lesions (risk of stenosis after subclavian vein catheters is 40%!).

PERIPHERAL VENOUS HYPERTENSION

Local swelling, skin pigmentation and even ulceration usually occur in side-to-side Brescia/Cimino AVFs with retrograde distal venous flow and proximal venous obstruction. Surgical correction is obtained by ligation of the distal vein, converting the side-to-side fistula in an end-to-side AVF. Graft bypass of an occluded proximal vein segment may be of additional value.

CENTRAL VENOUS HYPERTENSION

AVF creation in patients with unrecognized subclavian vein stenosis or occlusion may lead to swelling of the entire extremity with often prominent collateral veins in the shoulder region. The first treatment option is radiological intervention with PTA, recanalization or stent placement [23]. Surgical bypass from the upper arm veins to the ipsi- or contralateral jugular vein is an option, when interventional treatment has failed (Fig. 7). Jugular vein transposition is another elegant method to enhance venous outflow (Fig. 8) [24].

Aneurysm formation

False aneurysms may occur at the anastomosis when there has been an error in surgical technique or more commonly at a needling site which has been overused.

NATIVE AVFs

Dilatation of native AVFs is common. In general, no intervention is required but surgery is indicated if the overlying skin becomes very thin or if there is evidence of expansion. These lesions can be treated by resection with either direct end-to-end anastomosis or placement of an interposition graft. The incidence of true aneurysms in native AVFs

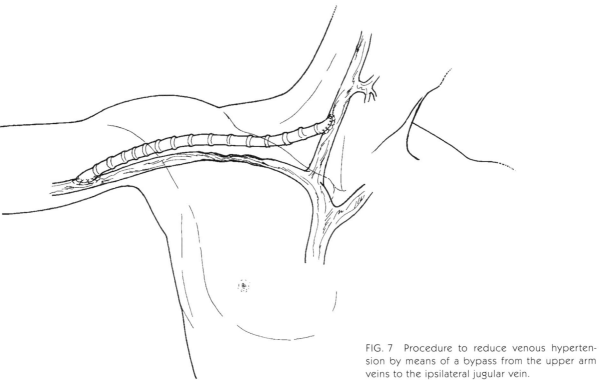

FIG. 7 Procedure to reduce venous hypertension by means of a bypass from the upper arm
veins to the ipsilateral jugular vein.

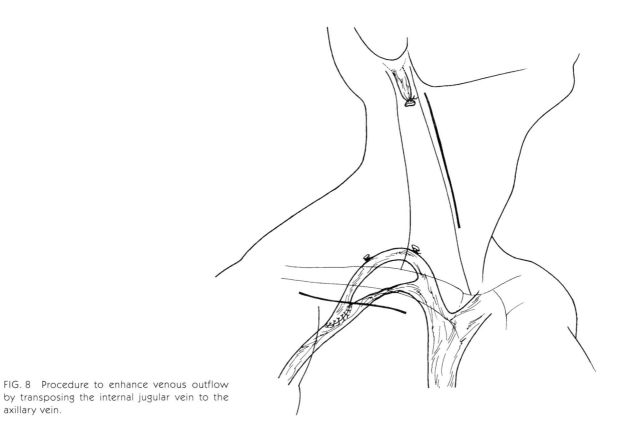

FIG. 8 Procedure to enhance venous outflow
by transposing the internal jugular vein to the
axillary vein.

is 2% [25]. Occult infection is common and local resection with bypass grafting is advocated.

PROSTHETIC GRAFT AVFs

The incidence of pseudoaneurysm is 10% for vascular access prostheses [26]. Usually they occur at needle puncture sites. If there is no infection, treatment simply consists of local suture repair of the small defect in the graft or interposition of a small segment of new graft.

Conclusion

Treatment of complications and salvage of the failing vascular access for hemodialysis remains a challenge for the vascular surgeon and interventional radiologist. Because prosthetic grafts have a high incidence of complications, attempts to create native AVFs as well as a plan for maximizing access sites, are indicated. A surveillance protocol in the dialysis unit is important as identification of a failing native or prosthetic graft AVF to allow early intervention with superior outcomes to those that have thrombosed. Surgical repair and radiological interventional techniques can provide durable patency rates. Arterial steal and venous hypertension can be devastating and efforts for adequate diagnosis and repair have high priority. Multidisciplinary approach of vascular access complications and intensive cooperation between nephrologists, surgeons and interventional radiologists are of utmost importance to achieve optimal results.

REFERENCES

1 Lemson MS, Leunissen KM, Tordoir JH. Does pre-operative duplex examination improve patency rates of Brescia-Cimino fistulas? Nephrol Dial Transplant 1998; 13: 1360-1361.

2 Reilly DT, Wood RF, Bell PR. Arteriovenous fistulas for dialysis: blood flow, viscosity, and long-term patency. World J Surg 1982; 6: 628 633.

3 Tordoir JH, Kwan TS, Herman JM et al. Primary and secondary access surgery for haemodialysis with the Brescia-Cimino fistula and the polytetrafluoroethylene (PTFE) graft. Neth J Surg 1983; 35: 8-12.

4 Palder SB, Kirkman RL, Whittemore AD et al. Vascular access for hemodialysis. Patency rates and results of revision. Ann Surg 1985; 202: 235-239.

5 Kherlakian GM, Roedersheimer LR, Arbaugh JJ et al. Comparison of autogenous fistula versus expanded polytetrafluoroethylene graft fistula for angioaccess in hemodialysis. Am J Surg 1986; 152: 238-243.

6 Simoni G, Bonalumi U, Civalleri D et al. End-to-end arteriovenous fistula for chronic haemodialysis: 11 years' experience. Cardiovasc Surg 1994; 2: 63-66.

7 Burger H, Kluchert BA, Kootstra G et al. Survival of arteriovenous fistulas and shunts for haemodialysis. Eur J Surg 1995; 161: 327-334.

8 Leapman SB, Boyle M, Pescovitz MD et al. The arteriovenous fistula for hemodialysis access: gold standard or archaic relic? Am Surg 1996; 62: 652-657.

9 Enzler MA, Rajmon T, Lachat M et al. Long-term function of vascular access for hemodialysis. Clin Transplant 1996; 10: 511-515.

10 Golledge J, Smith CJ, Emery J et al. Outcome of primary radiocephalic fistula for haemodialysis. Br J Surg 1999; 86: 211-216.

11 Turmel-Rodrigues L, Pengloan J, Rodrigue H et al. Treatment of failed native arteriovenous fistulae for hemodialysis by interventional radiology. Kidney Int 2000; 57: 1124-1140.

12 Munda R, First MR, Alexander JW et al. Polytetrafluoroethylene graft survival in hemodialysis. JAMA 1983; 249: 219-222.

13 Tordoir JH, Herman JM, Kwan TS et al. Long-term follow-up of the polytetrafluoroethylene (PTFE) prosthesis as an arteriovenous fistula for haemodialysis. Eur J Vasc Surg 1988; 2: 3-7.

14 Rizzuti RP, Hale JC, Burkart TE. Extended patency of expanded polytetrafluoroethylene grafts for vascular access using optimal configuration and revisions. Surg Gynecol Obstet 1988; 166: 23-27.

15 Puckett JW, Lindsay SF. Midgraft curettage as a routine adjunct to salvage operations for thrombosed polytetrafluoroethylene hemodialysis access grafts. Am J Surg 1988; 156: 139-143.

16 Schuman E, Quinn S, Standage B et al. Thrombolysis versus thrombectomy for occluded hemodyalisis grafts. Am J Surg 1994; 167: 473-476.

17 Beathard GA. Thrombolysis versus surgery for the treatment of thrombosed dialysis access grafts. J Am Soc Nephrol 1995; 6: 1619-1624.

18 Marston WA, Criado E, Jaques PF et al. Prospective randomized comparison of surgical versus endovascular management of thrombosed dialysis access grafts. J Vasc Surg 1997; 26: 373-381.

19 Polak JF, Berger MF, Pagan-Marin H et al. Comparative efficacy of pulse-spray thrombolysis and angioplasty versus surgical salvage procedures for treatment of recurrent occlusion of PTFE dialysis access grafts. Cardiovasc Intervent Radiol 1998; 21: 314-318.

20 Padberg FT Jr, Lee BC, Curl GR. Hemoaccess site infection. Surg Gynecol Obstet 1992; 174: 103-108.

21 Morsy AH, Kulbaski M, Chen C et al. Incidence and characteristics of patients with hand ischemia after a hemodialysis access procedure. J Surg Res 1998; 74: 8-10.

22 Berman SS, Gentile AT et al. Distal revascularization-interval ligation for limb salvage and maintenance of dialysis access in ischemic steal syndrome. J Vasc Surg 1997; 26: 393-404.

23 Vorwerk D, Bucker A, Alzen G et al. Chronic venous occlusions in haemodialysis shunts: efficacy of percutaneous treatment. Nephrol Dial Transplant 1995; 10: 1869-1873.

24 Tordoir JH, Leunissen KM. Jugular vein transposition for the treatment of subclavian vein obstruction in haemodialysis patients. Eur J Vasc Surg 1993; 7: 335-338.

25 Zibari GB, Rohr MS, Landreneau MD et al. Complications from permanent hemodialysis vascular access. Surgery 1988; 104: 681-686.

26 Nakagawa Y, Ota K, Sato Y et al. Complications in blood access for hemodialysis. Artif Organs 1994; 18: 283-288.

25

COMPLICATIONS OF SURGICAL TREATMENT FOR THORACIC OUTLET SYNDROME

ALAIN CARLIER, RAYMOND LIMET

Because of its multiple anatomic components, the thoracic outlet is an extremely complex surgical field. The surgeon entering this region should know precisely all the osseous and musculo tendineous components, and should be highly familiar with its nerve and vascular structures. This anatomic junction is of special interest for surgeons who accept the challenge of finding a correctable lesion in patients suffering from cervicobrachial pain syndromes, as well as in patients suffering from certain vascular symptoms in the upper extremities. Several pathologic entities find their origin in the thoracic outlet, however, it is difficult to objectively assess and diagnose these syndromes [1]. The tendency to prematurely diagnose a thoracic outlet syndrome (TOS) has led to many medical errors. Surgeons who perform a first rib resection in the treatment of a TOS preferably have had thoracovascular and peripheral nerve surgical training in order to avoid and, if necessary, to correct potential complications of this treatment.

The most frequent complication of surgery for TOS is the unsatisfactory outcome for the patient, which is less often related to intraoperative technical problems than to poor patient selection. In other words, the unsatisfactory outcome of TOS surgery might be partly due to insufficient preoperative diagnostic methods. This assertion determines the aim of this chapter, which is to describe the complications related to the surgical techniques.

Surgical techniques

Since resection of the first rib is one of the main techniques to decompress to thoracic outlet, different surgical approaches have been proposed: supraclavicular, transaxillary, and posterior access. Although complications can be encountered with all three surgical accesses, each individual access is susceptible to certain specific complications.

The most commonly adapted technique is the supraclavicular approach, offering complete exposure of the neurologic structures and, if necessary, allowing for vascular reconstruction. It appears to be more reliable and less traumatic than the other two approaches; however, it is not without risks.

The transaxillary access, popularized by Roos, requires traction manoeuvres and pushing of the brachial plexus, which can subsequently be damaged as a result. Several surgeons consider the transaxillary access as a relatively blind approach, causing technical difficulties and offering only mediocre exposure of the nerve and vascular structures. For these reasons, but in the absence of scientific proof, the transaxillary approach is assumed to cause more complications than the other techniques. The posterior access is associated with the inherent morbidity of its traumatic approach, risking the substantial diminishing of the force of the elevating muscles of the scapula.

The nerve roots can be relatively easy exposed, but the veins and arteries are difficult to approach. In this chapter we review the specific risks of each surgical access for TOS, and we have detailed the postoperative complications, of which it is important to distinguish between short-tem and long-term complications.

Incidence of complications

The exact incidence of minor and major complications is difficult to assess, because few studies have been devoted to evaluate these problems. The majority of the individual series do not report enough cases to allow any conclusions to be drawn, and often the postoperative complications are not mentioned. Therefore, the long-term results can not adequately be evaluated, which is a basic drawback of this functional surgery.

Sanders [2] reported a very large group of patients operated on for TOS: 111 rib resections by axillary access, and 278 by supraclavicular access. In the first group they encountered two brachial plexus complications, while in the second group they had two permanent and five temporary neurologic complications. The advantage of the series of Cormier and Kieffer [3] is the large number of patients and the detailed report of complications. Among 224 patients, all operated on by the supraclavicular approach, they observed 5 vascular, 29 neurologic, and 25 miscellaneous complications. The five vascular complications comprised three subclavian vein and two subclavian artery occlusions. The neurologic complications included 5 brachial plexus lesions (1 permanent), 16 phrenic nerve paralysis (1 permanent), and 8 Horner syndromes (1 permanent). The other complications were atelectasis (4), pneumothorax (1), pulmonary embolism (1), lymph leakage (8), sepsis (4), and second rib fracture (7).

Jamieson and Chinnick [4] observed eight major complications in a large group of 409 patients: 1 bleeding, 1 infection, 2 erroneous second rib resection requiring reoperation, 3 pneumothorax, and 1 radical nerve paralysis. Horowitz [5], a neurologist, reported four cases of causalgia with severe sensibility and motor function complaints, leading to a chronic depression in two patients, one of whom committed suicide.

These anecdotal and retrospective reports do not allow identification of the risk factors for major complications. However, their existence and incidence should be known and should serve to keep surgeons alert.

Two studies have been published which summarized the results of multicenter surveys. In 1981, Dale [6] conducted a survey among the members of the *International Society for Cardiovascular Surgery*, of whom 38% responded. The data collection revealed 102 complete brachial plexus paralyses, of which 22 with permanent complaints, and 171 partial neurologic deficits with 30 permanent aftereffects. In 1989, Mellière et al. [7] published the results of a survey which was organized among members of the *French Society of Vascular Surgery*, and which received responses from 66 surgeons. In ten cases the axillary artery was injured (in one case lethally), and in three patients the axillary-subclavian vein thrombosed, all during or after a rib resection by axillary access. A brachial plexus injury occurred in 19 cases: 16 underwent an axillary and 3 a subclavicular approach. Other neurologic complications included paralysis of the serratus anterior muscle with subsequent *scapula alata* (winged scapula) in 9 patients and phrenic nerve paralysis in 5 patients. It should be mentioned that in both studies the total number of patients operated for TOS were not provided.

Vascular complications

Surgical injury of the subclavian artery can even occur when operating through the supraclavicular approach, and in the worst scenario lead to complete damage and loss of the vessel, and even to loss of the patient. Predisposing risk factors for arterial injury are previous local irradiation or inflammatory process, surgical reintervention, or the presence of a cervical rib. Obviously, a subclavian artery aneurysm or poststenotic dilatation can cause additional difficulties during dissection.

Arterial bleeding most often occurs when a side branch is torn away from the subclavian artery, caused by faulty surgical dissection or excessive traction. If such arterial bleeding occurs during a transaxillary approach, the responsible side branch should be identified, clipped and transsected. This strategy, combined with external compression might gain some time, if necessary, to change surgical access.

In the most unfavorable cases, proximal arterial control can be achieved by means of vascular clamps, intra-arterial balloon or digital pressure. Vascular repair through the axillary route is technically difficult, and in most cases a supraclavicular or thoracic access is required. In life-threatening circumstances the only solution might be to ligate the subclavian artery, which in general is well tolerated due to the extensive collateral network. Gangrene of the fingers with subsequent amputation has been reported, albeit exceptionally. In case the subclavian artery is sacrificed, postoperative clinical surveillance should indicate the necessity for vascular reconstruction. Subclavian artery injuries might be restored through an extended supraclavicular approach (carotid-subclavian bypass) or a lateral thoracic access. Exceptionally, if the subclavian arterial or venous bleeding can not be controlled one might transsect or even resect the clavicula, however, this approach should only be applied if the above mentioned techniques are unsuccessful.

In addition to a torn side branch, surgical instruments used to perform the rib resection can also cause direct arterial or venous injury. After vascular repair it is important to have a strict postoperative surveillance, because seemingly successfully repaired injuries might bleed again and cause a significant extrapleural hematoma or, in case the pleura was opened, a hemothorax.

Besides the artery, the subclavian vein is also commonly found to be injured during first rib resections. It is located posterior and inferior to the clavicula and subclavian muscle and anterior to the insertion of the anterior scalenus muscle. The thin structure of the venous wall makes it vulnerable during hazardous manoeuvres. A tear or hole in the subclavian vein not only causes substantial bleeding but also increases the risk or air embolism, especially if a supraclavicular approach is used and a hydrostatic depression is induced by the half-sitting position of the patient.

If a venous tear occurs during an anterior or transaxillary approach, the bleeding can be controlled by external compression in most of the cases. A major injury obviously requires surgical repair.

The anatomic location of the main lymphatic pathways in the thoracic outlet should also be kept in mind. In particular, the supraclavicular access has been found to enhance the risk of transecting lymph channels. On the left side, the thoracic duct can be injured at the place where it crosses anterior to the transverse process C7 and anterior to the subclavian artery where it enters the left innominate vein. A lymphatic injury at this level should be recognized and immediately repaired. In other cases, it can lead to a lymphocele which can be treated by drainage or low lipid diet.

In summary, vascular problems determine a significant part of complications following surgery for TOS, potentially leading to loss of the upper extremity or even the life of the patient.

Nerve injuries

The thoracic outlet is highly vulnerable because of the high density of nerve structures present. The nerves are susceptible to injury by traction, compression, pulling, or dissection. In addition, they might be devascularized or embraced by fibrous tissue.

Damage to the complete brachial plexus can occur, particularly during the axillary approach, if traction of the arm by the assistant is too excessive.

Mechanical traction systems to pull up the arm and enhance the surgical exposure can even increase these risks and should therefore be prohibited. Plexus lesions can also be caused by metallic retractors which are placed too deep and excessively pulled. Direct injury of the brachial plexus, the inferior branches in particular, can occur during the *blind* phase of resecting the first rib at its posterior origin, using the ribscissors.

Brachial plexus injuries are dreadful because the long-term complaints can be catastrophic. Fortunately, the majority of plexus lesions are temporary, due to neuropraxia caused by excessive compression. The clinical consequences of a brachial plexus injury vary from moderate or severe pain to partial or total loss of sensibility or motor function of the upper extremity.

An individually adapted physiotherapeutic program can finally lead to full recovery in the majority of patients. Permanent disability due to crushing or transection is less frequent and occurs in approximately 1% of operations. In general, brachial plexus lesions are more often encountered after the transaxillary approach because traction is inevitable for adequate exposure.

Besides the brachial plexus, other nerves can be injured as well: the cubital nerve, long thoracic nerve, intercostobrachial nerve and phrenic nerve. Also, these nerves can suffer from temporary dysfunction due to manipulation and excessive traction or permanent failure after transection or major contusion. The phrenic nerve traverses the anterior side of the anterior scalenus muscle, both interior and exterior, and can be damaged during transection of the anterior scalenus tendon. However, most phrenic nerve injuries are caused by excessive traction. Postoperatively, a phrenic nerve lesion is most frequently discovered by a chest x-ray demonstrating elevation of the ipsilateral diaphragm.

The long thoracic nerve can be identified at the lateral border of the middle scalenus muscle and serves as a landmark to transect this muscle during the supraclavicular approach. The nerve might partially be embraced by the muscle and therefore potentially be damaged by transecting the middle scalenus muscle. The transaxillary approach does generally not expose the long thoracic nerve, but partial transection of the middle scalenus muscle to expose the posterior segment of the rib might still harm the nerve. The course of the long thoracic nerve comprises numerous anatomical variations, but in all cases it is the motoric nerve of the serratus

anterior muscle, which, if injured leads to *scapula alata* and limited abduction of the upper extremity.

The intercostobrachial nerve is an anastomotic connection between the accessory internal cutaneous brachial nerve and second intercostal nerve. It can be stretched or transected, sometimes deliberately, during the transaxillary approach.

The intercostobrachial nerve is partly responsible for the sensitive innervation of the axillary cavity. Damage to the nerve therefore explains the hypo- or anesthesia in the armpit and at the internal upper arm, sometimes extending to the elbow.

For the sake of completeness, however, rarely they may occur, damage to the vagus nerve and the stellate ganglion should be mentioned. In fact, the recurrent branch of the right vagus nerve might be injured where it traverses the anterior plane of the right subclavian artery. The stellate ganglion might eventually be damaged by traction during the transaxillary access, clinically expressed as Horner's syndrome.

Pulmonary complications

A parietal pleural lesion during a first rib resection often occurs and the subsequent pneumothorax can often be corrected with a pleural suture. However, if there is any doubt, placement of a thoracic drain is recommended. Some surgeons consider a pneumothorax not a complication but rather an anticipated risk of the surgical procedure.

Long-term complications

As described before, the immediate intra- and postoperative complications of a rib resection are significant with potential dramatic clinical outcome. Besides the persistent complaints of nerve injuries, the long-term complications are related to:
1 - inadequate resection of compressing structures around the brachial plexus,
2 - fibrous tissue formation due to hematoma or excessive local dissection,
3 - devascularization of plexus tissue.

Recurrence of symptoms can also occur if a stump of the supernumerary rib or first rib is left in-situ. Excessive fibrous tissue formation around the brachial plexus can occur soon after the operation. Early physiotherapy might prevent this complication. It should be emphasized that early and late physiotherapy plays an important role in the rehabilitation of patients operated for TOS.

Discussion

Resection of a first rib as a treatment for thoracic outlet syndrome is susceptible for serious complications like permanent brachial plexus paralysis, ischemic upper extremity, and even death. These complications, though fortunately rare, are observed regardless of the surgical approach and appear to be related to inexperience or inadequate equipment.

The type of complications seem to be related to the type of surgical access: the transaxillary approach predisposes for brachial plexus lesions and the supraclavicular approach increases the risk of vascular and phrenic nerve injuries.

The value of this surgery is still under debate. The surgical indications are fully based on subjective, clinical impressions and to date no objective method is available to assess a causal relation between the symptoms and compression. Furthermore, no methods can be applied to predict a successful clinical outcome. The majority of authors who have published their experience report good functional results in 80% to 85% of patients. Urschel [8], having a large experience with more than 3000 operated patients, reported good short-term results in 90% of cases and a recurrence rate of 12%-15%. In contrast, Cuypers et al. [9] only encountered a good result in 52% of 85 patients, using the principal criteria that patients should reach an activity level similar to their preoperative level, as judged by an independent observer.

In this context of functional surgery with uncertain outcome, the occurrence of complications with potential permanent damage is an unacceptable catastrophe. Therefore, it is extremely important to inform patients about these complications, which can be taken into the account of their final decision.

Conclusion

Based on our personal experience of the treatment of arterial or neurologic TOS, we prefer the supraclavicular approach because it renders fewer complications and allows for superior anatomic control of the subclavian artery in case of intraoperative incidents.

REFERENCES

1 Cherington M. Surgery for thoracic outlet syndrome? *N Engl J Med* 1986; 314: 322.

2 Sanders RJ. Traitement des syndromes de la traversée thoraco-brachiale par voie sus-claviculaire. In: Kieffer E (ed). *Les syndromes de la traversée thoraco-brachiale.* Paris; AERCV, 1989: pp 125-134.

3 Cormier F, Kieffer E. Résultats de la chirurgie des syndromes neurologiques de la traversée thoraco-brachiale par voie sus-claviculaire. In: Kieffer E (ed). *Les syndromes de la traversée thoraco-brachiale.* Paris; AERCV, 1989: pp 283-292.

4 Jamieson WG, Chinnick B. Thoracic outlet syndrome: fact or fancy? A review of 409 consecutive patients who underwent operation. *Can J Surg* 1996; 39: 321-326.

5 Horowitz SH. Brachial plexus injuries with causalgia resulting from transaxillary rib resection. *Arch Surg* 1985; 120: 1189-1191.

6 Dale WA. Thoracic outlet compression syndrome. *Arch Surg* 1982; 117: 1437-1445.

7 Mellière D, Kassab M, Salion C et al. Complications graves de la chirurgie des syndromes de la traversée thoraco-brachiale. In: Kieffer E (ed). *Les syndromes de la traversée thoraco-brachiale.* Paris; AERCV, 1989: pp 309-316.

8 Urschel HC. The transaxillary approach for treatment of thoracic outlet syndrome. *Seminars in thoracic and cardiovascular surgery* 1996; 8: 214-220.

9 Cuypers PW, Bollen ECM, van Houtte HP. Transaxillary first rib resection for thoracic outlet syndrome. *Acta Chir Belg* 1995; 95: 119-122.

26

Complications and Side Effects of Endoscopic Thoracic Sympathicotomy

LARS REX, C DROTT

The upper thoracic sympathetic chain runs parallel with the spine and close to the costovertebral junction on each side. The ganglia lye between the ribs and are connected by the interganglionic chain. The thoracic (T) 2 ganglion is located between the second and third ribs. Postganglionic branches innervate sweatglands, bloodvessels and pilomotor muscles, as well as lungs, heart and esophagus. The key ganglion in the upper thoracic part is the second ganglion, as the greatest number of sympathetic fibers pass through it (Figure) The sympathetic outflow to the upper extremity, head and neck are derived from T1 down to T6, but the distribution is approximate and variation can occur. The T2 ganglion is, however, the crucial level for the face and hands. Occasionally postganglionic fibers bypass the sympathetic chain to the brachial plexus and upper extremity via the so-called Kuntz nerve. Failure to interrupt this branch during surgery may result in an incomplete sympathectomy.

The first description of surgery on the sympathetic chain appeared in 1889 [1]. It was, however, not until 1920 when Kotzareff reported a case of palmar hyperhidrosis that the operation became more established [2]. Various open surgical approaches were described during the following decades. The thoracoscopic approach, which today is the standard procedure, was well described already in 1942 by Hughes [3]. Furthermore, over 1000 cases were described by Kux in 1954 [4]. For unknown reasons the endoscopic approach never became standard. During the general development of endoscopic surgery in the 1980´ies, the thoracoscopic approach to the sympathetic chain was popularized. This minimally invasive technique has led to an increasing number of procedures worldwide. The nerve may be endoscopically removed (sympathectomy) or just divided (sympathicotomy) (Table I).

Indications

Thoracic sympathetic ablation has been used for various indications during the previous century. Table II shows the current indications. Very good and durable results have been reported for palmar hyperhidrosis, facial hyperhidrosis, facial blushing, angina pectoris and the long Q-T syndrome. Endoscopic thoracic sympathicotomy (ETS) for pain syndromes and vasospastic disease often leads to immediate symptom relief, but long-term results are rather disappointing.

OPERATIVE TECHNIQUE

The procedure is performed under general anesthesia and standard single lumen intubation is appropriate. The most popular technique today is endoscopic thoracic sympathicotomy. Access to the pleural cavity is usually achieved by incision in the third intercostal space. Carbondioxide insufflation is used by most surgeons in order to partially deflate the lung. Our group has simplified the procedure by using a modified standard urological resectoscope of 7 mm diameter. This technique requires only one incision as the cutting electrode and optical system are combined in one instrument [5]. The sympathetic chain is transsected over the second and third rib thus excluding the T2 ganglion. Another new, but not yet established technique is to apply clips on the sympathetic chain thereby blocking the conduction [6]. The potential advantage of this method is the reversibility after clip removal. Solid data to support the possibility of nerve recovery is, however, still lacking.

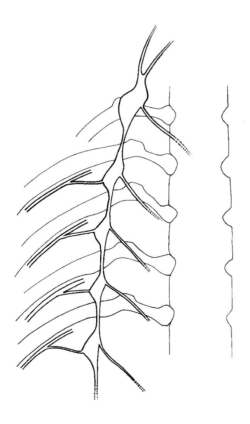
Figure - Schematic drawing of the sympathetic chain.

Table I	TECHNIQUES FOR THORACIC SYMPATHETIC ABLATION

1. **Open approach**
   Dorsal midline
   Anterior transthoracic
   Supraclavicular
   Transaxillary

2. **Endoscopic**
   Thoracoscopic sympathectomy/sympaticotomy

3. **Other procedures**
   Percutaneus radiofrequency sympathetic ablation
   CT guided chemical percutaneous sympathetic ablation

Table II	INDICATIONS FOR SYMPATHETIC ABLATION

➤ Palmar hyperhidrosis
➤ Facial blushing
➤ Facial hyperhidrosis
➤ Angina pectoris
➤ Long Q-T syndrome
➤ Raynaud´s syndrome

Complications

Riskfactors for complications are previous chest surgery or trauma, pleuritis, obesity and advanced age.

The main complications comprise Horner's syndrome (Table III) and pneumothorax/hemothorax (Table IV).

MORTALITY

Review of the literature only reports three cases with a fatal outcome. The reason was bleeding in one case, causing hypovolemia and subsequent irreversible brain damage. One patient died the first postoperative day without proven explanation, probably because of arrythmia [22]. The third case was due to sudden hypoxemia and hypovolemia, probably due to a mediastinal shift and delayed release of the insufflated gas. The patient never recovered and suffered from irreversible brain damage [23].

INFECTIONS

Wound infections are very rare. Occasional cases of postoperative pneumonia have been described.

PNEUMOTHORAX

The thoracoscopic technique requires partial lung collapse by artificial pneumothorax. The most common way to achieve this is insufflation of carbondioxide with a Veress needle. With this blind pleural cannulation the presence of adhesions may increase the risk for visceral pleural tears which subsequently could lead to air leaks. When the operation is finished the carbondioxide is exsufflated by

Table III	HORNER'S SYNDROME FOLLOWING DIFFERENT TECHNIQUES OF SYMPATHECTOMY/SYMPATHICOTOMY		
Technique	*1st author [ref.]*	*Number of patients*	*Number of Horner's syndrome*
Transaxillary	Atkins [7]	26	0
	Berguer [8]	22	0
Supraclavicular	Adar [9]	475	40
	Hashmonai [10]	85	5
	Conlon [11]	75	2
Anterior thoracic	Cloward [12]	82	3
	Shih [13]	457	0
Endoscopic sympathicotomy	Fritsch [14]	164	5 (2 transient)
	Malone [15]	17	3 (transient)
	Byrne [16]	112	3 (transient)
	Kopelman [17]	116	10
	Lai [18]	72	5
	Lin [19]	1360	NA
	Zacherl [20]	630	20
	Rex [21]	1152	5
Endoscopic clipping	Lin [6]	326	0

NA: not available

Table IV	PNEUMOTHORAX AND HEMOTHORAX FOLLOWING DIFFERENT TECHNIQUES OF SYMPATHECTOMY/SYMPATHICOTOMY			
Technique	1st author [ref.]	Number of patients	Number of pneumothorax	Number of hemothorax
Transaxillary	Atkins [7]	26	0	0
	Berguer [8]	22	4	0
Supraclavicular	Adar [9]	475	6	0
	Hashmonai [10]	85	1	3
	Conlon [11]	75	1	0
Anterior thoracic	Cloward [12]	82	4	0
	Shih [13]	457	1	3
Endoscopic sympathicothomy	Fritsch [14]	164	2	NA
	Malone [15]	17	0	NA
	Byrne [16]	112	1	NA
	Kopelman [17]	116	15*	
	Lai [18]	72	6	NA
	Lin [19]	1360	5	NA
	Zacherl [20]	630	8	1
	Rex [21]	1152	12	4
Endoscopic clipping	Lin [6]	326	0	0

NA: not available
* Including hemothorax + pneumonia

suction. The anesthesiologist facilitates lung expansion by applying continuous positive airway pressure. A postoperative chest X-ray should be performed. Any remaining carbondioxide will quickly be reabsorbed but a progressive pneumothorax should be treated by suction drainage.

BLEEDING

The two main reasons for bleeding are intercostal vessel injury or azygos vein branch injury. These veins are predominantly present adjacent to the third rib on the right side.

A rare cause of bleeding is a tear of vascularized apical adhesions. Small venous bleedings cease by compression or electrocautery in most cases. Another option is to use an extra port for endoclip application. Conversion to open thoracotomy is mandatory if endoscopic techniques fail to control the bleeding. If a substantial hemothorax is evident on the postoperative chest X-ray, evacuation by pleural suction drainage is important.

HORNER'S EYE SYNDROME

The cause of this complication is damage to the ocular sympathetic fibers from the stellate ganglion. Another explanation may be more caudally located ocular fibers than the normal T1 location. The open supraclavicular approach to the sympathetic chain allows access to the stellate ganglion and exposes it at risk for injury. During endoscopic surgery Horner´s eye syndrome can be the result of thermal injury to the stellate ganglion from coagulating the interganglionic fibers. For endoscopic procedures, the incidence varies between 0% and 23%. The majority is transient and approximately 6% of patients complain of permanent symptoms.

Reviewing the literature indicates that Horner's syndrome occurs more frequently after open, surgical procedures (up to 40%), however, this was never prospectively compared.

The triad of miosis, ptosis and enofthalmus is often associated with nasal congestion on the affected side.

CARDIAC COMPLICATIONS

Cardiac complications seem to be rare except a reduction of heart rate. Two perioperative cardiac arrests have, however, been described [24], the mechanism of which remains unclear. Hypothetically, sympathetic stimulation to the stellate ganglion by electrocautery may result in a reduction of ventricular fibrillation threshold, arrhythmia and subsequent cardiac arrest.

POST PROCEDURAL PAIN

Post sympathectomy pain, described as a dull, deep burning pain in the arm is described in few reports with an incidence up to 13%, but most authors do not mention this complication. There is seldom any distinction between postoperative somatic pain from traction or heat spread from diathermia to the brachial plexus and true sympathetic neuralgia. In our experience of more than 5000 cases with sympaticotomy we have not experienced more than a few cases with postoperative arm pain and therefore we believe that, in general, sympaticotomy does not cause postoperative neuropathic pain.

MISCELLANEOUS COMPLICATIONS

A few case reports have documented rare complication such as false aneurysms of an intercostal artery, intercostal neuralgia, injury to the long thoracic nerve, inferior brachial plexus injury, thoracic duct injury, and recurrent laryngeal nerve damage.

Side effects

COMPENSATORY SWEATING

The effect of upper thoracic sympathetic ablation on palmar hyperhidrosis is extremely good with up to 99% dry hands, however, the subjective satisfaction rate is normally lower. The explanation for this is usually caused by side-effects, predominantly compensatory hyperhidrosis, which affects the non-denervated area of the body with a prevalence of 30% to 100% of patients. The distribution of compensatory sweating (CS) is predominantly the back, lower chest, abdomen and groin areas. For the majority of patients, the CS is evident within the first postoperative months. The CS is often triggered by warm environment and physical activity. For most of the patients this is well tolerated but it may also be severe enough to cause regret of the operation [25]. There is no ideal treatment for compensatory sweating but various anticholinergic drugs and aluminium chloride solution can alleviate it to some extent. Botulinum toxin injection may cure excessive sweating in localized areas but are impractical in large body areas. The calcium-ion plays a key role for the function of the sweatglands and therefore, on theoretical grounds, calcium-channel-blockers could have a role in treating CS, but no clinical studies are published.

GUSTATORY SWEATING

A side effect of sympathicotomy may be increased sweating of the face from exposure to certain food components or smells. This is described by 10%–30% of patients but seldom cause any major discomfort.

PHANTOM SWEATING

Phantom sweating is a sensation of sweating or blushing but the hands remain dry or the face does not blush. This phenomenon is seldom of any major concern, however, the patient should be informed.

MISCELLANEOUS POTENTIAL SIDE EFFECTS

A number of symptoms have been claimed as side effects of ETS, although they are not supported by scientific studies. Arm fatigue has been described by a few patients but systematic studies have not supported causality to ETS. Impaired physical performance has been reported by a few patients after ETS. Studies by means of ergometer cycle before and after ETS have not been able to show any detoriation of maximal physical performance [26].

Finally, one case of transient abnormal suntanning has been reported.

Conclusion

Endoscopic transthoracic sympathicotomy or sympathectomy is a safe and efficient procedure, especially for palmar hyperhidrosis and facial blushing. The complication rate is low compared to open surgical sympathectomy. The side effects have, however, not decreased by the use of endoscopic techniques. Compensatory sweating is the major side effect and may be severe enough to cause regret of the procedure. Only patients with severe impairment of quality of life from their symptoms are candidates for ETS. Thorough disclosure of expected effects, side effects and complication risks are mandatory.

REFERENCES

1 Abadie. 1899.Cited by Kotzareff, ref no. 12.
2 Kotzareff A. Resection partielle du tronc sympathique cervical droit pour hyperhidrose unilatérale. *Rev Med Suisse Romande* 1920; 40: 111-113.
3 Hughes. Thoracoscopic sympathectomy. *Proc Roy Soc Med* 1942; 35: 585-586.
4 Kux E. Thorakoskopische Eingriffe am Nervensystem. Stuttgart: George Thieme Verl 1954.
5 Claes G, Göthberg G. Endoscopic transthoracic electrocautery of the sympathetic chain for palmar and axillary hyperhidrosis. *Br J Surg* 1991; 78: 760.
6 Lin CC, Mo LR, Lee LS et al. Thoracoscopic T2-sympathetic block by clipping – A better and reversible operation for treatment of hyperhidrosis palmaris: experience with 326 cases. *Eur J Surg* 1998; Suppl 580: 13-16.
7 Atkins HJB. Sypathectomy by the axillary approach. *Lancet* 1954; 1: 538-539.
8 Berguer R, Smit R. Transaxillary sympathectomy for relief of vasospastic- sympathetic pain of upper extremities. *Surgery* 1981; 89: 764-769.
9 Adar R, Kurchin A, Zweig A, Moses M. Palmar hyperhidrosis and its surgical treatment. *Ann Surg* 1977; 186: 34-41.
10 Hashmonai M, Kopelman D, Kein O, Schein M. Upper thoracic sympathectomy for primary palmar hyperhidrosis: long-term follow-up. *Br J Surg* 1992; 79: 268-271.
11 Conlon KC, Keaveny TV. Upper dorsal sympathectomy for palmar hyperhidrosis. *Br J Surg* 1987; 74: 651.
12 Cloward RB. Hyperhidrosis. *J Neurosurg* 1969; 30: 545-551.
13 Shih CJ, Wang YC. Thoracic sympathectomy for palmar hyperhidrosis: report of 456 cases. *Surg Neurol* 1978; 10: 291-296.
14 Fritsch A, Kokoschka R, Mach K. Ergebnisse der thorakoskopischer sympathectomie bei hyperhidrosis der oberen extremität. *Wien Klin Wochenschr* 1975; 87: 548-550.
15 Malone PS, Cameron AEP, Rennie JA. Endoscopic thoracic sympathectomy in the treatment of upper limb hyperhidrosis. *Ann R Coll Surg Engl* 1986; 68: 93-94.
16 Byrne J, Walsh TN, Hederman WP. Endoscopic transthoracic electrocautery of the sympathetic chain for palmar and axillary hyperhidrosis. *Br J Surg* 1990; 77: 1040-1049.
17 Kopelman D, Hashmonai M, Ehrenreich, Assalia A. Thoracoscopic sympathectomy for palmar hyperhidrosis. *Eur J Surg* 1998; Suppl 580 Abstr 31 : 58.
18 Lai YT, Yang LH, Chio CC et al. Complications in patients with palmar hyperhidrosis treated with transthoracic endoscopic sympathectomy. *Neurosurgery* 1997; 41: 110-113.
19 Lin TS, Fang HY. Transthoracic endoscopic sympathectomy in the treatment of palmar hyperhidrosis -with emphasis on perioperative management (1360 case analyses). *Surg Neurol* 1999; 52: 453-457.
20 Zacherl J, Huber ER, Imhof M et al. Long-term results of 630 thoracoscopic sympathicotomies for primary hyperhidrosis: the Vienna experience. *Eur J Surg* 1998; Suppl 580: 43-46.
21 Rex Lo, Drott C, Claes G et al. The Borås experience of endoscopic thoracic sympaticotomy for palmar, axillary, facial hyperhidrosis and facial blushing. *Eur J Surg* 1998; Suppl 580: 23-26.
22 Hedman A. Handsvett blev hans död. Orsaken var sympathicus-imbalans. *Läkartidningen* 1995; 92: 2310-2 (in Swedish).
23 Cameron A. Complications of endoscopic sympathectomy. *Eur J Surg* 1998; Suppl 580: 33-35.
24 Lin CC, Mo LR, Hwang MH. Intraoperative cardiac arrest: a rare complication of T2,3-sympathicotomy for treatment of hyperhidrosis palmaris. *Eur J Surg* 1994; Suppl 572: 43-45.
25 Fredman B, Zohar E, Shachor D et al. Video-assisted transthoracic sympathectomy in the treatment of primary hyperhidrosis: Friend or foe? *Surg Laparos Endosc* 2000; 10: 226-229.
26 Drott C, Claes G, Göthberg G, Paszkowski P. Cardiac effects of endoscopic electrocautery of the upper thoracic sympathetic chain. *Eur J Surg* 1994; Suppl 572: 65-70.

27

COMPLICATIONS AFTER RECONSTRUCTIVE SURGERY OF THE MAIN VENOUS TRUNKS

PETER GLOVICZKI, THOMAS C BOWER, KENNETH J CHERRY
JOHN W HALLETT, JEAN PANNETON, AUDRA A NOEL

Careful planning, perfect execution and effective postoperative surveillance are the hallmarks of success of any surgical procedure. Venous reconstructions are among the most demanding operations. Appropriate patient selection is essential and the decision to operate should be based on clinical symptoms, preoperative functional tests, and imaging studies. The conduct of the operation, atraumatic surgical technique, selection of proper graft material, and the use of adjuncts to maintain graft patency are all important components of the strategy to minimize peri-operative complications. Postoperative care is aimed at reducing the risk of thrombosis and graft surveillance will decrease late failure of venous grafts. Once complications have occurred, immediate recognition and effective treatment will assure good long-term results. In this chapter we will review the most important complications of open surgical reconstructions of the main venous trunks and suggest guidelines for their prevention, recognition, and treatment. We will also present current results of open surgical reconstructions of large veins.

Classification of complications

Complications of venous reconstructions, as of any other vascular procedures, include systemic and local, vascular and nonvascular complications. Of the systemic nonvascular complications, cardiac and pulmonary complications are the most severe and careful patient selection is important for prevention. In general, large vein reconstructions for benign disease are performed in good risk patients only, with a very low risk of systemic, nonvascular complications. Of the local, nonvascular complications, wound infection and lymphatic leaks (fistula, lymphocele) are the most frequent, and atraumatic surgical technique, antibiotic prophylaxis, and standard surgical principles are helpful in prevention.

Of the systemic vascular complications, deep venous thrombosis and pulmonary embolism are the most important and their prevention is crucial. Peri-operative anticoagulation with heparin and warfarin, the use of elastic stockings, intermittent pneumatic compression pumps and early ambulation help prevent both venous thrombosis and pulmonary embolism. Air embolism during vena caval reconstruction is a serious complication and it should be avoided by flushing all air out of the caval grafts before re-establishment of the circulation.

Local vascular complications are specific to venous reconstructions and include graft stenosis or venous thrombosis, peri-operative bleeding, graft infection, and injury to the surrounding vascular and nonvascular structures. A rare late complication is prosthetic graft fistulization, with bowel, ureter or the biliary tract. The most important local vascular complications, like early and late graft thrombosis, deep venous thrombosis and bleeding complications deserve detailed discussion.

Graft thrombosis

FACTORS AFFECTING GRAFT PATENCY

Grafts placed in the venous system have a higher rate of thrombosis than arterial grafts. Flow rate in venous grafts in general is lower than in arterial grafts placed at the same location, since significant collateral circulation develops to compensate for the venous obstruction. Pressure in the venous system is low; grafts can collapse because of increased abdominal pressure or when tunneled under the inguinal ligament, in the retrohepatic space, through the diaphragm or in the thoracic outlet. Obese patients are poor candidates for the Palma procedure using saphenous vein because external compression of the graft by the heavy adipose tissue in the groins can compress the vein graft. Infrainguinal venous obstruction and valvular incompetence further decrease inflow to the graft, and it is a major contributing factor to failure [1,2]. Thrombophilia is prevalent among patients undergoing venous reconstructions and many patients have absent circulating anticoagulants such as protein factor C, protein factor S, and antithrombin III, or they have Factor V Leiden mutation. The throm-

bogenic surface of any prosthetic graft also increases the risk of graft failure.

VENOUS GRAFTS

Autologous grafts have the lowest thrombogenicity, but for large vein reconstruction size mismatch is a problem as are low flow rates and low pressure in the grafts. The greater saphenous vein is used most frequently as a suprapubic femorofemoral bypass (Palma procedure) [3-12]. Other autologous grafts available include the superficial femoral vein, the basilic/axillary vein, and the internal jugular veins. The use of these, however, is limited either because the lack of adequate length or because these veins had previous thrombosis as well. The superficial femoral vein should not be harvested from a post-thrombotic leg and the patients should be made aware that there is a small but definite risk of late leg swelling in patients who undergo harvesting of the deep leg veins. Also, a neck incision in a young patient to harvest an internal or external jugular vein may be cosmetically unacceptable.

Our usual strategy for superior vena cava or innominate vein reconstruction is to use a spiral vein graft [1,13]. The graft is prepared from the saphenous vein, which can be harvested using the endoscopes technique to minimize skin incisions in the leg. Valves are excised and the vein is wrapped around a 32 Fr or 36 Fr polyethylene chest tube. The edges of the vein are then approximated with running 6-0 monofilament polypropylene sutures or, more recently, we have been using non-penetrating vascular clips (U.S. Surgical, Inc) (Fig. 1). Placement of clips rather than suturing reduces the time needed for graft preparation considerably. Of the available prosthetic grafts polytetrafluoroethylene (PTFE) has produced the best results for superior vena cava (SVC) or innominate vein replacement [13-17].

For inferior vena cava (IVC), iliocaval, or femorocaval bypass, as do most other authors we also prefer to use expanded PTFE grafts with external spiral or ring support [18-35]. Fresh human allograft, using the IVC or a longer, iliocaval segment, can be considered in those patients who receive immunosuppressive treatment for protection of another transplanted organ, e.g., kidney or liver [36]. Cryopreserved grafts have less antigenicity and usually do not require immuno-suppression. Graft thrombosis, at least at the femoral vein level, is significant, and long-term results for large vein reconstruction are not available.

Adjuncts to decrease thrombotic complications

ARTERIOVENOUS FISTULA

An arteriovenous fistula (AVF), first suggested by Kunlin in 1953, improves patency of grafts placed in the venous system [37,38]. Higher flow rate, especially for prosthetic grafts, decreases thrombosis rate. In experiments we found the optimal ratio between the diameters of the fistula and the prosthetic graft to be 0.3 [38]. Elevated intra-operative pressure in the femoral vein after placement of a fistula indicates increased outflow obstruction and if possible, it should be avoided. In patients who undergo Palma procedure, this may not be possible, since the size of the graft is usually equivalent with the size of the fistula. Improvement in venous function in these patients cannot be expected before closure of the fistula. Disadvantages of an AVF include an increased operating time and the inconvenience of a second procedure to ligate the fistula at a later date. A potential side effect is a high cardiac output.

We use either the side branch of the greater saphenous vein or a 4-mm prosthetic graft for fistula and place the venous end right onto the hood of the prosthetic graft. The arterial anastomosis is usually made to the superficial femoral artery. A small silastic sheet is placed around the fistula to avoid any healing and to permit easy dissection and ligation of the fistula at the second operation. Percutaneous closure of the fistula with transcatheter embolization is also an option.

Grafts for IVC replacement are usually placed without a fistula. We add an AVF, however, for all prosthetic grafts anastomosed to the femoral vein and for all longer (more than 10 cm) iliocaval grafts. The fistula is kept open for at least six months postoperatively, but in patients without any side effects, it is kept open for as long as possible to help maintain patency. A fistula is used for Palma grafts selectively, for a period of three months, if flow is less than 100 cc through the graft.

Duplex scan on the first postoperative day or contrast venography is performed to confirm graft patency. Stenosis or thrombosis is corrected immediately after recognition. If thrombosis occurred in a graft without fistula, thrombectomy is done with addition of a fistula. Grafts stenosis discovered during surveillance in the late postoperative period is treated with angioplasty or venous stenting (Fig. 2 A-C). Late graft thrombosis, if diagnosed within a few days or weeks, is treated with thrombolysis, angioplasty and stenting.

THROMBOSIS PROPHYLAXIS

Intra-operative full heparinization is done in all patients and protamine is avoided at the completion of the procedure. Low dose heparin (500 to 800 units/hour) is administered locally through a small polyethylene catheter (Fig. 3 A-B) and it is continued until complete systemic heparinization is achieved by 48 hours. The catheter is then removed, but full dose low molecular weight heparin is continued subcutaneously for another 3-5 days, given simultaneously with oral anticoagulation. Intermittent pneumatic compression pump, leg elevation, and elastic bandages are routine and early ambulation is encouraged. The patients are fitted with 30-40 mmHg compression stockings before discharge. Warfarin is continued indefinitely in most patients with prosthetic grafts and in all with a known underlying coagulation abnormality.

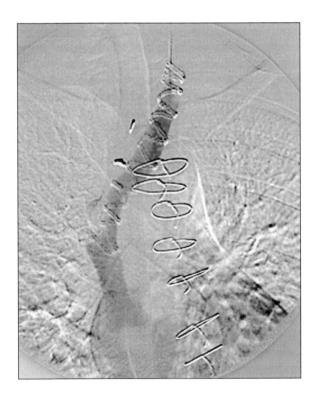

FIG. 1 Left internal jugular vein-right atrial appendage spiral saphenous vein graft, patent at three months after surgery. Note the vascular clips, used to prepare the graft from clipping the edges of the saphenous vein.

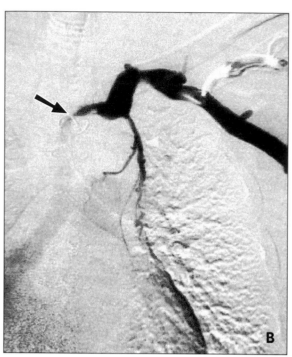

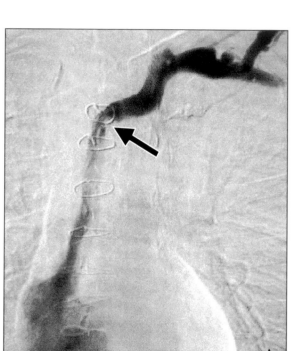

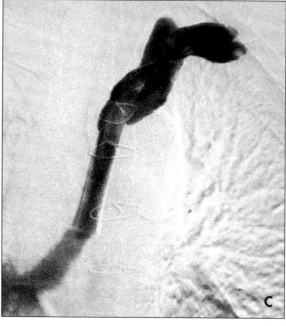

FIG. 2   A - Venogram six months after placement of left innominate-vein atrial appendage spiral saphenous vein graft in 46-year-old man revealed mild stenosis at proximal anastomosis (*arrow* indicates stenosis). B - Venogram at 10 months reveals severe stenosis at proximal anastomosis. Note presence of mediastinal collaterals *(arrowhead)* indicating partial obstruction of flow in graft. C - Venogram six months after Wallstent placement confirms widely patent stent and graft. *(From Alimi YS, Gloviczki P et al. Reconstruction of the superior vena cava: benefits of postoperative surveillance and secondary endovascular interventions. J Vasc Surg 1998; 27: 287-301, with permission).*

BLEEDING COMPLICATIONS

The incidence of postoperative bleeding is between 5% and 10%, mainly as a result of anti-coagulation. All larger hematomas, and any small hematoma that has the potential to compress the graft, are managed aggressively, with surgical evacuation.

Results of large vein reconstructions

PALMA PROCEDURE (SUPRAPUBIC SAPHENOUS VEIN TRANSPOSITION)

Analysis of results of 398 operations, published in 9 series revealed clinical improvement in 78% and a patency rate of 74% (Table I) [3-12]. However, follow-up was variable and objective graft assessment with imaging was rarely done.

We recently reported results of 44 femoral or iliocaval reconstructions, performed in 42 patients

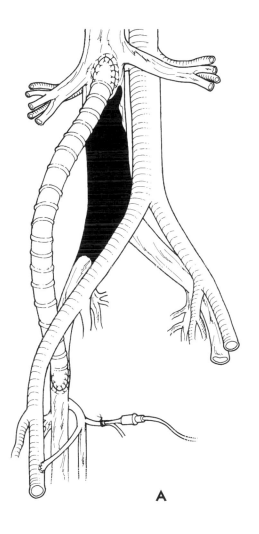

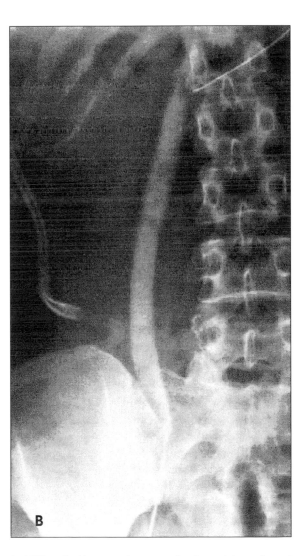

FIG. 3   A - Illustration of right iliac vein-IVC externally supported ePTFE graft. Note arteriovenous fistula at right groin and 20-gauge catheter, which is introduced through tributary of saphenous vein for postoperative heparin infusion. B - Postoperative venogram confirms patency of graft. *(From Gloviczki P, Pairolero PC, Toomey BJ et al. Reconstruction of large veins for nonmalignant venous occlusive disease. J Vasc Surg 1992; 16: 750-61, with permission).*

| Table I | RESULTS OF FEMOROFEMORAL SAPHENOUS VEIN CROSSOVER BYPASS GRAFTS (PALMA PROCEDURE) |

1st author [ref.]	Year	Number of limbs	Follow-up (years)	Patency %	Clinical improvement %
Palma [3]	1960	8	Up to 3	NA	88
Dale [4]	1969	48	Up to 12	NA	77
May [5]	1981	66	NA	73	NA
Dale [6]	1983	56	NA	NA	80
Husni [7]	1983	85	0.5-15	70	74
Halliday [8]	1985	47	Up to 18	75 (5 years)	89
Danza [9]	1991	27	NA	NA	81
AbuRahma [10]	1991	24	5.5	75 (7 years)	63
Gruss [11]	1997	19	NA	71	82
Jost [12]	In press	18	0.1-9.1	82 (4 years)	67
Total		**398**		**74 (mean)**	**78 (mean)**

NA: not available

with benign venous thrombosis or trauma [12]. Thirty-six patients had limb swelling or venous claudication, and 38 patients had pain. Fourteen patients had healed or active ulcers. The etiology of venous obstruction was congenital in 2 patients and secondary to other causes in 40: of these, deep vein thrombosis was the etiology in 25, trauma in 5, retroperitoneal fibrosis in 4, caval occlusion devices in 4, and others in 2. Eighteen reconstructions were femorofemoral Palma procedures using the greater saphenous vein (Fig. 4). Four-year patency of the 18 Palma grafts was 83%. (Fig. 5) Edema decreased, usually after take down of the arteriovenous fistula. Improvement in clinical signs and symptoms correlated with graft patency.

PROSTHETIC FEMOROFEMORAL BYPASS GRAFTS

Early graft thrombosis in our limited experience with this graft was frequent and we favor in-situ femorocaval grafts. The experience of Eklof et al. [18,19] with PTFE Palma grafts used in 7 patients with acute DVT was only slightly better. Although all six surviving patients reported only minimal leg

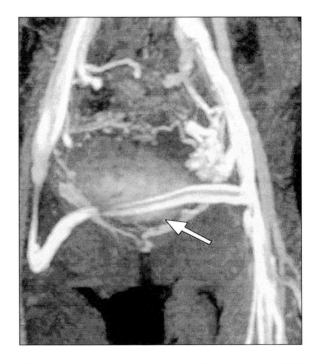

FIG. 4 Magnetic resonance venography showing a patent left to right Palma saphenous vein graft at nine years and six months after operation.

swelling, five grafts had thrombosed within 31 months, and only one graft remained patent at 36 months.

The best results have been reported by Sottiurai et al. [20]. They observed a 100% patency of suprapubic PTFE grafts in 26 patients, maintained during follow-up that ranged from 11 to 139 months. Gruss and Hiemer have a large experience with ePTFE grafts in this position, and with an 85% (27/32) patency rate in a long-term follow-up study [11].

INFERIOR VENA CAVA, ILIOCAVAL OR FEMOROCAVAL RECONSTRUCTIONS

Table II shows the results observed in the main series published in the literature. In our recent review of 44 large vein reconstructions for benign disease, 24 patients had direct in-situ reconstruction for iliocaval, iliac, or femoral occlusions [12]. Seventeen patients had ePTFE grafts (8 femorocaval [Fig. 6], 5 iliocaval [Fig. 3], 3 cross-femoral, 1 cavoatrial), 6 had spiral vein grafts (5 iliofemoral and 1 cavoatrial), and one femoral vein patch angioplasty was performed. Follow-up with imaging studies averaged 2.6 years (median 1.6), clinical follow-up averaged 3.5 years (median 2.5). Three patients died of unrelated causes, two with patent grafts. Most patients with prosthetic iliocaval replacement remained on long-term oral anticoagulation. Secondary patency rate of ilio/femorocaval ePTFE bypasses at 2 years was 54% (Fig. 5).

Secondary patency was lower in patients with an arteriovenous fistula (p = 0.023), although these data likely reflect the more extensive disease in those patients, who required a fistula to maintain patency.

In a recent report from our institution, Bower et al. [32] found excellent patency of IVC grafts placed following resection of a primary or metastatic tumor. Large diameter (greater than 14 mm) externally supported PTFE grafts were used in 28 patients and a panel graft of superficial femoral vein in one. IVC replacement was at the suprarenal segment in 15 patients, at the infrarenal segment in 10 patients, and in both in 4 patients.

Thirteen of these patients underwent major hepatic resections and this explains why complications in patients who undergo caval reconstruction for malignant disease occur much more frequent than in those who have post-thrombotic syndrome. In this series two deaths occurred, for an overall peri-operative mortality rate of 6.9%. One patient died intra-operatively of coagulopathy during attempted resection of a large central liver tumor and the retrohepatic IVC. The other in-hospital death occurred at 4 months, from multisystem organ failure and duodenal perforation. Only 16 patients (55.2%) recovered without complication. Major morbidity included cardiopulmonary problems in five patients, with one major myocardial infarction and bleeding in patients, of whom two required

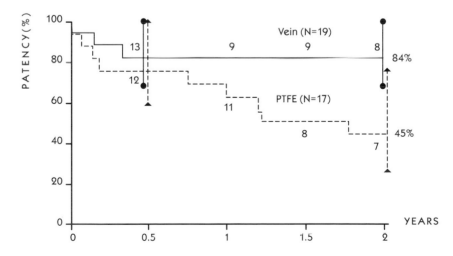

FIG. 5 Cumulative secondary patency rates of ePTFE ilio/femorocaval bypasses and saphenous vein crossover bypass grafts (Palma procedure). Palma grafts maintained same patency at four years. (From Jost CJ, Gloviczki P, Cherry KJ et al. Surgical reconstruction of iliofemoral veins and the inferior vena cava for nonmalignant occlusive disease. J Vasc Surg 2001; in press, with permission).

Table II		RESULTS OF FEMOROCAVAL/ILIOCAVAL PROSTHETIC BYPASS GRAFTING			
1st author [ref.]	*Year*	*Number of limbs*	*Follow-up* (months)	*Patency* %	*Clinical improvement* %
Husfeldt [21]	1981	4	4-30	100	100
Dale [22]	1984	3	1-30	100	100
Ijima [23]	1985	5	22-36	60	60
Eklof [18]	1985	7	2-31	29	86
Plate [24]	1985	3	1-11	33	67
Okadome [25]	1989	4	17-48	100	100
Gloviczki [1]	1992	12	1-60	58	67
Alimi [26]	1997	8	10-45	88	88
Jost [12]	In press	13	1-150	54	49
Sottiurai [20]	In press	19	80-113	84	84
Total		**78**		**71 (mean)**	**49-100**

re-operation and one needed percutaneous drainage of the hematoma. Chylous ascites or large pleural effusions developed in two patients each; and bile leak, leg edema with tibial vein thrombosis, and wound infection in one patient each. The patient with the autologous caval graft had a bile leak and a hematoma that compressed the graft. The bile leak was drained and the graft stenosis was treated successfully with a 16-mm self-expanding stent. Thrombosis rate has been low, and patency of the grafts in the 27 early survivors was 92% at a mean follow-up of 2.8 years (range: 2.7 months - 6.3 years). Other authors reported similar good patency of IVC grafts as well [28-35].

RESULTS OF RECONSTRUCTIONS FOR SUPERIOR VENA CAVA (SVC) SYNDROME

Patency of short SVC or innominate vein-atrial grafts have been excellent, with both spiral vein graft or PTFE grafts. PTFE grafts, however, have a higher failure rate, if they have to be anastomozed with the internal jugular vein and cross the thoracic outlet. Of the early reports, Doty et al. reported on long-term results in nine patients who underwent spiral vein grafting for superior vena cava syndrome, caused by benign disease [39]. Seven of nine grafts remained patent during follow-up that extended from one to 15 years and all but one of

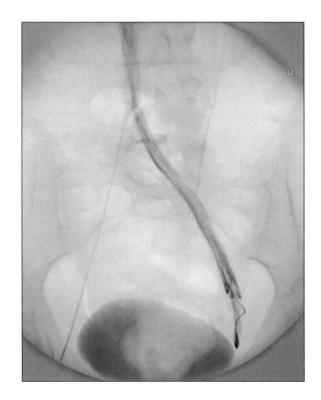

FIG. 6 Patent left femorocaval ePTFE bypass graft in a 54-year old female 11.7 years after graft placement. *(From Jost CJ, Gloviczki P, Cherry KJ et al. Surgical reconstruction of iliofemoral veins and the inferior vena cava for nonmalignant occlusive disease. J Vasc Surg 2001; in press, with permission).*

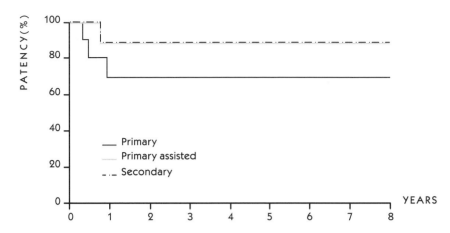

FIG. 7 Cumulative patency rates of 12 straight spiral saphenous vein grafts used for superior vena cava reconstructions. *(From Alimi YS, Gloviczki P, Vrtiska TJ, et al. Reconstruction of the superior vena cava: benefits of postoperative surveillance and secondary endovascular interventions. J Vasc Surg 1998; 27: 287-301, with permission).*

the patients became asymptomatic. A more recent report from the *Mayo Clinic* included 19 patients who underwent SVC reconstruction for benign SVC syndrome [13]. Spiral vein grafts (n = 14), ePTFE grafts with external support (n = 4), and one human allograft (n = 1) were implanted. No early death or pulmonary embolism occurred. Four early graft stenoses or thromboses (2 spiral vein grafts and 2 ePTFE grafts) required thrombectomy, with success in three. Four of 19 grafts occluded during follow-up (2 ePTFE, 2 spiral vein grafts). The primary, primary-assisted, and secondary patency rates were 53%, 70%, and 74% at 5 years, respectively. Straight spiral vein grafts had a 90% secondary patency rate at 5 years (Fig. 7). Most secondary interventions included endovascular therapy, angioplasty or stenting.

Dartevelle et al. observed excellent patency in 20 of 22 ePTFE grafts, with a mean follow-up of 23 months [14]. Moore and Hollier observed no graft occlusion at a mean follow-up of 30 months among 10 patients who underwent large central vein reconstruction [17]. In 8 of these 10 patients an additional arteriovenous fistula at the arm was used to increase flow and maintain patency. Reviewing other series from the literature, we found that patency of ePTFE grafts at 2 years was approximately 70%. Although spiral vein graft continues to be our first choice for superior vena cava replacement, short, large diameter ePTFE is an excellent alternative for SVC replacement.

Conclusion

Large vein reconstructions can be performed effectively with a low rate of nonvascular complications for benign disease, if the patients are carefully selected. The most feared complication, pulmonary embolism, is fortunately very rare and graft thrombosis is usually not followed by extensive deep venous thrombosis. Failure rate of grafts, implanted in the venous system is still high and further research should be focused to improve results of surgical treatment for large vein obstruction in those patients who are not candidates for endovascular revascularization, or who failed venous stenting. Endovascular techniques are helpful adjuncts to prolong patency of grafts used for large vein reconstruction.

REFERENCES

1 Gloviczki P, Pairolero PC, Toomey BJ et al. Reconstruction of large veins for nonmalignant venous occlusive disease. *J Vasc Surg* 1992; 16: 750-761.
2 Schanzer H, Skladany M. Complex venous reconstruction for chronic iliofemoral vein obstruction. *Cardiovasc Surg* 1996; 4: 837-840.
3 Palma EC, Esperon R. Vein transplants and grafts in the surgical treatment of the postphlebitic syndrome. *J Cardiovasc Surg* 1960; 1: 94.
4 Dale WA, Harris J. Cross-over vein grafts for iliac and femoral venous occlusion. *J Cardiovasc Surg* 1969; 10: 458-462.

5 May R. The Palma operation with Gottlob's endothelium preserving suture. In: May R, Weber J (eds), *Pelvic and abdominal veins: progress in diagnostics and therapy*. Amsterdam, Excerpta Medica, 1981; pp 192-197.

6 Dale WA. Crossover vein grafts for iliac and femoral venous occlusion. *Resident and staff physician* 1983; 3: 58.

7 Husni EA. Reconstruction of veins: the need for objectivity. *J Cardiovasc Surg* 1983; 24: 525-528.

8 Halliday P, Harris J, May J. Femoro-femoral crossover grafts (Palma operation) : a long-term follow-up study. In: Bergan JJ, Yao JST (eds), *Surgery of the Veins*. Orlando, Grune & Stratton, inc. 1985; pp 241-254.

9 Danza R, Navarro T, Baldizan J. Reconstructive surgery in chronic venous obstruction of the lower limbs. *J Cardiovasc Surg* 1991; 32 : 98-103.

10 AbuRahma AF, Robinson PA, Boland JP. Clinical, hemodynamic, and anatomic predictors of long-term outcome of lower extremity venovenous bypasses. *J Vasc Surg* 1991; 14: 635-644.

11 Gruss JD, Hiemer W. Bypass procedures for venous obstruction: Palma and May-Husmi bypasses, Raju perforator bypass, prosthetic bypasses, and primary and adjunctive arteriovenous fistulae. In: Raju S, Villavicencio JL (eds), *Surgical management of venous disease*. Baltimore: Williams & Wilkins, 1997; pp 289-305.

12 Jost CJ, Gloviczki P, Cherry KJ Jr et al. Surgical reconstruction of iliofemoral veins and the inferior vena cava for nonmalignant occlusive disease. *J Vasc Surg*, in press.

13 Alimi YS, Gloviczki P, Vrtiska TJ et al. Reconstruction of the superior vena cava: benefits of postoperative surveillance and secondary endovascular interventions. *J Vasc Surg* 1998; 27: 287-301.

14 Dartevelle PG, Chapelier AR, Pastorino U et al. Long-term follow-up after prosthetic replacement of the superior vena cava combined with resection of mediastinal-pulmonary malignant tumors. *J Thor Cardiovasc Surg* 1991; 102: 259-265.

15 Bergeron P, Reggi M, Jausseran J et al. Our experience in superior vena cava surgery (in French). *Ann Chir: Chir Thorac Cardiovasc* 1985; 39: 485-491.

16 Herreros J, Glock Y, De la Fuente A et al. The superior vena cava compression syndrome. Our experience of twenty six cases (in French). *Ann Chir: Chir Thorac Cardiovasc* 1985; 39: 495-512.

17 Moore WM Jr, Hollier LH. Reconstruction of the superior vena cava and central veins. In: *Venous Disorders*, Bergan JJ, Yao JST (eds), Philadelphia, WB Saunders, 1991; pp 517-527.

18 Eklof B, Albrechtson U, Einarsson E, Plate G. The temporary arteriovenous fistula in venous reconstructive surgery. *Int Angio* 1985; 4: 455-462.

19 Eklof BG, Kistner RL, Masuda EM. Venous bypass and valve reconstruction: long-term efficacy. *Vasc Med* 1998; 3: 157-64.

20 Sottiurai VS, Gonzales J, Cooper M et al. A new concept of arteriovenous fistula in venous bypass requiring no fistula interruption: surgical technique and long-term results. *Cardiovasc Surg*, in press.

21 Husfeldt KJ. Venous replacement with Gore-Tex prosthesis: experimental and first clinical results. In: May R, Weber J (eds), *Pelvic and abdominal veins: progress in diagnostics and therapy*. Amsterdam, Excerpta Medica, 1981; pp 249-258.

22 Dale WA, Harris J, Terry RB. Polytetrafluoroethylene reconstruction of the inferior vena cava. *Surgery* 1984; 95: 625-630.

23 Ijima H, Kodama M, Hori M. Temporary arteriovenous fistula for venous reconstruction using synthetic graft: a clinical and experimental investigation. *J Cardiovasc Surg* 1985; 26: 131-136.

24 Plate G, Einarsson E, Eklof B et al. Iliac vein obstruction associated with acute iliofemoral venous thrombosis. Results of early reconstruction using polytetrafluoroethylene grafts. *Acta Chir Scand* 1985; 151: 607-611.

25 Okadome K, Muto Y, Eguchi H et al. Venous reconstruction for iliofemoral venous occlusion facilitated by temporary arteriovenous shunt. Long-term results in nine patients. *Arch Surg* 1989; 124: 957-960.

26 Alimi YS, DiMauro P, Fabre D, Juhan C. Iliac vein reconstructions to treat acute and chronic venous occlusive disease. *J Vasc Surg* 1997; 25: 673-681.

27 Bower TC, Nagorney DM, Cherry KJ Jr et al. Replacement of the inferior vena cava for malignancy: an update. *J Vasc Surg* 2000; 31: 270-281.

28 Victor S, Jayanthi V, Kandasamy I et al. Retro-hepatic cavo-atrial bypass for coarctation of inferior vena cava with a polytetrafluoroethylene graft. *J Thorac Cardiovasc Surg* 1986; 91 : 99-105.

29 Rhee RY, Gloviczki P, Luthra HS et al. Iliocaval complications of retroperitoneal fibrosis. *Am J Surg* 1994; 168: 179-183.

30 Dzsinich C, Gloviczki P, van Heerden JA et al. Primary venous leiomyosarcoma: a rare but lethal disease. *J Vasc Surg* 1992; 15: 595-603.

31 Bower TC, Nagorney DM, Toomey BJ et al. Vena cava replacement for malignant disease: is there a role? *Ann Vasc Surg* 1993; 7: 51-62.

32 Wang ZG, Zhu Y, Wang SH et al. Recognition and management of Budd-Chiari syndrome: report of one hundred cases. *J Vasc Surg* 1989; 10: 149-156.

33 Risher WH, Arensman RM, Ochsner JL, Hollier LH. Retro-hepatic vena cava reconstruction with polytetrafluoroethylene graft. *J Vasc Surg* 1990; 12: 367-370.

34 Kieffer E, Bahnini A, Koskas F. Nonthrombotic disease of the inferior vena cava: surgical management of 24 patients. In: Bergan JJ, Yao JST (eds), *Venous Disorders*. Philadelphia, WB Saunders, 1991; pp 501-516.

35 Sarkar R, Eilber FR, Gelabert HA et al. Prosthetic replacement of the inferior vena cava for malignancy. *J Vasc Surg* 1998; 28: 75-83.

36 Rhee RY, Gloviczki P, Steers JL et al. Superior vena cava reconstruction using an iliocaval allograft. *Vasc Surg* 1996; 30 : 77-83.

37 Yamaguchi A, Eguchi S, Iwasaki T, Asano K. The influence of arteriovenous fistulae on the patency of synthetic inferior vena caval grafts. *J Cardiovasc Surg* 1968; 9: 99-103.

38 Menawat SS, Gloviczki P, Mozes G et al. Effect of a femoral arteriovenous fistula on lower extremity venous hemodynamics after femorocaval reconstruction. *J Vasc Surg* 1996; 24: 793-799.

39 Doty DB, Doty JR, Jones KW. Bypass of superior vena cava. Fifteen years' experience with spiral vein graft for obstruction of superior vena cava caused by benign disease. *J Thorac Cardiovasc Surg* 1990; 99: 889-895.

28

COMPLICATIONS OF VENA CAVAL FILTER PROCEDURES

HEIKE LORCH

Fatal pulmonary embolism (PE) is a major cause of death. Probably more than 250 000 patients are hospitalized annually in the US with venous thromboembolism. The mortality rate of PE is high, with a 3-month mortality rate of 17.5% [1]. In approximately 90% of cases, deep vein thrombosis (DVT) of the leg or pelvic veins is the source of the emboli.
Sufficient anticoagulation decreases the risk of PE. The perioperative prophylactic administration of low doses of subcutaneous unfractioned heparin reduces the rate of fatal PE by at least 60% [2]. However, if anticoagulation is contraindicated or ineffective, a mechanical barrier in the vena cava is a rational attempt to prevent PE.

History

It was John Hunter in 1784 who first ligated the femoral vein in order to reduce PE. In 1868, Trousseau suggested to place a barrier into the inferior vena cava (IVC). Bottini, in 1883, ligated the IVC. Surgical ligation, plication or clipping of the IVC remained the method of choice for vena cava interruption until the early seventies, bound with a mortality rate of 12%. In the 60s, the Mobin-Uddin filter, an inverted umbrella filter with six flat stainless steel spokes, covered with a silastic membrane, was developed. As caval occlusion occurred in 65%, the application of this filter was soon abandoned, but the idea of an endoluminal caval obstruction device was born. In 1973, Greenfield et al. [3] presented a stainless steel device, consisting of six stainless steel wires in a conical shape extending from a central hub. The tips form a circular base with a maximal diameter of 30 mm. The conical geometry allows a progressive vertical filling of the device while maintaining circumferential blood flow. The filter was inserted via a 24F carrier catheter requiring venotomy.

The first filter which could be inserted percutaneously without venotomy was the bird's nest filter, released in 1983. It was the breakthrough for the development of a variety of percutaneously insertable filters. Today, sheath diameters can be as small as 6F.

Permanent vena cava filters (pVCF)

Permanent vena cava filters are inserted into the vena cava and remain there for the duration of the patient's lifetime. Table I summarizes the currently available filter devices, Fig. 1 shows three representative permanent vena cava filters. Clinical experiences with vena cava filters are limited to 20-30 years only. To date, only one randomized and controlled trial evaluating the effectiveness and safety of vena cava filters has been performed [4]. Our knowledge about vena cava filters is based on a bundle of clinical observation studies and case reports, which, in general, do not fulfill the recently published guidelines for vena cava filter evaluation [5]. Nevertheless, in the United States, 30 000 – 40 000 permanent vena cava filters are implanted per year, a number which is still increasing [6]. Complication rates of permanent vena cava filters are estimated to be low.

Table I		CHARACTERISTICS OF WIDELY USED PERMANENT, RETRIEVABLE AND TEMPORARY VENA CAVA FILTERS						
	Producer	*Design*	*Size of sheath*	*Characterization of hooks*	*Number of struts*	*Material*	
Stainless steel Greenfield	Boston Scientific	Conical	12F	6 hooks (at the end of struts)	6	Titanium alloy	p
LGM	Braun	Conical	12F	6 hooks at the fixation struts (parallel to caval wall)	6	Phynox	p
Keeper	Cordis	Conical	12F	2x6, two at each strut, apical and caudal direction	6	Phynox	p
Bird´s nest	Cook	Bird's nest	14F	4 hooks, variable and different fixation levels	4	Stainless steel	p
Simon nitinol	Bard	Umbrella + conical	9F	6 hooks (at the end of struts)	6	Nitinol	p
Antheor	Boston Scientific	Basket	9.5/10.5F	6 hooks struts, (eccentrically at the two fixation levels)	6	Phynox	p
Trap Ease	Cordis	Conical	6F	12 hooks, two fixation levels	6	Nitinol	p
Tempofilter	Braun	Conical	12F	No hooks	8	Phynox	r
Günther tulip	Cook	Conical	10F	4 hooks (at the end of struts)	4	Elgiloy	r
Antheor temporary filter	Boston Scientific	Basketlike	7/8F	No hooks	6	Phynox	t
Prolyser	Cordis	Basketlike	8.5F	No hooks	8	Teflon	t
Günther	Cook	Basketlike	6.5F	No hooks	10	Stainless steel	t

p: permanent
r: retrievable
t: temporary

C.R. Bard GmbH, Wachhausstr. 6, 76227 Karlsruhe, Germany
Boston Scientific Corporation, 480 Pleasant Street, Watertown, MA 02172, USA
B Braun Melsungen AG, Sieversufer 8, 12359 Berlin, Germany
William Cook Europe, Sandet 6, Bjaeverskov, Denmark
Cordis, Oosteinde 8, 9300 AA Roden, Netherlands

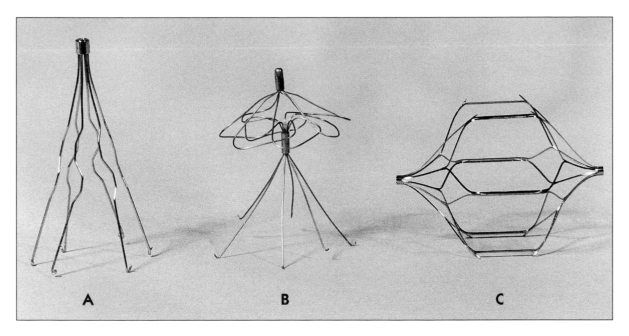

FIG. 1 Permanent vena cava filters. A - Stainless steel Greenfield filter. B - Simon nitinol filter. C - Trap Ease filter.

So, besides classical indications, contraindications to anticoagulation, complications of anticoagulation or ineffective anticoagulation, there is a trend to liberalize permanent filter insertion for other indications like prophylactic insertion in orthopedic or neurosurgical patients without a proven DVT [6], resulting in a shift towards the application of pVCF in younger patients. There are only a few absolute contraindications for insertion of a pVCF, such as inability to gain venous access or complete thrombosis of the IVC. In 2000, two large studies about pVCF were published: a clinical observation study [6], reporting the 26-year single-center experience with 1765 filters, and a review article [7], summarizing and evaluating the results of previously published clinical studies. These publications are the main references of this part of this chapter.

Complications with permanent vena cava filters can be distinguished into complications caused by a filter failure, which means recurrent PE, and complications caused by the filter device itself, so-called filter-related complications. Besides a correct indication, which remains controversial, cavography must be performed prior to filter implantation in every case to rule out anatomic variations like a megacava or significant venous anomalies. Venocavography reveals anatomic variants like a double cava and multiple renal veins in 11% of patients. The only vena cava filter on the market suitable for insertion in a vena cava with a diameter over 28 mm is the bird's nest filter.

Complications of permanent vena cava filters

PULMONARY EMBOLISM (PE)

No filter protects completely against PE. According to the study of Athanasoulis et al. [6], the total prevalence of observed postfilter PE was 5.6%, of which 3.7% was fatal. In most cases, fatal PE occurred soon after filter insertion (median, 4.0 days). According to Streiff [7], no superiority of any filter can be indicated with respect to the incidence of recurrent PE because of the lack of randomized studies (Table II). Although not proven, the current opinion is that recurrent PE is generally due to filter failure, and not to thrombus formation at the filter.

PROCEDURAL PROBLEMS

Technical problems with filter insertion are rare. In a report of 320 cases, Ferris et al. [8] describe a 9.7% rate of insertion problems which were all of minor impact, delivery problems, incomplete opening, difficulties because of tortuous anatomy. Magnant et al. [9] report one fatal procedural complication after placement of a bird's nest filter due to an acute IVC occlusion. Incomplete filter opening, potentially compromising filter function and predisposing to migration, is reported by Wittenberg et al. [10] in 8% of the LGM and 12% of the titanium Greenfield filter insertions. In his meta-analysis, Streiff [7] reports that procedural complications during the delivery of the stainless steel Greenfield filter are rare: 2 cases of pneumothorax, 1 case of a cerebrovascular accident, 3 deaths. Difficulties to release the Simon nitinol filter are reported in 0.3%, incomplete opening of the LGM filter in 5.2%. Streiff reports 1 myocardial infarction, 1 cardiac tamponade and 1 death [7].

FILTER MISPLACEMENT AND TILTING

Filter misplacement means filter delivery in a different than the intended anatomic region, which is usually the inferior infrarenal vena cava. Filter misplacement can lead to filter function loss, filter embolization or tissue damage caused by the filter struts. Filter misplacement rarely occurs and can be of minor importance (misplacement into the iliac vein, suprarenal IVC), sometimes requiring the placement of a second filter. However, misplacement can be significant, like filter displacement into the renal vein or the right atrium. Lahey et al. [11] report

the case of a misplaced filter into the right atrium, causing pericardiac tamponade, requiring emergency surgery. Athanasoulis et al. report one case of a Greenfield filter prematurely released into the right atrium which was explanted by cardiotomy [6].

Filter tilting reduces the clot trapping efficiency of filters in vitro [12], the clinical impact of which remains still unclear. Streiff [7] reports a 5.3% rate of Greenfield filter tilting, a 12.4% of titanium Greenfield filter tilting and a 4.7% of LGM filter tilting. In none of these cases clinical sequelae were obvious.

FILTER MIGRATION

Significant filter migration is defined as caudal or cranial filter movement in excess of one centimeter. Short migration may not be clinically significant. Caudal migration becomes significant if the function of the filter is compromised, which may necessitate the placement of a second filter above. Cranial migration may be fatal or require surgical intervention. Athanasoulis et al. [6] report central migration in 0.1% (2 out of 1731 patients). Two filters (first generation bird's nest, Simon nitinol) which had migrated into the right atrium were retrieved percutaneously. The study of Ferris et al. [8] reports a 6% total rate of migration; some filters were found in the heart or the pulmonary arteries. No surgical interventions were performed and no clinical symptoms were caused by the filters left there. Poillaud

Table II	COMPILATION OF VENA CAVA FILTER STUDY DATA, ACCORDING TO STREIFF [7]					
	PE %	Fatal PE %	New DVT %	IVCT %	PPS %	AST %
Stainless steel Greenfield filter	2.6	0.9	5.9	3.6	19	23
Titanium Greenfield filter	3.1	1.7	22.7	6.5	14.4	28
Bird's nest filter	2.9	0.9	6	3.9	14	23
Simon nitinol	3.8	1.9	8.9	7.7	12.9	31
Vena Tech LGM	3.4	0.3	32	11.2	41	36

AST: access site thrombosis
DVT: deep venous thrombosis
IVCT: inferior vena caval thrombosis
PE: pulmonary embolism
PPS: postphlebitic symdrome

Numbers indicate average percentage rates of patients who were evaluated
Numbers for AST are rates found with routine surveillance for AST

et al. [13] described a case of a sudden death caused by filter migration into the heart. Villard et al. [14] reported ten cases of Greenfield filters which had migrated into the heart. Wittenberg et al. [10] report a 11% rate of LGM filter migration and a 15% rate of titanium Greenfield filter migration. In his overview, Streiff [7] found Greenfield filter migration in 5.3% (clinical sequelae in 0.4%), titanium Greenfield filter migration in 12.8%, bird's nest filter migration in 1.9%, Simon nitinol filter migration in 2.2% and LGM filter migration in 8.3%.

There are no general guidelines how to prevent migration and how to assess migration during follow-up. Mismatch between the filter and caval size should be avoided. After filter implantation, a plain abdominal x-ray should be performed to document the filter position. Filter position should be controlled in every case of suspected recurrent PE and symptoms like sudden onset of cardiac arrhythmia.

CAVAL WALL PERFORATION AND PENETRATION

Caval wall penetration and perforation can either be regarded as a complication or a beneficial mechanism that fixes filters firmly in the IVC. In the editorial *Vena cava filters: prevalent misconceptions* [15], Simon points out that in general, filter struts become incorporated into the caval wall and may extend as much as 5-10 mm outside the imaged vein lumen. This mechanism fixates the filter within the caval wall, prevents migration and is usually asymptomatic. He indicates acute caval wall perforation during filter delivery as a true complication, although asymptomatic in most cases.

Streiff [7] reports a rate of filter strut perforation through the caval wall in 4.4% of the Greenfield filters (0.4% symptomatic), 3.5% of the titanium Greenfield filter, 37.9% of the bird's nest filter (all asymptomatic), and 36.9% of the Simon nitinol filter (one patient symptomatic). Athanasoulis et al. report a 0.1% rate of caval wall perforation, all clinically insignificant [6]. Ferris et al. report one case of filter penetration into the duodenum, one into the iliac artery and two into the aorta, all asymptomatic [8]. Appleberg et al. [16] describe one case of a Greenfield filter perforation into the duodenum, requiring surgery and Kupferschmid et al. [17] report on a small bowel obstruction as a consequence of Greenfield filter migration. A retroperitoneal hemorrhage was caused by the penetration of a Greenfield filter according to Taheri et al. [18].

FILTER FRACTURE

Filter fracture is a relatively rare event in modern filters and usually clinically asymptomatic. No data were found about recurrent PE caused by broken filters. Athanasoulis et al. [6] report filter fracture in 0.2%, Ferris et al. [8] in 2% (no symptoms), and Streiff [7] in 1.3% for the Greenfield filter, 0% for the titanium Greenfield filter, 2.8% for the bird's nest filter, 14.1% for the Simon nitinol filter and 1.7% for the LGM filter.

ACCESS SITE THROMBOSIS (AST), NEW OR INCREASED DVT

Access way thrombosis is a quite common event, which might be dependent on the filter introducer size. It has to be emphasized that venous patency after venotomy is estimated to be less than 60%. Furthermore, 70% of the patients with DVT who do not undergo filter placement or anticoagulant therapy will develop post-thrombotic syndrome (PTS).

Ferris et al. [8] report a 22% rate of new or increased DVT after filter insertion. Athanasoulis et al. [6] report AST, new or worse leg edema, or episodes of new DVT in 3.1% of 1731 patients within 30 days and in 4.0% beyond 30 days. The rates reported by Streiff [7] are summarized in Table II.

CAVAL THROMBOSIS, FILTER THROMBOSIS

Filter thrombosis may have four theoretical causes: the filter device itself may be thrombogenic; the device may be too effective and catch small, harmless clots; iliac thrombi may have propagated into the caval vein and occlude the device; and the filter might have trapped large, potentially life-threatening thrombi, which is the only purpose to insert filters. Filters are made of biocompatible material, so that the chance of thrombi developing at the filter itself should be minimal. The very first vena cava filter, the Mobin-Uddin filter, led to caval occlusion in more than 60% and was subsequently withdrawn from the market. Modern filters try to keep a balance between filtration rates and caval occlusion. A caval occlusion caused by trapped large thrombi should not be considered as a complication of the device, but as a life-saving event. One has to be aware of the fact that before the time of vena cava filters the vena cava was surgically interrupted or narrowed. Numbers of postfilter caval thrombosis vary according to the methods of observation and definition. Athanasoulis et al. [6] report an overall rate of 3.2%, which decreases to 2.7% when the

Mobin-Uddin filter is excluded in the statistics. Rates evaluated by Streiff [7] are shown in Table II.

Besides post-thrombotic syndrome and, in very rare cases, phlegmasia cerulea dolens, one complication of caval occlusion can be the development of large collateral veins which can allow recurrent PE.

RARE COMPLICATIONS

Anecdotal reports of rare complications often concern the 24F original stainless steel Greenfield filter, which is no longer on the market. With this filter, severe hypotension after venotomy, large groin hematomas and a hypertrophic scar at the neck have been reported. Other rare complications of filter insertion include the development of an arteriovenous fistula in the groin, arterial pseudoaneurysms, incidental puncture of the carotid artery followed by the development of a mediastinal hematoma, and chronic right heart failure after formation of an arteriovenous fistula.

THE DECOUSUS STUDY

In 1988, Decousus et al. published the first randomized, controlled study of permanent vena cava filters in the prevention of PE [4]. Vena caval filters were associated with a significant decrease in the incidence of PE compared with anticoagulation alone at 8 to 12 days of follow-up. After 2 years, however, this difference was no longer statistically significant. In contrast, vena cava filters were associated with significantly more recurrent DVT than anticoagulation alone. No difference in bleeding or overall mortality was documented.

Retrievable vena cava filters

Retrievable filters are filters which have the potential to be removed, by means of a snaring hook or a catheter. Experiences with retrievable filters are very limited and little is known about the time frame in which the filter has to be retracted without injuring the caval wall.

TEMPOFILTER

The Tempofilter (Fig. 2) is a conical filter which remains attached to the insertion catheter. During filter use, the tip of the catheter is fixed subcuta-

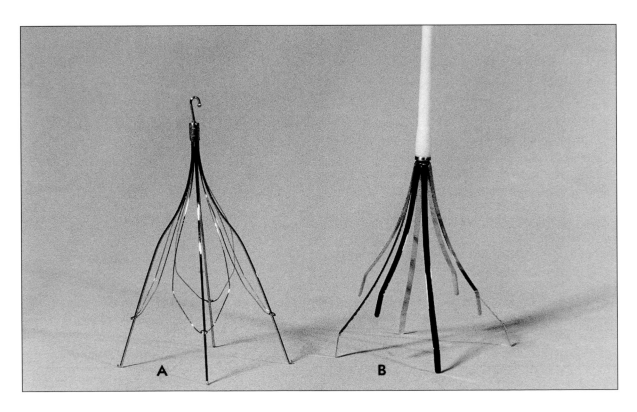

FIG. 2   Retrievable vena cava filters. A - Günther tulip filter. B - Tempofilter.

neously at the neck nearby the insertion site. If the filter has to be removed, it can be extracted under local anesthesia after performing a small incision at the neck.

In 1995, Kuszyk et al. performed an animal filter test in swine [19]. They used the soft catheter prototype which led to cephalic migration in 100% of cases and later on a somewhat stiffer catheter which allowed cephalic migration in 83%. Caval stenosis developed in 40% of the soft catheter pigs and 100% of the stiff catheter pigs. Thrombi at the tethering catheter developed in 20% of the soft and 83% of the stiff catheters, filter cone thrombus was seen in 0% of the soft and 67% of the stiff catheters. Pulmonary embolism occurred in 0% of the soft and 50% of the stiff catheters and death in 0% of the soft and 17% of the stiff catheter pigs. Retraction was possible until 6 weeks after insertion. Kuszyk et al. concluded that *substantial cephalic migration should be expected with this device.* Bovyn et al. reported successful removal of a Tempofilter 55 days after insertion [20]. One filter had to be surgically extracted because of organized thrombi. In 3%, migration to the right atrium was observed.

In 1999, Rossi et al. [21] reported three cases of death after atrial migration of a Tempofilter: two patients died from massive recurrent PE, one patient because of cardiac tamponade. In five patients (3%) atrial migration of the filter occurred. The Tempofilter was withdrawn from the market and the potential of life-threatening complications of the Tempofilter had obviously been underestimated.

GÜNTHER TULIP FILTER

The Günther tulip filter is a conic-shaped filter with a hook at its top which can be retracted with a snare if intended as a temporary filter. Experiences with the retraction of a Günther tulip filter are still very limited: Neuerburg et al. [22] retrieved 2 of 83 filters on day 6 and 11. In a recent report [23], in 9 patients filters were successfully retrieved after a mean implantation period of 8.6 days (range 5-13 days).

Temporary vena cava filters

Temporary filters are attached to a catheter or guide wire which projects from the insertion site, indicating that removal of the filter will be required after a maximum of 14 days. These filters are commercially available in Europe, but not in the USA, because they are not FDA-approved yet. Fig. 3 shows temporary vena cava filters.

The rationale to use temporary vena cava filters is the fact that in specific situations the risk of PE is transient and does not require the insertion of a permanent filter, an indication which should increasingly be considered in young patients. Another argument for the insertion of retrievable or temporary filters are the data of Decousus et al. [4], showing a statistically significant reduction of the rate of recurrent PE only until day 12 after filter insertion, and the study of Athanasoulis et al. [6], reporting a mean time between filter placement and fatal post-filter PE of only 4 days.

Experiences with temporary vena cava filters are limited. There are no controlled, randomized trials signifying that safety and efficacy of temporary vena cava filters have been proven in vivo to date. Patient collectives are inhomogeneous, as indications range from purely prophylactic insertion to implantation in patients with DVT undergoing surgery, patients with transient contraindications for anticoagulation and patients undergoing thrombolysis therapy for DVT. Implantation of vena cava filters seems to be feasible in patients with pelvic or caval thrombosis undergoing ultra-high dose streptokinase thrombolysis, as the rate of fatal PE during this therapy is 15% in case of right-sided iliac vein thrombosis and 6.25% in case of left-sided iliac vein thrombosis [24].

Complications of temporary vena cava filters

PULMONARY EMBOLISM

Systematic screening for recurrent PE during the insertion time of a temporary filter has not been performed in any of the present clinical studies and is a rarely reported complication [25,26]. However, fatal PE occurs in approximately 2% of patients [25,27,28], in most cases during thrombolytic therapy. Although temporary vena cava filters seem to reduce the rate of fatal PE as compared to the PE rates without a filter [24], statistical prove is lacking until now.

FILTER IMPLANTATION PROBLEMS

Problems with filter implantation are rare. In a large multicenter registry [25], implantation problems are reported in 2.2%, all of minor importance:

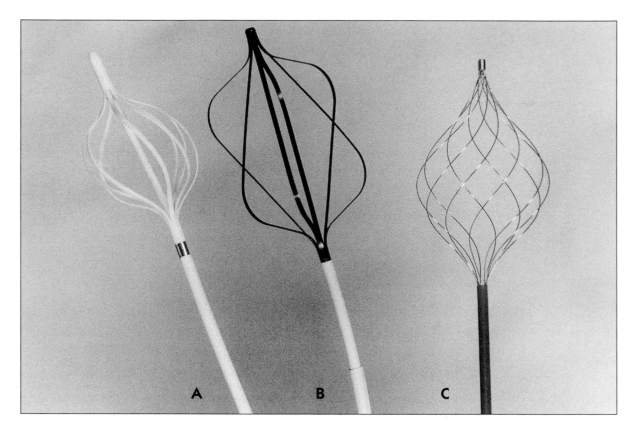

FIG. 3   Temporary vena cava filters. A - Prolyser filter. B - Antheor filter. C - Günther filter.

defect material, one subintimal injection of contrast medium without clinical sequelae, one hemorrhage during thrombolysis after accidental puncture of the brachial artery during insertion. Kunisch et al. reported one case of a incidental puncture of the carotid artery [28].

ACCESS-RELATED COMPLICATIONS

Local complications at the insertion site occur in 2%-46% of cases, the majority of which are hematomas during thrombolysis [27], thrombophlebitis (2.1% [25]), and access vein thrombosis (1-2% [25,27]).

FILTER DISLOCATION

Filter dislocation is reported in 4%-13% of cases and can be clinically insignificant in case of minor dislocation within the caval vein; or significant in case of dislocation into other anatomic regions like the iliac or femoral vein, the right atrium or the superior vena cava. Dislocated filters may allow thrombi to pass [26,27].

ENDOTHELIALISATION

According to the recommendations of the manufacturers, temporary vena cava filters should be removed as soon as possible, but can remain in place for up to 14 days. However, one case of a temporary Günther filter was reported by Burbridge et al. [29], which had been incorporated into the caval wall after 12 days. As the risk of endothelialization is supposed to rise with filter implantation time, early filter removal is essential to avoid this complication.

FILTER THROMBOSIS

If thrombi are found in or at the vena cava filter (Figs. 4,5) before explantation, these thrombi might either have been captured by the filter or have developed at the filter itself. According to an informal recommendation by the filter manufacturers, thrombi smaller than one square cm can be retracted with the filter without any risk. If the thrombus mass is larger, there are several possibilities to solve the problem:
- thrombolysis through the filter;

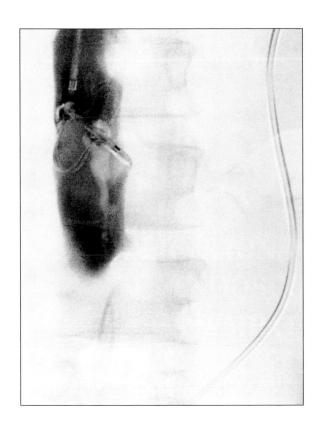

FIG. 4 Thrombi in and at a prolyser temporary filter in a young patient after Cesarean section. The filter is tilted in the inferior vena cava. The thrombus was retracted together with the filter and the sheath without complications.

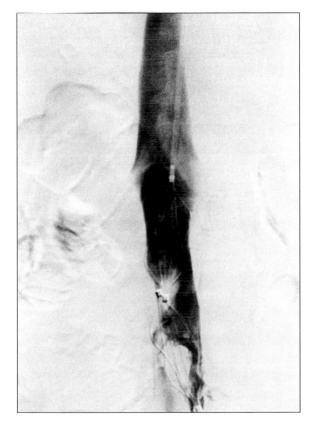

FIG. 5 This patient was submitted from another hospital with two temporary vena cava filters in situ. The first filter had been placed postoperatively via the femoral vein. No thrombolysis was performed. After 14 days, the filter was clotted and the thrombus had propagated into the inferior caval vein. A second filter was placed from a jugular access. No additional therapy was performed. Ten days later, this filter was also thrombosed. We cautiously retracted first the femoral, than the jugular filter without any clinically apparent complications. This example illustrates the need for clear indications for filter insertion and shows that temporary filters should not remain in place longer than absolutaly necessary.

- implantation of a second filter, permanent or temporary;
- cautious retraction with special retraction sets or into a large-size sheath;
- surgical filter explantation.

Thrombi in the filter are found in 16% of cases in the pre-explantation cavography [25].

In this study, 66.6% could be retracted without complications, additional thrombolysis was performed in 16.7%, a second temporary filter was placed in 3.3%, a second permanent filter in 6.7%, and thrombus aspiration was successful in 6.7%. No clinically significant PE was noted during these procedures.

Linsenmaier et al. report a 18% incidence of filter thrombosis, requiring surgery in 2 of 9 patients [30]. Scholz et al [26] found a rate of 7.6% of filter thrombosis (9/118); filters were surgically removed in two patients. After thrombolysis, thrombi were found in the filter in 4.4% (2/45), the filters could be retracted without complications [27].

How to manage thrombus material found in or at the filter before explantation remains an important question and is the main argument against the use of temporary vena cava filters. The situation is paradoxical because the problem rises at the moment when the filter does what it is supposed to do: to catch thrombi. The clinical situation becomes even more uncomfortable if thrombolysis is contraindicated. So, in our opinion, the use of temporary vena cava filters should be limited to very strict indications and the duration of filter implantation should be as short as possible. At our hospital, temporary vena cava filters are used only in case of proven pelvic or caval vein thrombosis if thrombolysis therapy is intended and, in rare cases, during surgery. Filters are removed immediately after termination of thrombolysis or after surgery.

Conclusion

Vena cava filters are endoluminal devices which are inserted percutaneously to prevent potentially life-threatening pulmonary embolism. Because randomized controlled trials are lacking, the indication for filter insertion remains controversial. Whereas the number of permanent filter implantations is continuously rising in the USA, temporary filters are not yet FDA-approved and its use debated in Europe. The definite solution of the filter problem might be the development of retrievable filters, which can be used either as permanent or temporary devices. These filters should be easy and safe to retrieve within a defined period of time, for example 6 weeks.

The best method, of course, to avoid the complications of vena cava filters, is to reduce the incidence of DVT by mechanical and pharmacological methods. In special situations, however, if other methods fail, vena cava filters can be life-saving devices. Their complications have then to be compared with those of the surgical interruption of the vena cava.

REFERENCES

1 Goldhaber SZ, Visani L, De Rosa M. Acute pulmonary embolism: clinical outcome in the International Cooperative Pulmonary Embolism Registry. *Lancet* 1999; 353: 1386-1389.
2 Collins R, Scrimgeour A, Yusuf S et al. Reduction in fatal pulmonary embolism and venous thrombosis by perioperative administration of subcutaneous heparin: overview of results of randomized trials in general, orthopedic and urologic surgery. *N Engl J Med* 1988; 318: 1162-1173.
3 Greenfield LJ, McCurdy JR, Brown PP et al. A new intracaval filter permitting continued flow and resolution of emboli. *Surgery* 1973; 73: 599-606.
4 Decousus H, Leizorovicz A, Parent F et al. A clinical trial of vena caval filters in the prevention of pulmonary embolism in patients with proximal deep-vein thrombosis. *N Engl J Med* 1998; 338: 409-415.
5 Greenfield LJ, Rutherford RB et al. Recommended reporting standards for vena caval filter placement and patient follow-up. Vena cava filter consensus conference. *J Vasc Interv Radiol* 1999; 10: 1013-1019.

6 Athanasoulis CA, Kaufman JA, Halpern EF et al. Inferior vena caval filters: review of a 26-year single-center clinical experience. *Radiology* 2000; 216: 54-66.
7 Streiff MB. Vena caval filters: a comprehensive review. *Blood* 2000; 95: 3669-3677.
8 Ferris EJ, McCowan TC, Carver DK, McFarland DR. Percutaneous vena caval filters: follow-up of seven designs in 320 patients. *Radiology* 1993; 188: 851-856.
9 Magnant JG, Walsh DB, Juravski LI et al. Current use of inferior vena cava filters. *J Vasc Surg* 1992; 16: 701-706.
10 Wittenberg G, Kueppers V, Tschammler A et al. Long-term results of vena cava filters: experiences with the LGM and the titanium greenfield devices. *Cardiovasc Intervent Radiol* 1998; 21: 225-229.
11 Lahey SJ, Meyer LP, Karchmer AW et al. Misplaced caval filter and subsequent pericardial tamponade. *Ann Thor Surg* 1991; 51: 299-301.
12 Greenfield LJ, Proctor MC. Experimental embolic capture by assymetric Greenfield filters. *J Vasc Surg* 1992; 16: 436-444.

13 Pouillaud C, Ollitrault J, Paillard F et al. Proximal migration of a caval filter: apropos of a case. *Ann Cardiol Angiol* 1988; 37: 129-131.

14 Villard J, Detry L, Clermont A, Pinet F. Eight cases of Greenfield filters in the right heart cavities: their surgical treatment. *Ann Radiol* 1987; 30: 102-104.

15 Simon M. Vena cava filters: prevalent misconceptions. *J Vasc Interv Radiol* 1999; 10: 1021-1024.

16 Appleberg M, Crozier JA. Duodenal penetration by a Greenfield caval filter. *Aust N Z J Surg* 1991, 61: 957-960.

17 Kupferschmid JP, Dickson CS, Townsend RN et al. Small-bowel obstruction from an extruded Greenfield filter strut: an unusual late complication. *J Vasc Surg* 1992; 16: 113-115.

18 Taheri SA, Kulaylat MN, Johnson E et al. A complication of the Greenfield filter: fracture and distal migration of two struts – a case report. *J Vasc Surg* 1992; 16: 96-99.

19 Kuszyk BS, Venbrux AC, Samphilipo MA et al. Subcutaneously tethered temporary filter: pathologic effects in swine. *J Vasc Interv Radiol* 1995; 6: 895-902.

20 Bovyn G, Gory P, Reynaud P, Ricco JB. The Tempofilter: a multicenter study of a new temporary caval filter implantable for up to six weeks. *Ann Vasc Surg* 1997; 11: 520-528.

21 Rossi P, Arata FM, Bonaiuti P et al. Fatal outcome in atrial migration of the Tempofilter. *Cardiovasc Intervent Radiol* 1999; 22: 227-231.

22 Neuerburg JM, Gunther RW, Vorwerk D et al. Results of a multicenter study of the retrievable tulip vena cava filter: early clinical experience. *Cardiovasc Intervent Radiol* 1997; 20 : 10-16.

23 Millward SF, Bhargava A, Aquino J Jr et al. Günther tulip filter: preliminary clinical experience with retrieval. *J Vasc Interv Radiol* 2000; 11: 75-82.

24 Martin M. Phleko-/Phlefi-Studien. *VASA* 1997; S 49: 1-39.

25 Lorch H, Welger D, Wagner V et al. Current practice of vena cava filter insertion: a multicenter registry. *J Vasc Interv Radiol* 2000; 11: 83-88.

26 Scholz KH, Just M, Buchwald AB et al. Experiences with temporary vena cava filters in 114 at-risk patients with thrombosis or thromboembolism. *Dtsch Med Wochenschr* 1999; 124: 307-313.

27 Lorch H, Zwaan M, Siemens HJ et al. Temporary vena cava filters and ultrahigh streptokinase thrombolysis therapy: a clinical study. *Cardiovasc Intervent Radiol* 2000; 23: 273-278.

28 Kunisch M, Rauber K, Bachmann G et al. Temporary cava filter: effective prophylaxis of pulmonary embolism in venous thrombosis in the region of the pelvic vascular system and of the inferior vena cava? *Fortsch Röntgenstr* 1995; 163: 523-526.

29 Burbridge BE, Walker DR, Millward SF. Incorporation of the Günther temporary inferior vena cava filter into the caval wall. *J Vasc Interv Radiol* 1996; 7: 289-290.

30 Linsenmaier U, Rieger J, Schenk F et al. Indications, management and complications of temporary vena cava filters. *Cardiovasc Intervent Radiol* 1998; 21: 464-469.

29

COMPLICATIONS OF SURGERY
FOR VARICOSE VEINS

CHRISTOS D LIAPIS, JOHN D KAKISIS

Although varicose veins are a disease of western civilization, there is good evidence that they have afflicted humans since antiquity. An ancient Greek bas-relief shows a patient, probably asking for a cure, presenting a votive tablet of a leg with a large varicosity to Asclepios (Fig. 1). The operative treatment of varicose veins was described much later by Celcus (25 B.C. to A.D. 50). The Byzantine surgeon Orivasius (4th century A.D.) described in detail the operative techniques for varicose veins, including preoperative tourniquet testing and stab incisions that were rediscovered 1 500 years later [1]. Injection therapy was introduced in 1853 by Cassaignac. Nowadays, continuing advances in technology have led to a new era, where a lot of information about varicose vein surgery is available on numerous Internet web sites [2].

Incidence of complications

Surgery for varicose veins appears on the top of the list of the most frequently performed procedures (50 000 per year in the UK) [3]. Despite the significant progress in medicine and technology, complications of varicose vein surgery as well as recovery expectations continue to be among the main focuses of interest of both the surgeons and the patients. In general, varicose vein surgery is considered to be a safe procedure. However, it has a broad variety of complications ranging from minor ones (such as bleeding, hematoma, wound infection, and saphenous nerve injury), to limb-threatening conditions such as injury to the femoral artery or vein, and even life-threatening situations such as pulmonary embolism.

The overall incidence of complications in varicose vein surgery ranges between 2% and 58% [4-8]. There are two main reasons accounting for the wide variation in the reported incidence of complications. The first reason is that most of the studies referring to complications are retrospective. This fact leads to an underestimation of the complication risk, since some minor complications will not be recorded. The second reason is that many papers focus exclusively on specific complications such as vascular or nerve injuries, making the estimation of the overall incidence of complications impossible. Whichever the exact incidence, major complications are undoubtedly rare. On the other hand, minor complications gain particular importance not only because they are more frequent, but also because they develop on the grounds of an operation often performed for cosmetic reasons only.

Complications of varicose vein surgery can be divided into two categories: local and distant. Local complications include hematomas, wound infections, vascular injuries, lymphatic complications, nerve injuries, venous thromboses, and recurrent varices, while distant complications include pulmonary embolism and sexual complications (Table).

This chapter addresses the problems associated with these complications, with emphasis on methods of prevention and treatment.

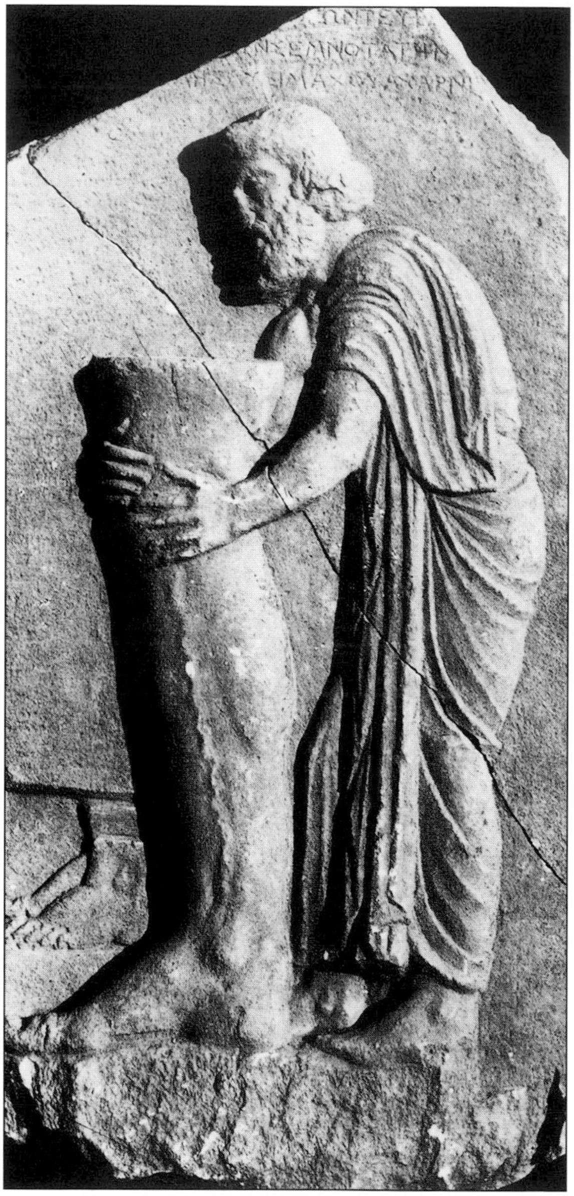

Hematomas

Hematomas are the most frequent of all complications, occurring almost constantly after saphenous vein stripping. They are usually caused by avulsion of perforating veins of the thigh or the accessory saphenous vein. Their occurrence is so common and (to some degree) expected, that many authors do not consider them as complications but as a normal consequence of the stripping procedure [9].

Hematomas are more spectacular in obese patients, since diffusion of blood in the fatty tissue is easier. Spinal anesthesia is also associated with a higher risk of postoperative hematoma due to the

FIG. 1 Ancient Greek bas-relief showing a patient presenting a votive tablet of a leg with a large varicosity to Asclepios (*National Archeological Museum of Athens*).

Table	COMPLICATIONS OF VARICOSE VEIN SURGERY	
	Local	*Distant*
	Hematomas	Pulmonary embolism
	Wound infections	Sexual complications
	Vascular injuries	
	Lymphatic complications	
	Nerve injuries	
	Venous thromboses	
	Recurrent varices	

vascular paralysis caused by the sympathetic block. On the contrary, general anesthesia is believed to be helpful in diminishing the risk of hematoma formation due to its stimulatory effects on the coagulation system [9]. Similarly, the injection of xylocaine plus adrenaline at the level of perforating veins, in cases of local anesthesia, results in fewer and smaller hematomas. As regards the technique of stripping, it seems that a violent and rapid traction of the stripper is related to an increased incidence of hematomas, while several procedures that have been proposed in order to reduce that risk, such as stripping with mesh or invagination [10-13] or cryosurgery [14-15], have not proved advantageous [9,13].

Several devices have also been used for the purpose of reducing intra-operative blood loss and postoperative bruising. Corbett and Jayakumar [16] showed a significant decrease in mean blood loss with the use of an Esmarch tourniquet. Similarly, Thompson et al. [17] found that blood loss was significantly less and postoperative cosmetics significantly improved with the use of a pneumatic tourniquet, while no difference was found in the extent of bruising. In a recent trial by Sykes et al. [18], both the peri-operative blood loss and the extent of bruising were significantly reduced when the autoclavable Lofquist cuff was used as a tourniquet in varicose vein surgery. Using the same cuff, Robinson et al. [19] reported that the blood loss from the avulsion sites during routine varicose vein surgery was significantly reduced, and this encouraged the surgeons to perform more avulsions.

Postoperatively, the standard way of preventing these hematomas consists of the compression of the operated limb with elastic bandages from the ankle to groin. The main problem with this type of bandaging is that the duration of effective compression is short due to slipping of the bandage. As Raj et al. [20] have demonstrated, this is especially true in the case of ambulatory treatment of varicose veins, since the exerted pressure falls to 0-15 mmHg after 6-8 hours of normal activity. In order to overcome this difficulty, Travers et al. [21] have proposed the application of a high-compression short-stretch adhesive bandage, which was shown to achieve symptomatic improvement with less bruising postoperatively. For the same purpose, Raso et al. [22] introduced a two-part device functioning as an elastic and pneumatic bandage. The authors report complete disappearance of postoperative hematomas with the use of this device.

Despite their frequency, hematomas do not constitute any major concern, since they are almost always completely absorbed without any further action except for the elastic bandage. Non-steroid anti-inflammatory drugs might also be used in some cases to prevent hypodermitis. Only on very rare occasions, where the hematoma continues to enlarge or becomes infected, should it be evacuated and drained [23]. In a series of 1 250 patients operated on over 19 years in our department, transfusion was required once, in a female patient with a previously undiagnosed coagulation disorder.

Wound infections

The meticulous application of general concepts and techniques of asepsis and antisepsis as well as the employment of single-use strippers have made wound infections, cellulites, and abscesses quite rare, with a reported incidence of less than 1% [9]. Concomitant pathologic situations and limb infections increase the risk, while obesity does not seem to play an important role. In order to minimize the risk of infection, venous ulcers and fungus infections of the toes and feet should be treated before the operation. Preferably, the operation should be delayed 4 to 6 weeks after healing [22]. When infection does occur, it can usually be managed by routine principles of wound care. Unless the patient becomes febrile or develops a spreading cellulitis, antibiotics are seldom necessary. In cases of abscesses, open drainage is required with the only adverse but inevitable sequel being an unsightly scar. In our series of 1 250 operations, we encountered only 4 wound infections requiring prolonged antibiotic treatment.

Vascular injuries

Injuries to the femoral vessels are among the most serious complications of varicose vein surgery. They occur in about 0.1%-4% of cases, with the venous injuries being five times more common than arterial injuries [24,25]. The causes of such injuries include:
1 - inadequate exposure of the saphenofemoral junction;
2 - erroneous identification of the vessels in the surgical field;

3 - blind grasping with artery forceps in cases of bleeding;

4 - excessive traction of the saphenous vein during exposure of the saphenofemoral junction.

Anatomic variations, surgery for recurrent disease, and operations performed by inexperienced surgeons with poor surgical technique and inadequate knowledge of anatomy, are additional factors contributing to the occurrence of vascular complications [25].

As a general rule, we should always keep in mind that clamping, transection, ligation, and stripping should be avoided before positive identification of vascular structures. Adequate exposure is mandatory. There is no justification for keyhole surgery in this area, since cosmetic reasons can never outweigh the risk of vascular injury [26]. Additional care should be taken in thin patients, where both the common femoral artery and vein are superficially located and can be easily mistaken for the long saphenous vein [25,27]. Such a confusion is facilitated by the fact that the artery may become spastic during dissection and appear bluish like a vein. An extremely rare (0.02%) anatomic variation, where the femoral vein and artery are transposed in the region of the fossa ovalis, has also been described [28].

As in any other case in medicine, the best way of treatment is prevention. If, however, a vascular injury occurs, prompt recognition and immediate repair are usually followed by a good outcome, while failure to note occlusive damage is catastrophic. Postoperative diagnosis of arterial injury is often delayed because the pain of ischemia may be mistaken for the pain of the surgical trauma. Accurate differential diagnosis of postoperative pain is therefore mandatory [29]. Pain arising from the surgical trauma is tolerable; pulses are present and skin is normal. Unusually severe pain accompanied by numbness, paleness and coldness of the foot must be considered as ischemic until proven otherwise. A tight bandage is a common cause of peripheral ischemia but it is easily ruled out, since the pain is immediately relieved on relaxation of the bandage. The presence of edema and a doppler examination will also rule out deep venous thrombosis.

The choice of the optimal arterial reconstruction will be based on an angiography, which will determine the extent of damage and provide a mapping of the residual arterial tree. Basic principles of such a reconstruction are the following ones.

1 - The deep femoral artery is the first to be revascularized.

2 - The anterior tibial artery is in place and never damaged by the stripper due to its off-course direction.

3 - The long saphenous vein is frequently intact and usable. In such cases, it is the vascular conduit of choice for a femoral-distal bypass. When, on the other hand, the long saphenous vein is not suitable, the contralateral long saphenous vein should be used.

4 - Revascularization of a single tibial artery is sufficient for good long-term results.

Based on these principles, Ramsheyi et al. [29] reported two cases of limb salvage after inadvertent arterial stripping during varicose vein surgery. Four more cases of successful arterial reconstruction are reported by Natali [27], in a series of seven arterial strippings. In the remaining three patients, a major amputation was required. Pegoraro et al. [30] report a limb salvage with the use of a composite bypass between the femoral artery and the posterior tibial artery. No arterial injuries occurred in our series. There was only one case of arterial stripping referred to our department, which required a below-knee amputation due to late recognition.

As regards venous injuries, profuse bleeding and marked edema of the limb are the main manifestations of injury to the deep venous system. Inadvertent stripping of the femoral vein is undoubtedly the most serious of such injuries, the reconstruction of which is extremely demanding. When the saphenous vein remains intact, venous outflow may be restored by reconstruction of the junction between the common femoral vein, the deep femoral vein and the saphenous vein below the inguinal ligament and by surgical connection between the deep and superficial venous system below the knee [31].

Nerve injuries

Injury to the saphenous nerve is one of the most common and well-known complications of varicose vein surgery. The saphenous nerve arises from the femoral nerve at the level of the femoral triangle and enters the adductor canal (canal of Hunter) along with the superficial femoral artery and vein (Fig. 2). It then pierces the fascia lata between the tendons of the sartorius and gracilis muscles and becomes subcutaneous on the medial aspect of the leg. From this point on, it gradually approaches the great saphenous vein and courses along with it to the level of the medial malleolus.

Due to its close proximity to the long saphenous vein [32], the saphenous nerve is frequently damaged during stripping of the saphenous vein, with resulting troublesome paresthesia, anesthesia, or hyperesthesia in the medial aspect of the lower third of the thigh and the medial aspect of the leg and the foot, including the great toe. The reported incidence of such injuries ranges between 23% and 58% [7,8,33]. Stripping the vein through the ankle incision rather than the groin incision has reduced the incidence but not eliminated it [34-37]. In any case, the numbness usually greatly diminishes in area or disappears within a year.

Several authors have suggested that the incidence of injury to the saphenous nerve may be further reduced if the long saphenous vein is stripped from the groin to the upper calf only. Preservation of the distal long saphenous vein not only reduces nerve damage but also retains enough vein for use, should coronary artery bypass or peripheral vascular grafting be necessary in the future. This procedure reduces the risk of saphenous nerve injuries to about 4%-7%, while it does not increase the risk of recurrence [33,38].

Indeed, Holme et al. [6] found, in a long-term randomized study of classical (total) versus partial (i.e., only of the femoral part) stripping of the long saphenous vein, that 29% of the patients who were submitted to total stripping had permanent lesions of the saphenous nerve, whereas only 5% of the patients who were submitted to partial stripping had lasting nerve lesions (p<0.01). Recurrent varicosities developed in 10% of patients in both groups. The authors conclude that total stripping of the long saphenous vein should be abandoned as a routine in varicose vein stripping, since it increases the permanent nerve damage six-fold without reducing long-term recurrence. Our incidence of saphenous nerve injury in cases of stripping to the ankle was 25%; with just below-knee stripping it was 6%.

The femoral nerve is almost never injured during saphenous vein stripping since it does not lie in close vicinity to the vein. The femoral nerve exits the greater pelvis through the muscular compartment inferior to the inguinal ligament, coursing lateral to the femoral artery, which lies laterally to the femoral vein. Complications regarding the femoral nerve are more likely to occur as consequences of locoregional anesthesia. Residual paresthesia at the distribution of the femoral nerve as well as transient quadriceps palsy after femoral nerve block have been reported [39,40].

On the contrary, injury to the common peroneal nerve after varicose vein surgery is a well-known complication. The common peroneal nerve arises in the popliteal fossa as the sciatic nerve bifurcates into the common peroneal and tibial nerves (Fig. 3). The common peroneal nerve diverges laterally, passes posterior to the head of the fibula, and laterally across the neck of that bone it divides into the superficial peroneal and the deep peroneal nerves.

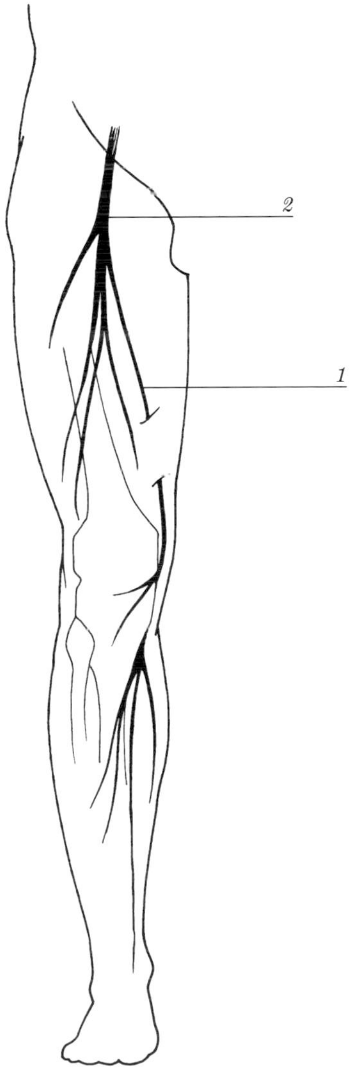

1. Saphenous nerve
2. Femoral nerve

FIG. 2   Course and distribution of the saphenous nerve.

Due to these anatomic relations, the common peroneal nerve can be injured either by attempts at blind avulsion of varices through stab incisions or by excessive retraction of the nerve in order to expose the saphenopopliteal junction [33]. Re-explorations of the popliteal fossa for previous inadequate saphenopopliteal ligation, as well as primary operations when the saphenopopliteal junction is higher than usual above the knee crease, carry a particular risk of injury to the common peroneal nerve.

Such an injury results in foot-drop (inability to dorsiflect the foot or to stand back on the heels) as well as in loss of sensation along the lateral aspect of the leg and dorsum of the foot. Peroneal nerve palsy produces a characteristic gait with *foot-slap*. Dissection of the short saphenous vein might also result in damage of the sural nerve with subsequent loss of sensation along the posterior aspect of the leg. The sural nerve is formed by contributions from the tibial and common peroneal nerves and is damaged in 0%-21% of the operations performed for the treatment of varicose veins [33,38].

Lymphatic complications

Injury to the lymphatic vessels is an inevitable consequence of varicose vein surgery. During exposure of the saphenofemoral junction, numerous microscopic lymphatic vessels that are not visible, are destroyed. Similarly, stripping of the long saphenous vein causes destruction of the perivascular lymphatic plexus, even if less traumatic techniques, such as stripping with invagination or mesh, are employed. Despite these unavoidable injuries to the lymphatics, postoperative complications develop in less than 1% of the patients. This contradiction is due to the remarkable regeneration ability of the lymphatics. Animal studies have shown that half of the lesions to the lymhatics are repaired within eight days from the operation, while one month after the surgical injury complete restoration has been achieved [41].

There are four major categories of lymphatic complications: lymphorrhea, lymphocele, lymphangitis, and lymphedema. The first three are transient, while the fourth is usually permanent.

Lymphorrhea is undoubtedly the most common lymphatic complication. In a multicenter retrospective review of 184 182 patients, based on personal communication, Ouvry et al. [41] reported a 0.54%

incidence of lymph leakage after variceal surgery. They note, however, that this number may be an underestimate of the true incidence of lymphorrhea due to the inherent disadvantages of a retrospective study. In the series of Critchley et al. [4], leakage of lymph from the groin incision occurred only in re-explorations with an incidence of 4.5%, while lymph leak from the phlebectomy sites was very rare, occurring in only 0.3% of the patients. The authors remark that re-exploration of the groin for recurrence is a potentially dangerous procedure, carrying a higher risk of hematoma formation, infection, lymphatic fistula, and venous injury.

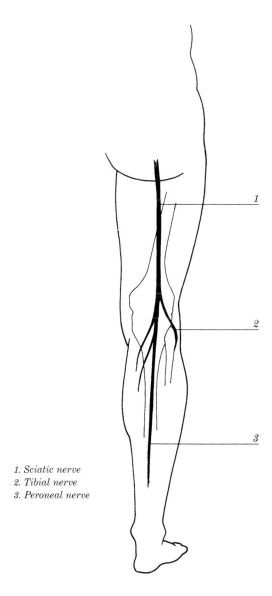

1. *Sciatic nerve*
2. *Tibial nerve*
3. *Peroneal nerve*

FIG. 3 Branches of the sciatic nerve.

Fortunately, lymphedema, which is the most serious of all lymphatic complications, is much more rare. Critchley [4] reported only one lymphedema out of 973 operated limbs; it occurred in a patient operated on for the third time in the groin. In the review of Ouvry et al. [41], the incidence was 0.05%, indicating that the risk of lymphedema in a normal patient who is submitted to varicose vein surgery is minimal. If, however, there is a pre-existing lymphatic insufficiency resulting either from aplasia, hypoplasia, or dysplasia of the lymphatics, it would be prudent to avoid stripping of the long saphenous vein and use sclerotherapy instead. A careful preoperative clinical examination is therefore mandatory and, if lymphatic insufficiency is suspected, radionuclear lymphangiography should be performed.

Management of lymphatic complications is sometimes difficult. Compression is the mainstay of treatment in cases of lymphedema, lymphocele and lymphorrhea, while lymphangitis requires antibiotic administration.

Thrombo-embolic complications

The incidence of thrombo-embolic complications in varicose vein surgery is very low. In the series of Critchley et al. [4], the risk of deep vein thrombosis was 1:200 and for pulmonary embolism 1:600. Similarly, Miller et al. [5] reported an incidence of 0.7% for deep vein thrombosis and 0.2% for pulmonary embolism. By comparison of unilateral surgery versus bilateral surgery, he concluded that an increased length of time on the operating table does not increase the incidence of thrombo-embolic complications, while early mobilization may play a role, as may the prolonged use of elastic stockings. The low incidence of deep thrombophlebitis (0.6%) in the series of Keith and Smead [23] was also attributed to the early and frequent postoperative ambulation, while the authors report their doubts on whether these cases represent true complications or reactivation of unrecognized previous disease.

An even lower incidence at 0.15% for deep vein thrombosis and 0.06% for pulmonary embolism was suggested by Hagemuller [24], while Baccaglini et al. [39] had no thrombo-embolic complications in their series of 2 568 patients being submitted to outpatient surgery of varices. Likewise, a prospective study of the thrombotic risk of varicose vein stripping, which was conducted by Bohler et al. [42], disclosed no postoperative deep vein thrombosis in 100 limbs investigated.

Taking into consideration the very low risk of thrombo-embolic complications and, on the other hand, the high incidence of hematomas, most surgeons suggest that routine anticoagulant prophylaxis in a patient submitted to varicose vein surgery is not justified. Other methods of antithrombotic prophylaxis should be used instead. Keeping the duration of the operation short, tilting the operating table head-down and the use of graduated compression stockings after operation may be helpful, while early mobilization is essential. Anticoagulant prophylaxis should be reserved for high-risk patients, such as patients with history of thrombo-embolic disease or other risk factors for deep vein thrombosis [9,43-45]. These factors include obesity, advanced age, particularly long operations, and the contraceptive pill [44].

There are, however, some authors advocating routine anticoagulation in all patients undergoing varicose vein surgery [46-49]. In a large retrospective series of 19 161 patients who were operated on for various diseases, Huber et al. [47] found a 0.56% incidence of postoperative pulmonary embolism after varicose vein stripping, which was similar to the incidences of 0.40% that was observed after biliary surgery and 0.60% after laparotomy. Based on these findings, the authors recommend routine prophylactic anticoagulation in all patients undergoing varicose vein surgery. In this study, however, no attempt was made in order to discriminate patients according to obesity, age, or prior deep venous disease.

On the other hand, we should not forget that heparin itself can be associated with side effects as shown in the report of Parvulesco [50] on the use of heparin employed in the prevention of deep vein thrombosis in 60 varicose vein surgery patients. Hemorrhagic complications were noted in 13.3% of the patients treated with unfractionated heparin and in 3.3% treated with low molecular weight heparin. This rate of complications far exceeded the risk of postoperative thromboembolism shown in this study.

In order to examine current surgical practice in the prophylaxis of thromboembolism by vascular specialists undertaking varicose vein surgery, Campbell and Ridler [44] sent a questionnaire to members of the *Vascular Surgical Society* of Great

Britain and Ireland. The results of the survey showed that subcutaneous heparin prophylaxis was always used by 12% of the surgeons, selectively by 71%, and never by 17%. A similar study by Lees et al. [45] showed that 27% of the surgeons used deep vein thrombosis prophylaxis in patients undergoing varicose vein surgery routinely, 62% selectively, and 11% never. In our department, we encountered no thrombo-embolic complications in 1250 patients with a rate of 5% prophylaxis used in selected cases. In the era of evidence-based medicine, the strategy of selective anticoagulant prophylaxis seems to be justified.

Sexual complications

Another complication of varicose vein surgery, which is often ignored and only occasionally reported, is postoperative erectile dysfunction [51]. It is undoubtedly rare, however, there are certain cases where impotence develops in a patient immediately after saphenous vein stripping. It is known from the anatomy that the erectile tissue (corpora cavernosa) of the penis is supplied by the internal pudendal arteries, while the superficial skin of the penis is supplied by both the internal as well as the external pudendal arteries, which arise from each femoral artery. In cases of congenital malformation or other obstructive lesions of the internal pudendal arteries, a collateral circulation develops through the external pudendal arteries, which, in this way, become the main arteries supplying the corpora cavernosa. It should be noted that even in such cases, the external pudendal artery is about 1.5 millimeter in diameter and is therefore easily sacrificed by the surgeon in his attempt to achieve better access to the saphenofemoral junction. This is more likely to happen when the external pudendal artery crosses the femoral and the saphenous vein at a level immediately below the saphenofemoral junction (30%-35% of the patients). In cases where the erectile function is based on the external pudendal artery, ligation of this artery will have devastating consequences for the sexual potency of the man who is submitted to saphenous vein stripping. Unfortunately, there is no way for the surgeon to know that beforehand.

Recurrent varicose veins

Varicose vein surgery is associated with a substantial rate of recurrence, ranging from 7% to 65% [8,38,52,53]. Different surgical techniques, follow-up periods and ways of assessment account for this wide variation in the reported rates of recurrence. In any case, recurrence rates of varicose vein surgery remain unacceptably high. This fact represents a great problem both for the patient, who will have to be re-operated on, as well as for the surgeon, who will have to face his failure to provide lasting relief from varicose veins. In addition, it is a heavy burden for the healthcare system, which will see its cost-effectiveness decreasing and the waiting lists enlarging. Indeed, it has been demonstrated by the Lothian surgical audit database that 20% of varicose vein surgery currently performed is for the treatment of recurrences [54].

Several studies have been performed in order to clarify the reasons why varicose veins recur. These reasons can be divided into two major categories (Fig. 4), according to a classification proposed by Stonebridge et al. [55]. Type 1 recurrences result from failure to deal adequately with the saphenofemoral venous complex. This group can be further divided into type 1A recurrences, where the main stem of the long saphenous vein has been left intact, type 1B, where the reflux ensues from residual saphenofemoral complex tributaries connecting the deep and the superficial system, and type 1C, where the communication between the deep and the superficial system is restored due to neovascularization. On the contrary, in type 2 recurrences, the saphenofemoral venous complex has been adequately obliterated. In these cases, the recurrence arises either from direct connections with abdominal and perineal veins (2A) or as a result of an incompetent thigh perforator (2B). Short saphenous vein incompetence represents an additional cause of recurrence.

Type 1 is the most frequent type of recurrence, accounting for 61%-72% of the cases [55-58]. An intact long saphenous vein (type 1A) is found in 12%-66% [55,58-61], intact tributaries (type 1B) in 44%-46% [55,59,60] and neovascularization (type 1C) in 3%-54% [55,58]. It should be noted that while neovascularization has been accepted as a major cause of recurrent connections between the femoral vein and the retained long saphenous vein [58-60,62-64], there are authors who dissent with this mechanism of recurrence [65]. Alternatively, they suggest that these connections are due to a residual rather than a newly formed network of interconnecting veins.

Type 2 recurrences account for 28%-32% of the cases [55,56]. A mid-thigh perforator (type 2B) is found in 11%-53% of limbs with recurrent varicose veins [55,57,59-61], while cross-groin recurrence (type 2A) is uncommon, occurring in only 4% [55].

The short saphenous vein contributes to the recurrence of varicose veins in 6%-33% of the cases [57,66,67]. This can either be due to failure to identify this vein as a source of the varicosity at the time of the original surgery, or to the development of saphenopopliteal incompetence after the original surgery.

The classification described by Stonebridge et al. is treatment-oriented, allowing identification of the type of recurrence with respect to the type of surgical procedure required. All type 1 recurrences require full re-exploration of the saphenofemoral junction, while type 2 recurrences do not require

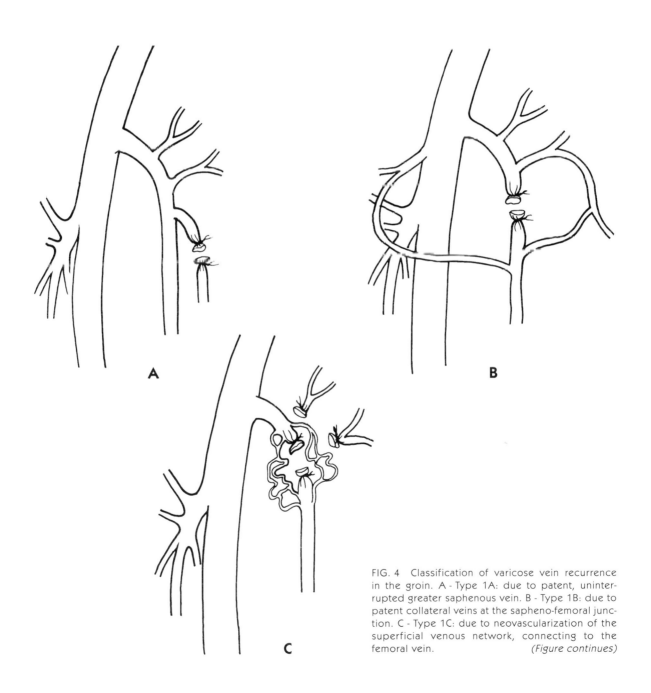

FIG. 4 Classification of varicose vein recurrence in the groin. A - Type 1A: due to patent, uninterrupted greater saphenous vein. B - Type 1B: due to patent collateral veins at the sapheno-femoral junction. C - Type 1C: due to neovascularization of the superficial venous network, connecting to the femoral vein.   *(Figure continues)*

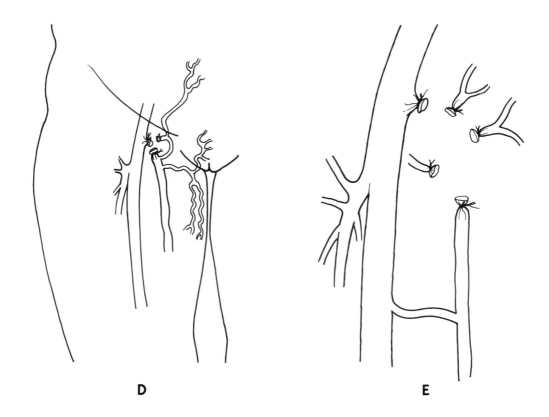

D   E

FIG. 4 (continued) D - Type 2A: adequate resection of sapheno-femoral junction, however, reflux established through perineal and abdominal veins. E - Type 2B: adequate resection, however, remaining perforating vein(s) in the mid-thigh.

groin re-exploration; they require local excision of veins. Minor residual or recurrent veins can be controlled with sclerosing injections of sodium tetradecyl sulfate.

Several studies have been performed in order to determine the treatment of choice for varicose veins, with respect to the lower recurrence rate. Surgery has been found to be associated with improved long-term results than injection sclerotherapy alone [68-70]. As regards the type of surgical procedure, it has been shown that stripping of the long saphenous vein confers a significant advantage over saphenofemoral ligation alone. Three prospective randomized studies by Sarin et al. [71], Rutgers et al. [7], and Neglen et al. [72] showed that the cosmetic results, both judged by the patient and the surgeon, were significantly better in the stripped limbs than in the limbs with high saphenofemoral ligation combined with sclerotherapy or multiple avulsions. In all three studies, clinical examination, doppler or duplex ultrasound testing, and photo-plethysmography verified the superiority of long saphenous stripping. Similarly, Jones et al. [63] found that stripping of the long saphenous vein reduced the rate of recurrence from 43% to 25%, while Dwerryhouse et al. [73] reported that stripping of the long saphenous vein reduced the risk of re-operation by two-thirds after five years.

In accordance with these findings, a double-blind controlled trial by Munn et al. [8] showed that the results of treatment, judged solely by the incidence of varicosities at follow-up, were significantly better in limbs from which the long saphenous vein had been stripped. However, the increased incidence of paresthesia in stripped limbs biased patient opinion against stripping. The authors comment that, in the patients' view, the complications produced by ankle to groin stripping outweighed the advantage of a lessened incidence of varicosities after treatment.

Taking into account that:
1 - saphenofemoral dissection combined with stripping provides the best results,

2 - and stripping to the ankle does not appear to confer any additional benefit over stripping to the knee but does significantly increase the number of saphenous nerve injuries, we could say that stripping to the knee or just below, combined with multiple avulsions, is the treatment of choice for varicose veins.

It is a choice strongly supported by level I evidence. The procedure should be complemented by suturing the fascia over the cribriform opening, in order to avoid recurrences due to neovascularization [74]. Alternatively, the long saphenous vein could be removed by sequential avulsion from the groin to below the knee, as Khan et al. [75] have suggested. According to these authors, sequential avulsion is less painful, reduces bruising, and avoids a significant scar below the knee.

Contrary to the results of the above mentioned randomized studies, there have been two comparative trials by Woodyer and Dormandy [76] and Hammarsten, et al. [77] showing no differences between stripped and non-stripped limbs after three and four years, respectively. However, in both studies saphenous vein sparing surgery was based on a thorough preoperative ultrasonographic or phlebographic mapping of all insufficient perforators followed by ligation of such at surgery. Whether such a strategy is justified in terms of practicability, simplicity, cost and effectiveness is questionable.

Miscellaneous

Poor quality of the stripper may result in rupture during the stripping procedure. Although such a mishap cannot normally elude observation, there have been cases where components of vein strippers were left behind in the leg at the primary procedure and later recovered, having presented as a mass or a sinus [26]. Careful inspection of the stripped vein and the stripper will guarantee that no such complication will be left unnoticed.

Chest infections, anesthetic complications, and keloid scars after varicose vein surgery are also reported occasionally.

Conclusion

Varicose vein surgery is by all means a safe procedure if performed lege artis. Most of the complications are minor and inherited with the procedure and the anatomy of the vein system. However, particular attention has to be devoted to both:
1 - the preoperative diagnosis and planning as well as patient *education* about the disease and the outcome,
2 - and careful following of the details in the execution of the operation.

Scientific information regarding rate of complications and outcome, including patient satisfaction, cannot be obtained unless we all agree, patients included, on what should be named a complication and what the expectations of this surgical procedure are.

ACKNOWLEDGEMENTS
The authors wish to thank Ms. Maria Kouvaraki, MD, for the drawings.

R E F E R E N C E S

1 Lascaratos J, Liapis C, Kouvaraki M. Surgery on varix in Byzantine times (324-1453 AD). *J Vasc Surg* 2000; 33: 197-203.
2 Libertiny G, Perkins JM, Magee TR et al. Varicose veins on the Internet. *Eur J Vasc Endovasc Surg* 2000; 20: 386-389.
3 Anonymous. Department of Health and Social Security. Hospital episode statistics 1987-1988. London: DHSS, 1988.
4 Critchley G, Handa A, Maw A et al. Complications of varicose vein surgery. *Ann R Coll Surg Engl* 1997; 79: 105-110.
5 Miller GV, Lewis WG, Sainsbury JR et al. Morbidity of varicose vein surgery: auditing the benefit of changing clinical practice. *Ann R Coll Surg Engl* 1996; 78: 345-349.
6 Holme JB, Skajaa K, Holme K. Incidence of lesions of the saphenous nerve after partial or complete stripping of the long saphenous vein. *Acta Chir Scand* 1990; 156: 145-148.
7 Rutgers PH, Kitslaar PJ. Randomized trial of stripping versus high ligation combined with sclerotherapy in the treatment of the incompetent greater saphenous vein. *Am J Surg* 1994; 168: 311-315.
8 Munn SR, Morton JB, Macbeth WA et al. To strip or not to strip the long saphenous vein? A varicose vein trial. *Br J Surg* 1981; 68: 426-428.
9 Millien JP, Coget JM. Complications of superficial venous surgery of the legs: thigh hematomas and abscess. *Phlebologie* 1993; 46: 583-590.
10 Fullarton GM, Calvert MH. Intraluminal long saphenous vein stripping: a technique minimizing perivenous tissue trauma. *Br J Surg* 1987; 74: 255.
11 Van der Stricht PJ. Saphénectomie par invagination sur fil. *La Presse Médicale* 1963; 71: 1081-1082.
12 Goren G, Yellin AE. Invaginated axial saphenectomy by a semirigid stripper: perforate-invaginate stripping. *J Vasc Surg* 1994; 20: 970-977.
13 Durkin MT, Turton EPL, Scott DJ et al. A prospective randomized trial of PIN versus conventional stripping in varicose vein surgery. *Ann R Coll Surg Engl* 1999; 81: 171-174.
14 Cheatle TR, Kayombo B, Perrin M. Cryostripping the long and short saphenous veins. *Br J Surg* 1993; 80: 1283.

15 Milleret R. Mon expérience de la cryochirurgie des varices. *Phlebologie* 1989; 42: 573-577.

16 Corbett R, Jayakumar K. Clean up varicose vein surgery - use a tourniquet. *Ann R Coll Surg Engl* 1989; 71: 57-58.

17 Thompson JF, Royle GT, Farrands PA et al. Varicose vein surgery using a pneumatic tourniquet: reduced blood loss and improved cosmesis. *Ann R Coll Surg Engl* 1990; 72: 119-122.

18 Sykes TC, Brookes P, Hickey NC. A prospective randomised trial of tourniquet in varicose vein surgery. *Ann R Coll Surg Engl* 2000; 82: 280-282.

19 Robinson J, Macierewicz J, Beard JD. Using the Boazul cuff to reduce blood loss in varicose vein surgery. *Eur J Vasc Endovasc Surg* 2000; 20: 390-393.

20 Raj TB, Goddard M, Makin GS. How long do compression bendages maintain their pressure during ambulatory treatment of varicose veins? *Br J Surg* 1980; 67: 122-124.

21 Travers JP, Rhodes JE, Hardy JG et al. Postoperative limb compression in reduction of haemorrhage after varicose vein surgery. *Ann R Coll Surg Engl* 1993; 75: 119-122.

22 Raso AM, Rispoli P, Maggio D et al. A new device for prevention of postoperative haematoma in the surgery of varicose veins. *J Cardiovasc Surg* 1997; 38: 177-180.

23 Keith LM Jr, Smead WL. Saphenous vein stripping and its complications. *Surg Clin North Am* 1983; 63: 1303-1312.

24 Hagmuller GW. Komplikationen bei der Chirurgie der Varikose. *Langenbecks Arch Chir* Suppl (Kongressbericht) 1992; 470-474.

25 Jantet G. Vascular lesions of the groin after variceal surgery. *Phlebologie* 1993; 46: 559-561.

26 Tennant WG, Ruckley CV. Medicolegal action following treatment for varicose veins. *Br J Surg* 1996; 83: 291-292.

27 Natali J. Medico-legal consequences of complications of superficial venous surgery of the legs. *Phlebologie* 1993; 46: 613-618.

28 Nabatoff RA. Anomalies encountered during varicose vein surgery. *Phlebologie* 1981; 34: 21-27.

29 Ramsheyi A, Soury P, Saliou C et al. Inadvertent arterial injury during saphenous vein stripping. Three cases and therapeutic strategies. *Arch Surg* 1998; 133: 1120-1123.

30 Pegoraro M, Baracco C, Ferrero F et al. Successful vascular reconstruction after inadvertent femoral artery "stripping." *J Cardiovasc Surg* 1987; 28: 440-444.

31 Flis V. Reconstruction of venous outflow after inadvertent stripping of the femoral vein. *Eur J Vasc Endovasc Surg* 1995; 10: 253-255.

32 Holme JB, Holme K, Sorensen LS. The anatomic relationship between the long saphenous vein and the saphenous nerve. *Acta Chir Scand* 1988; 154: 631-633.

33 Negus D. Complications of superficial venous surgery: nerve lesions in the leg and the popliteal fossa. *Phlebologie* 1993; 46: 601-602.

34 Cox SJ, Wellwood JM, Martin A. Saphenous nerve injury caused by stripping of the long saphenous vein. *Br Med J* 1974l: 415-417.

35 Docherty JG, Morrice JJ, Bell G. Saphenous neuritis following varicose vein surgery. *Br J Surg* 1994; 81: 695-698.

36 Jacobsen HB, Wallin L. Proximal or distal extraction of the internal saphenous vein? *VASA* 1975; 4: 240-242.

37 Ramasastry SS, Dick GO, Futrell JW. Anatomy of the saphenous nerve: relevance to saphenous vein stripping. *Am Surg* 1987; 53: 274-277.

38 Koyano K, Sakaguchi S. Selective stripping operation based on Doppler ultrasonic findings for primary varicose veins of the lower extremities. *Surgery* 1988; 103: 615-619.

39 Baccaglini U, Spreafico G, Sorrentino P et al. Outpatient surgery of varices of the lower limbs: experience of 2,568 cases at four universities. *Int Angiol* 1995; 14: 397-399.

40 Goren G, Yellin AE. Ambulatory stab evulsion phlebectomy for truncal varicose veins. *Am J Surg* 1991; 162: 166-174.

41 Ouvry PA, Guenneguez H, Ouvry PA. Lymphatic complications from variceal surgery. *Phlebologie* 1993; 46: 563-568.

42 Bohler K, Baldt M, Schuller-Petrovic S et al. Varicose vein stripping - A prospective study of the thrombotic risk and the diagnostic significance of preoperative color coded duplex sonography. *Thromb Haemost* 1995; 75: 597-600.

43 Lofgren EP, Coates HL, O'Brien PC. Clinically suspect pulmonary embolism after vein stripping. *Mayo Clin Proc* 1976; 51: 77-80.

44 Campbell WB, Ridler BM. Varicose vein surgery and deep vein thrombosis. *Br J Surg* 1995; 82: 1494-1497.

45 Lees TA, Beard JD, Ridler BM et al. A survey of the current management of varicose veins by members of the Vascular Surgical Society. *Ann R Coll Surg Engl* 1999; 81: 407-417.

46 Bentley PG. Varicose veins. *Br Med J* 1990; 300: 1586.

47 Huber O, Bounameaux H, Borst F et al. Postoperative pulmonary embolism after hospital discharge. An underestimated risk. *Arch Surg* 1992; 127: 310-313.

48 Hach-Wunderle V. Thromboseprophylaxe nach chirurgischen Eingriffen am Venensystem. *VASA* Suppl 1992; 35: 110-114.

49 Bounameaux H, Huber O. Postoperative deep vein thrombosis and surgery for varicose veins. *Br Med J* 1996; 312: 1158.

50 Parvulesco J. La prévention des complications thrombo-emboliques postopératoires par Clexane (héparine des bas poids moléculaires) dans la chirurgie des varices. *VASA* Suppl 1989; 27: 117-119.

51 Henriet JP. Sexual complications from superficial venous surgery. *Phlebologie* 1993; 46: 569-575.

52 Rivlin S. The surgical cure of primary varicose veins. *Br J Surg* 1975; 62: 913-917.

53 Royle JP. Recurrent varicose veins. *World J Surg* 1986; 10: 944-953.

54 Davies GC. The Lothian surgical audit. *Medical Audit News* 1991; 1: 26-27.

55 Stonebridge PA, Chalmers N, Beggs I et al. Recurrent varicose veins: a varicographic analysis leading to a new practical classification. *Br J Surg* 1995; 82: 60-62.

56 Bradbury AW, Stonebridge PA, Callam MJ et al. Recurrent varicose veins: assessment of the saphenofemoral junction. *Br J Surg* 1994; 81: 373-375.

57 Redwood NF, Lambert D. Patterns of reflux in recurrent varicose veins assessed by duplex scanning. *Br J Surg* 1994; 81: 1450-1451.

58 Khaira HS, Parnell A. Patterns of reflux in recurrent varicose veins assessed by duplex scanning. *Br J Surg* 1995; 82: 564.

59 Bradbury AW, Stonebridge PA, Ruckley CV et al. Recurrent varicose veins: correlation between preoperative clinical and hand-held doppler ultrasonographic examination, and anatomical findings at surgery. *Br J Surg* 1993; 80: 849-851.

60 Bradbury AW, Ruckley CV. Patterns of reflux in recurrent varicose veins assessed by duplex scanning. *Br J Surg* 1995; 82: 424-425.

61 Labropoulos N, Touloupakis E, Giannoukas AD et al. Recurrent varicose veins: investigation of the pattern and extent of reflux with color flow duplex scanning. *Surgery* 1996; 119: 406-409.

62 Glass GM. Neovascularization in recurrence of varices of the great saphenous vein in the groin: phlebography. *Angiology* 1988; 39: 577-582.

63 Jones L, Braithwaite BD, Selwyn D et al. Neovascularisation is the principal cause of varicose vein recurrence: results of a randomized trial of stripping the long saphenous vein. *Eur J Vasc Endovasc Surg* 1996; 12: 442-445.

64 Nyamekye I, Shephard NA et al. Clinicopathological evidence that neovascularisation is a cause of recurrent varicose veins. *Eur J Vasc Endovasc Surg* 1998; 15: 412-415.

65 Bergan JJ. New technology and recurrent varicose veins. *The Lancet* 1996; 348: 210-211.

66 Lees T, Singh S, Beard J et al. Prospective audit of surgery for varicose veins. *Br J Surg* 1997; 84: 44-46.

67 Darke SG. The morphology of recurrent varicose veins. *Eur J Vasc Surg* 1992; 6: 512-517.

68 Hobbs JT. Treatment of varicose veins. A random trial of injection-compression therapy versus surgery. *Br J Surg* 1968; 55: 777-780.

69 Jakobsen BH. The value of different forms of treatment for varicose veins. *Br J Surg* 1979; 66: 182-184.
70 Eklof B. Modern treatment of varicose veins. *Br J Surg* 1988; 75: 297-298.
71 Sarin S, Scurr JH, Coleridge-Smith PD. Stripping of the long saphenous vein in the treatment of primary varicose veins. *Br J Surg* 1994; 81: 1455-1458.
72 Neglen P, Einarsson E, Eklof B. The functional long-term value of different types of treatment for saphenous vein incompetence. *J Cardiovasc Surg* 1993; 34: 295-301.
73 Dwerryhouse S, Davies B, Harradine K et al. Stripping the long saphenous vein reduces the rate of re-operation for recurrent varicose veins: five-year results of a randomized trial. *J Vasc Surg* 1999; 29: 589-592.
74 Glass GM. Prevention of recurrent saphenofemoral incompetence after surgery for varicose veins. *Br J Surg* 1989; 76: 1210.
75 Khan B, Khan S, Greaney MG et al. Prospective randomized trial comparing sequencial avulsion with stripping of the long saphenous vein. *Br J Surg* 1996; 83: 1559-1562.
76 Woodyer AB, Dormandy JA. Is it necessary to strip the long saphenous vein? *Phlebology* 1986; 1: 221-224.
77 Hammarsten J, Pedersen P, Cederlund CG et al. Long saphenous vein saving surgery for varicose veins. A long-term follow-up. *Eur J Vasc Surg* 1990; 4: 361-364.

29